60·00

369 0240167

D1766751

Clinical Trials in Rheumatology

Rüdiger Müller • Johannes von Kempis

Clinical Trials in Rheumatology

Volume 2

Second Edition

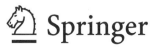 Springer

Authors
Rüdiger Müller, M.D.
Division of Rheumatology
and Rehabilitation
Department of Internal Medicine
Kantonsspital St. Gallen
Switzerland

Johannes von Kempis, M.D.
Division of Rheumatology
and Rehabilitation
Department of Internal Medicine
Kantonsspital St. Gallen
Switzerland

ISBN 978-1-4471-2869-4   ISBN 978-1-4471-2870-0   (eBook)
DOI 10.1007/978-1-4471-2870-0
Springer Dordrecht Heidelberg New York London

Library of Congress Control Number: 2012943694

To our parents, wives and children.

Rüdiger Müller
Johannes von Kempis

Foreword (Second Edition)

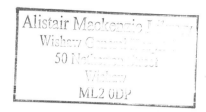
Who does not recognize the trouble to keep an integrated overview of all the existing and new evidence for the medical treatment of the rheumatic diseases? You may be inclined – like me – to make comprehensive short summaries of the studies to keep the overview, but fail to carry on with this because of the abundance of published studies. You do not have to worry anymore! This book *Clinical Trials in Rheumatology* is the perfect book to find the summaries of all the important trials in rheumatology. In the era of evidence-based medicine, 'early treatment' and 'treat to target strategies,' it is very important to get a good insight into the trials as to the clinical outcomes as well as the patients characteristics of the study population. Direct comparison of treatments is often not possible due to lack of head-to-head trials. The authors of this book, however, offer us the essential information of all trials in a comprehensive and well-organized way. They present publication details, inclusive study acronym, study design, study population, intervention, clinical outcomes, and adverse events. By presenting all trials in a preset format, the risk of biased information is minimized, and for the reader, it is easier to interpret the results in relation to comparable trials.

All doctors working in rheumatology, clinicians, trainee's, supervisors and clinical researchers alike, will love this book as it will render them easy access to all trials in rheumatology of the past 40 years. It proofed to be a very frequently consulted book not only by me but also by my staff and trainees. It does not discharge us, however, from the obligation to follow the literature. The amount of clinical data is constantly growing, and 174 new trials have been added to this second edition since 2011. The book is conveniently divided into two parts in one volume: one for the trials in arthritic disease and one for the connective tissue diseases.

Knowing that books are always behind as to the most recent information, *Clinical Trials in Rheumatology* will be invaluable to providing a comprehensive overview of all trials in rheumatology to date.

Prof. Dr. J.M.W. Hazes, M.D.
Erasmus University Medical Center,
Rotterdam, The Netherlands

Foreword (First Edition)

Over the past 20 years, rheumatologists have developed and witnessed many paradigmatic changes not only in the medication of rheumatoid arthritis (RA) but also in other autoimmune rheumatic diseases. With regard to RA, less joint damage and better physical function has been demonstrated as a consequence of an early institution of disease-modifying anti-rheumatic drugs. Furthermore, the definition of core set variables and developments of composite measurements to assess RA have allowed disease activity to be assessed reliably. Finally, new biologic active agents have shown to be of major importance for fulfilling the aim of low disease activity or even remissions, specifically if treatment is commenced at a very early stage of the disease.

These obvious significant advances in the treatment options for RA and other autoimmune rheumatic diseases would not have been made possible without a new culture for conducting clinical trials starting in the mid-1980s.

The book Clinical Trials in Rheumatology provides a comprehensive overview of trials in different rheumatic diseases. It presents many important clinical trials conducted over the last 40 years, ranging from complex, double-blinded or open multicentric trials, e.g., the BeSt study, to case studies in situations where real trials are still missing.

The different clinical trials to rheumatologic disease entities as listed in the book are not directly comparing outcome and clinical efficacy, or giving therapeutic recommendations. (For therapeutic decisions, the authors recommend to follow national and international guidelines and ongoing discussions concerning different treatment strategies in different autoimmune rheumatic diseases.) Instead, the book presents a well-founded and comprehensive selection of the most important studies. The authors present the relevant information concerning study design, medications, patient populations, clinical end points and adverse events, thus offering a quick overview on the clinical trials conducted in different autoimmune rheumatic diseases.

This new form of presenting the significant data of the most important studies in a comparable form renders this book a valuable help in the constantly growing multitude of clinical data in rheumatology.

Prof. J.R. Kalden
University of Erlangen,
Erlangen, Germany

Preface (Second Edition)

We would like to thank the readers of this book's first edition. A very satisfying number of people were interested in the first edition. We received a lot of very positive feedback from many rheumatologists and other colleagues working in the field.

The fast recent development of clinical rheumatology has made it necessary to prepare a second edition. For this new edition which additionally covers the period between January 2010 and 2012, we have selected and added 177 studies to the ones from the first edition. Most of these studies were published in the period between January 2010 and December 2011, but also older ones which appeared to be valuable additions have been included. Due to the added content and the consequently growing size, *Clinical Trials in Rheumatology* is now published in two volumes: the first on arthritic diseases and the second on connective tissue diseases/vasculitis.

We have improved the clarity of the presentation by replacing the former simple lists presenting the clinical results and side effects of each trial by tables. We have further tried to eliminate as many of the mistakes of the first edition as possible.

In the chapter on rheumatoid arthritis, '… patients with rheumatoid arthritis' in the 'Patients' section implies a diagnosis based on the 1987 ACR criteria.

The chapters on polymyalgia rheumatica and giant cell arteritis have now been merged. The respective disease entity and substance are indicated in the page header.

The chapter name "ANCA-associated vasculitis, Churg Straus Syndrome, and other vasculitic entitities" in the first edition has been renamed since it did not fit the generally accepted Chapel Hill classification of vasculitis. The part '… combination trials of Churg Strauss Syndrome and Panarteriitis nodosa' in the new title was necessary because of Guillevain's studies which combined patients with these two disorders on the basis of the older Fauci classification. In addition, page headers naming the respective disease and substance have been added.

February 2012, St. Gallen

Rüdiger Müller, M.D.
Johannes von Kempis, M.D.

Preface (First Edition)

This book wants to provide a comprehensive overview of clinical trials in rheumatology.

The driving force behind it was the constantly growing and increasingly confusing multitude of clinical trials in inflammatory rheumatic diseases. The great number of trials has been rendered possible by a steep increase in therapeutic options, such as the new therapeutic group of biologics, over roughly the last decade and by the development of more generally accepted response parameters. Many of the studies presented here were part of the clinical development programme of biologics such as the TNF inhibitors for different rheumatic diseases. They are complemented by studies with the same and older drugs, many of them investigator initiated, in different disease stages, e.g., in RA, or clinical situations, e.g., in vasculitis.

The main idea of this survey in the beginning simply was to set up a list of studies which had been named with an acronym, such as ATTAIN, ATTRACT, BeSt, in inflammatory joint disorders. We wanted to have such an acronym finder ready at hand at all times during the clinical day, in the laboratory and at scientific meetings. But during the selection process, more and more trials without an acronym either came to mind or appeared during online searches on public databases including others about non-biologic DMARD in arthritis, autoimmune connective tissue diseases, and vasculitis which seemed equally important.

The result of all this is the present compilation. Its major goal was to generate short summaries of the most relevant studies in a certain disease, without interpretation or valuation of the data. All types of studies are included, controlled prospective as well as observational ones – case studies even where real studies are still missing. We did, however, exclude analyses of cohort data except for some prominent examples. We have concentrated on autoimmune inflammatory disorders and have not included studies on inflammatory metabolic diseases.

Some of the studies in this book, e.g., in Sjögren's syndrome, do not fulfill the requirements of a modern drug trial, mostly due to the lack of accepted and specific response criteria. Our intention, however, was to list the relevant trials for every immunomodulatory drug in a certain disease, regardless of the trial's characteristics. For every study listed, we tried to present the relevant information with regard to authors, study design and substances used, patient population, clinical end points and adverse events, and nevertheless to stay within a one-study-one-page format wherever possible. Our focus was set on clinical, not laboratory, outcomes. Changes in laboratory parameters are presented in some studies, however, but only if absolute numbers – as opposed to values presented in graphs only – were available. Studies mainly represent the time span between the late 1980s and the beginning of 2010, but some historically interesting ones dating back to the 1970s or even earlier are included. To hold up a simple survey principle, data are neither interpreted nor commented on. Sometimes, however, details not mentioned in the original publication, such as changes in a certain parameter in percent, are added. The studies are listed by disease and compound; at the end of the book, a list of acronyms and of abbreviations, respectively, used throughout the text is provided.

We have made considerable efforts to reach all holders of copyright material and received permissions from all those we have been able to make contact with. In only very few, our repeated efforts have remained without answer.

We would like to emphasize that we are not comparing studies. We are furthermore definitely not giving therapeutic recommendations. For precise therapeutic decisions, we recommend to follow national or international guidelines and the ongoing discussion concerning treatment strategies for the different diseases.

This book presents our personal selection, and we may well have missed important studies. We are planning to regularly update this book and welcome any suggestions, including for additional studies to be included, if they help improving the present format, preferably by e-mail.

April 2010, St. Gallen   Rüdiger Müller, M.D.
                                                                    Johannes von Kempis, M.D.

Trials are listed by disease according to the table of contents. In the chapters on ANCA-associated vasculitis and giant cell arteritis/polymyalgia rheumatica, at the beginning of a trial summary, different disease entities are listed if the trial investigated a mixture of vasculitides affecting vessels of different sizes according to the Chapel Hill definitions.

The trial sequence within a disease/group of diseases is:
- Corticosteroid trials at the beginning
- Non-biologic DMARDs in alphabetical order
- Trials with biologics, again alphabetically
- Trials on small molecules

Several trials with one substance are presented in chronological order, beginning with the earliest.

Trial	Title of the publication as published Acronym: In case of an acronym, its meaning is explained
Substance	Name of substances (biologic or pharmaceutic), doses used and patient numbers in each treatment group, according to study design, e.g.,:
	X mg new drug. every X weeks (n = 175)
	X mg new drug. every X (n = 163)
	Placebo (n = 160)
	Only trials of registered substances or substances with far advanced registration process
	Concomitant medication:
	Additional medication permitted in the trial – if mentioned
	Previous medication:
	Medication before start of trial – if mentioned
	Name of substances (biologic or pharmaceutic), doses used and patient numbers in each treatment group, according to study design, e.g.:
Result	The main results are shortly summarized, mostly in compliance with the authors' conclusions. Speculations the authors may have based on their findings are left out

Patients	The number of patients, the disease/diseases treated, and if adding to the clinical meaning of the study, details of the patient disposition at study entry are specified
	The use of terms such as rheumatoid arthritis or SLE, if not specified otherwise, implies that these patients fulfilled the most generally accepted international classification criteria, e.g., the ACR criteria for SLE
	Important inclusion and exclusion criteria are listed in most cases
Authors	Names according to original publication
Publication	Original citation
Follow up	Total follow-up of the trial as defined or seen in the publication
	In many trials, the follow-up differed from the duration of the trial's treatment arms. In many of those trials, the duration of the trial can be seen under "Substance" sometimes under "Note".
ACR 20/50/70	In RA trials with these end points, the ACR response criteria are listed
Note	The data defined by the authors as study end points are presented as percentages or precise numbers, depending on their description in the publication, for every treatment group
	Changes from baseline, if available, are listed for every group
	Definitions of clear primary or secondary end points are restricted to more recent, controlled trials. For the sake of a standardized description of all trials and to keep the trial summaries as short as possible, they are not named
	The same applies to information on statistical significance, standard deviations, other methodologic details, definitions of remission, disease activity or relapse/flair and dropout rates. For all these, please refer to the original publications
	Numbers either as absolute values (e.g., $n = 1$) or means (e.g., duration of symptoms: 40 months), if not mentioned otherwise
Adverse events	Adverse events are listed as described for every study drug or therapy regimen

Contents

Acronym Finder

BLISS	Belimumab in Subjects With Systemic Lupus Erythematosus *Belimumab*: *SLE*	p. 796, 801, 804
BREATHE-1	Bosentan: Randomized trial of endothelin receptor antagonist therapy for pulmonary arterial hypertension *Bosentan in PAH*: *Systemic sclerosis > > other connective tissue diseases*	p. 866
CanACT	Canadian Standard of Care for the Treatment of Rheumatoid Arthritis *Adalimumab*: *RA*	p. 260
CANDLE	CANaDian evaluation of Low dosE infliximab in ankylosing spondylitis *Infliximab*: *Ankylosing Spondylitis*	p. 635
CAPRA	Circadian administration of prednisone in rheumatoid arthritis *Modified-release prednisone*: *RA*	p. 15
CESAR	Randomized Therapeutic Study of Steroid vs. Steroid Plus Cyclosphosphamide for Severe Viscera Henoch-Schoenlein Purpura *Cyclophosphamide*: *Purpura Schoenlein Henoch*	p. 1151
CHANGE	Clinical investigation in highly disease affected rheumatoid arthritis patients in Japan with adalimumab applying standard and general evaluation *Adalimumab*: *RA*	p. 250
CHARISMA	Chugai humanized anti-Human recombinant interleukin-6 monoclonal antibody *Tocilizumab*: *RA*	p. 471
CHUSPAN	Churg Straus polyarteritis nodosa trial *Cyclophosphamide*: *Churg Strauss/Polyarteritis nodosa*	p. 1069
CIMESTRA	Ciclosporin, methotrexate, steroid in RA *Methotrexate/Ciclosporin*: *RA*	p. 147, 149, 151
COBRA	Combinatietherapie bij reumatoide arthritis Combination of DMARDs in rheumatoid arthritis	p. 124, 130, 134, 161
COMET	Combination of methotrexate and etanercept in early rheumatoidarthritis *Etanercept + methotrexate*: *RA*	p. 321, 327

Systemic Lupus Erythematosus

Corticosteroids

Trial	A double-blind controlled trial of methylprednisolone infusions in systemic lupus erythematosus using individualized outcome assessment
Substance	**Methylprednisolone (MP), 3 daily infusions of 100 mg** (n = 10) **Methylprednisolone, 3 daily infusions of 1 g** (n = 11) *Alternative dose*: Nine patients who did not respond satisfactorily to the first set of infusions were treated with a second set of infusions at the alternative dose *Concomitant medication*: No limitations for any other drug Oral corticosteroids were withdrawn on the day of infusion
Result	Half of patients with severe episodes of systemic lupus erythematosus treated with infusions of methylprednisolone showed improvement, without additional effect of the higher dose
Patients	21 SLE patients with active disease • Failed to chloroquine (no precise number of patients) • Failed to oral prednisolone ($\leq$ 15 mg/day, n = 21) *Various features*: • Febrile without evidence of infection • Cerebral or renal problems • Rash or arthralgia • Hematological or serositis
Authors	Edwards JC, Snaith ML, Isenberg DA
Publication	*Ann Rheum Dis.* 1987 Oct;46(10):773–776
Follow-up	3 months

(continued) ➔

R. Müller, J. von Kempis, *Clinical Trials in Rheumatology*,
DOI 10.1007/978-1-4471-2870-0_4, © Springer-Verlag London 2013

Note	*Outcome parameters*:				
		1 g MP	100 mg MP	1 g MP alternative dose	100 mg MP, alternative dose
	Ideal outcome	n = 2	n = 1	–	–
	Useful outcome	n = 3	n = 5	n = 2	n = 2
	Static outcome	n = 4	n = 2	n = 3	n = 2
	Worsened outcome	n = 2	n = 2	–	–
Adverse events	(No percentages are listed)				
	No gastrointestinal bleeding				
	No osteonecrosis				
	Blood pressure rose temporarily in some patients				
	Headache, mood swings, and other nonspecific symptoms				
	Plasma urea levels rose in many cases				
	Raised serum glucose levels were transient				

FLOAT-Trial	Flares in lupus: Outcome Assessment Trial (FLOAT), a comparison between oral methylprednisolone and intramuscular Triamcinolone FLOAT: Flares in lupus: Outcome Assessment Trial
Substance	**Triamcinolone 100 mg** i. m. (n = 26) **Methylprednisolone p. o. tapered** and discontinued in 1 week (n = 24) *Concomitant medication*: Prednisone, cytotoxic agents or DMARDs and NSAIDs were all permitted to treat flares
Result	Triamcinolone and oral methylprednisolone treatment of SLE patients suffering from a mild or moderate flare equally reduced clinical signs and symptoms of the disease. Triamcinolone leads to a more rapid response than oral methylprednisolone
Patients	50 patients fulfilling the ACR criteria presenting with both: mild or moderate flare: • SELENA-SLEDAI score of > 3 points, total score < 12 • New or worsening discoid, photosensitive, or other lupus rash, nasopharyngeal ulcers, pleuritis, pericarditis, arthritis, or fever not attributable to infection • Increase in prednisone, but not to > 0.5 mg/kg/day • Initiation of either hydroxychloroquine or NSAIDS • Change in the physician's global assessment by ≥ 1.0 but remaining ≤ 2.5
Authors	Danowski A, Magder L, Petri M
Publication	*J Rheumatol.* 2006 Jan;33(1):57–60
Follow-up	4 weeks
Note	*Outcome parameters*:

	Methylprednisolone (%)	Triamcinolone (%)
Lupus flare gone	25	38
Lupus flare much better	29.1	23.8
Lupus flare a little better	20.8	23.5
No change	16.6	9.5
Lupus flare even worse	8.3	0
SF 36 improved	66.6	73.9
Rapid response	41.6	69.5

Adverse events	No side effects were seen with either treatment

Trial	The effect of moderate dose corticosteroids in preventing severe flares in patients with serologically active, but clinically stable, systemic lupus erythematosus: findings of a prospective, randomized, double-blind, placebo-controlled trial
Substance	**Prednisone 30 mg/day** for 2 weeks Prednisone 20 mg/day for 1 week Prednisone 10 mg/day for 1 week (n = 21) **Placebo** (n = 20) *Concomitant medication*: Prednisone ≤ 15 mg/day at study entry DMARDs were continued at stable doses (≥ 2 months prior randomization) Cyclophosphamide was permitted
Result	Short-term, moderate dose corticosteroid treatment seemed to prevent severe flares in patients with serologically active but clinically stable disease
Patients	154 patients fulfilling the ACR criteria, with inactive disease • History of anti DNS antibodies SLEDAI score ≤ 4 *Serologic flare (n = 41)*: • Elevations of C3a levels > 50% • Elevations of anti-dsDNA levels > 25% *Clinically stable*: ⇨ Randomization
Authors	Tseng CE, Buyon JP, Kim M, Belmont HM, Mackay M, Diamond B, Marder G, Rosenthal P, Haines K, Ilie V, Abramson SB
Publication	*Arthritis Rheum.* 2006 Nov;54(11):3623–3632
Follow-up	12–18 months
Note	*Outcome parameters*:

	Placebo	Prednisone
Mean prednisone dose (mg)	350	135
Severe flares	n = 6	n = 0

Adverse events		Placebo	Prednisone
	Hypertension	n = 0	n = 0
	Glucose intolerance	n = 0	n = 0
	Dyspepsia	n = 0	n = 1
	Total	n = 11	n = 12

Trial	Long-term survival of lupus nephritis patients treated with Azathioprine and prednisone
Substance	**Azathioprine** Loading dose 10, 8, 6 mg/kg/day for 2 days resp. Maintenance dose 1–4 mg/kg/day **Plus 30–60 mg prednisone/day**, tapered to an alternate day regimen *Escape therapy if worsening of renal parameters*: 60 mg prednisone/day *Concomitant medication*: No information provided *Previous treatment*: DMARDs were permitted Azathioprine was permitted
Result	Treatment of severe renal disease with initial high dose corticosteroids followed by combination of azathioprine with corticosteroids and a rapid reduction in corticosteroid dosage led to improved survival
Patients	47 patients with SLE and severe renal disease • Renal biopsy: Diffuse proliferative or membranous glomerulonephritis • Nephrotic syndrome
Authors	Barnett EV, Dornfeld L, Lee DB, Liebling MR
Publication	*J Rheumatol*. Fall 1978;5(3):275–287
Follow-up	12 years
Note	*Outcome parameters*:

	Survivorship	82% (5 years) 74% (10 years)
	Death	n = 8
	Hemodialysis	n = 2
	Improvement in creatinine	n = 21
	Decreased proteinuria	n = 35
Adverse events	Hypertension	n = 13
	Herpes zoster	n = 3
	Sepsis	n = 10

Trial	Treatment of pure membranous lupus nephropathy with prednisone and azathioprine: an open-label trial
Substance	**Prednisone 0.8–1 mg/kg/day** Tapered by 5 mg every week To maintenance dose 5–10 mg/day **Plus azathioprine 1 mg/kg/day** Increased to 2 mg/kg/day *Concomitant medication*: Hypertension: beta-blockers or calcium channel blockers Persisting proteinuria after 12 months: ACE inhibitors Hyperlipidemia: HMG CoA reductase inhibitors *Previous medication*: Prednisone 66% Azathioprine 18% Hydroxychloroquine 21% Cyclophosphamide 5%
Result	A combination of prednisone and azathioprine had some effect in the initial treatment of pure membranous lupus nephritis. Severe adverse effects were uncommon
Patients	38 consecutive SLE patients • Biopsy proven pure membranous glomerulonephritis
Authors	Mok CC, Ying KY, Lau CS, Yim CW, Ng WL, Wong WS, Au TC
Publication	*Am J Kidney Dis.* 2004 Feb;43(2):269–276
Follow-up	12 months

(continued)

Note	*Outcome parameters*:	
	Complete/partial remission	n = 32
	No remission	n = 4
	Withdrawal	n = 2
	Change of:	
	Proteinuria (g/day)	-2.72
	Urinary casts	-14%
	Serum creatinine (mg/dL)	0
	Creatinine clearance (mL/min)	+11.9
	Serum albumine (g/dL)	+10.2
	Nephrotic syndrome	-50%
	Hypertension	+3%
	Anti dsDNA	-25%
	Depressed serum C3	-31%
	Depressed serum C4	-16%
	SLEDAI score	-8.5
Adverse events	Cerebrovascular accident	5%
	Cardiovascular disorder	3%
	Amaurosis fugax	3%
	Pulmonary embolism	3%
	Avascular necrosis of the hips	8%
	Agranulozytosis	3%
	Leucopenia	5%
	Hepatitis	0%
	Azathioprine hypersensitivity	3%
	Herpes zoster	3%
	Severe infections	0%
	Malignancy	0%

Trial	A randomized pilot trial comparing Ciclosporin and Azathioprine for maintenance therapy in diffuse lupus nephritis over 4 years
Substance	Induction/Flare Treatment: **Cyclophosphamide p. o. 1–2 mg/kg/day** for 3 months **Methylprednisolone i. v. pulse** for 3 days (0.5 g ≤ 50 kg body weight; 1 g > 50 kg body weight) Followed by oral prednisone 1 mg/kg/day for 10–15 days Tapered to 0.7 mg/kg/day for the next 10–15 days Then tapered to 0.5 mg/kg/day up to the end of 2 months *Subsequently, patients were randomly assigned either to*: *Ciclosporin arm*: **Ciclosporin 4 mg/kg/day** (n = 36, blood level ≤ 200 ng/mL) Dose reduction 2.5–3 mg/kg/day If proteinuria persists > 1 g/day: Dose was reduced slower *Azathioprine arm*: **Azathioprine 2 mg/kg/day** (n = 33) Optional reduction to 1.5 mg/kg/day after 1 month Neither ciclosporin nor azathioprine was increased if renal or Extrarenal signs of lupus activity occurred *Concomitant medication*: Prednisone 0.2–0.5 mg/kg/day Prednisone was increased at clinical discretion of the clinician (maximum 25 mg/day)
Result	Maintenance therapy with azathioprine or ciclosporin combined with corticosteroids after initial high dose corticosteroid and cyclophosphamide treatment demonstrated equal efficacy in the prevention of flares in patients with diffuse proliferative lupus nephritis
Patients	75 patients with diffuse proliferative lupus biopsy-proven WHO class IV, Vc, or Vd nephritis • Chronicity index of ≤ 4 • Active urine sediment (≥ 5 erythrocytes/high power field) • Proteinuria > 1 g/day in the case of newly diagnosed nephritis or • > 2 g/day in the case of a new renal flare • Serum creatinine levels of ≤ 4 mg/dL
Authors	Moroni G, Doria A, Mosca M, Alberighi OD, Ferraccioli G, Todesco S, Manno C, Altieri P, Ferrara R, Greco S, Ponticelli C
Publication	*Clin J Am Soc Nephrol.* 2006 Sep;1(5):925–932
Follow-up	2 years (core study) Treatment continued for up to 4 years (follow-up study)

Note	Outcome parameters (24 months):		
		Ciclosporin	Azathioprine
	Mean prednisolone dose (mg/day)	7.5	7.2
	Cumulative Prednisone dose (mg)	7,667	7,377
	Mean systolic blood pressure (mmHg)	120/78	124/79
	Flares	n = 7	n = 8
	Proteinuria decreased (g/day)	2.8 → 0.4	2.2 → 0.5
	Proteinuria (after 4 years, g/day)	0.2	0.3
	Change of:		
		Ciclosporin	Azathioprine
	Prednisone dose (mg/day)	-16.7	-15.7
Adverse events		Ciclosporin (%)	Azathioprine (%)
	Leucopenia	11.1	30.3
	Anemia	13.9	15.2
	Hypertension	19.4	15.2
	Hypercholesterolemia	5.6	12.1
	Gum hyperplasia	5.6	0
	Hypertrichosis	5.6	0
	Diabetes	0	3.0
	Hyperkalemia	2.8	0
	Hypertensive crisis	2.8	0
	Infections	19.4	42.4
	Arthralgias	38.9	9.1
	Gastrointestinal disorders	30.6	9.1

Dutch Lupus Nephritis Study	Long-term follow-up of a randomized controlled trial of azathioprine/methylprednisolone versus cyclophosphamide in patients with proliferative lupus nephritis
Substance	*Azathioprine (Aza/MP, n = 37)*: **Azathioprine 2 mg/kg/day** Methylprednisolone 1,000 mg for 3 consecutive days Repeated after 2 and 6 weeks Prednisolone 20 mg/day Then tapered to 10 mg/day after 5 months *Cyclophosphamide (Cyc, n = 50)*: **Cyclophosphamide 6 × i. v. 750 mg/m² every 4 weeks** Followed by 7 pulses every 12 weeks 1 mg/kg prednisolone/day Then tapered to 10 mg/day after 6 months After 2 years, treatments were identical in both groups: Azathioprine 2 mg/kg/day 10 mg prednisolone/day
Result	Induction treatment with intravenuous cyclophosphamide was superior to azathioprine in preventing renal relapses. Other parameters for renal function did not differ
Patients	87 patients with biopsy-proven proliferative lupus nephritis fulfilling the ACR criteria for SLE • Creatinine clearance > 25 mL/min (Cockcroft–Gault formula) • Biopsy-proven proliferative LN (WHO Class III, IV, Vc, or Vd)
Authors	Arends S, Grootscholten C, Derksen RH, Berger SP, de Sévaux RG, Voskuyl AE, Bijl M, Berden JH; on behalf of the Dutch Working Party on systemic lupus erythematosus
Publication	*Ann Rheum Dis.* 2012 Jun;71(6):966–973
Follow-up	9.6 years (median)

Note		Aza/MP	Cyc
	Patients with sustained doubling of serum creatinine	n = 6	n = 4
	End-stage renal disease	n = 2	n = 2
	Mortality	n = 6	n = 5
	Renal relapses	n = 14	n = 5

Trial	A randomized study of the effect of withdrawing Hydroxychloroquine sulfate in systemic lupus erythematosus. The Canadian Hydroxychloroquine Study Group		
Substance	**Hydroxychloroquine sulfate 100–400 mg/day** (n = 25) **Placebo** (n = 22), dusted with 1 mg of hydroxychloroquine (HCQ) to give the same unfavorable taste *Concomitant medication*: Prednisone was continued *Previous medication*: No patients treated with HCQ > 6.5 mg/kg		
Result	Hydroxychloroquine treatment in patients with quiescent systemic lupus erythematosus decreased the occurrence of flares		

Patients	47 patients with clinically stable SLE diagnosed by the ACR criteria
	  • In remission or minimal disease activity
	  • Treated with 100–400 mg hydroxychloroquine for minimum 6 months, discontinued at trial entry		

Authors	The Canadian Hydroxychloroquine Study Group		
Publication	*N Engl J Med*. 1991 Jan 17;324(3):150–154		
Follow-up	24 weeks		
Note	*Outcome parameters*:		
		Placebo	HCQ
	New flare	73%	36%
	New objective manifestations	n = 16	n = 9
	Severe exacerbations of the disease	n = 5	n = 1
	Increasing prednisone dose	n = 22 (+2.7 mg/day)	n = 25 (+0.4 mg/day)
	Withdrawal because of flairs	n = 5	n = 1
Adverse events		Placebo	HCQ
	Light-headedness and loss of appetite	n = 1	–
	Bruising	–	n = 1
	Nausea	–	n = 1
	Diaphoresis	–	n = 1

Trial	Comparison of Hydroxychloroquine and Placebo in the treatment of the arthropathy of mild systemic lupus erythematosus
Substance	**Hydroxychloroquine 2×200 mg/day** (n = 40) **Placebo** (n = 31) *Concomitant medication*: Prednisone ≤ 10 mg/day at stable doses NSAIDs were continued *Previous medication*: NSAIDs were permitted No antimalarials < 6 weeks prior to randomization
Result	Treatment of the articular manifestations of SLE with hydroxychloroquine lead to some improvement of joint pain but of no other joint variables
Patients	71 patients with mild SLE, diagnosed by the ACR criteria • Requiring ≤ 10 mg of prednisone • With arthritis or arthralgia ≥ 4 joints • Treated unsuccessfully with NSAIDs • No cerebral, nephritic or other manifestations requiring corticosteroids • No information on other DMARDs
Authors	Williams HJ, Egger MJ, Singer JZ, Willkens RF, Kalunian KC, Clegg DO, Skosey JL, Brooks RH, Alarcón GS, Steen VD, Polisson RP, Ward JR
Publication	*J Rheumatol.* 1994 Aug;21(8):1457–1462
Follow-up	48 weeks

Note	*Change of*:	HCQ	Placebo
	Painful swollen joint count	-5.7	-1.1
	Painful swollen joint score	-7.1	-3.1
	Swollen joint count	-0.5	-2.2
	Swollen joint score	-1.1	-2.2
	Grip strength right (mmHg)	-2	-25
	Grip strength left	+1	-15
	General assessment (VAS 1–5)	-0.1	+0.1
	General pain assessment (VAS 1–5)	-0.2	+0.1
	Severity of pain (VAS 1–5)	-0.5	0
	ESR (mm/h)	-9	+3
	ANA titer	+40	+40
	Complement C3 (mg/dL)	-31	+12

Adverse events		HCQ	Placebo
	Rash	n = 1	n = 0
	Dizziness	n = 1	n = 0
	Lack of articular response	n = 4	n = 4
	Lack of nonarticular response	n = 1	n = 3

Trial	Controlled trial with Chloroquine diphosphate in systemic lupus erythematosus
Substance	**Chloroquine diphosphate 250 mg/day** (CDP, n = 11) **Placebo** (n = 12) *Concomitant medication*: Prednisone ≤ 0.5 mg/kg/day *Previous medication*: No immunosuppressive therapy
Result	Chloroquine treatment of patients with non–life-threatening systemic lupus erythematosus prevented disease exacerbation and reduced the required prednisone dose
Patients	24 SLE patients fullfilling the ACR criteria • No life-threatening manifestation • Fever n = 1 (CDP), n = 3 (placebo) • General symptoms n = 0 (CDP), n = 1 (placebo) • Articular complaints n = 0 (CDP), n = 8 (placebo) • Skin lesions n = 1 (CDP), n = 5 (placebo) • Serositis n = 0 (CDP), n = 2 (placebo) • Alopecia n = 1 (CDP), n = 1 (placebo) • Renal involvement n = 1 (CDP), n = 0 (placebo) • Central nervous system involvement n = 0 (CDP), n = 2 (placebo) • Hematological involvement n = 0 (CDP), n = 2 (placebo) • Hypocomplementemia n = 1 (CDP), n = 3 (placebo) • Anti-DNA antibodies n = 2 (CDP), n = 1 (placebo)
Authors	Meinão IM, Sato EI, Andrade LE, Ferraz MB, Atra E
Publication	*Lupus*. 1996 June;5(3):237–241
Follow-up	12 months
Note	*Outcome parameters*:

	CDP	Placebo
Exacerbation of disease	n = 2	n = 10
Decrease of prednisone dose	n = 9	n = 3
SLEDAI (12 months)	ca. 0	ca. 3

Adverse events	CDP	Placebo
Dyspepsia	n = 0	n = 1

HELP-trial	Hydroxychloroquine Effects on Lipoprotein Profiles (the HELP trial): a double-blind, randomized, placebo-controlled, pilot study in patients with systemic lupus erythematosus HELP: Hydroxychloroquine Effects on Lipoprotein Profiles
Substance	**Hydroxychloroquine 400 mg/day** (HCQ, n = 6) **Hydroxychloroquine 800 mg/day** (n = 6) **Placebo** (n = 5) *Concomitant medication*: Prednisone ≤ 20 mg/day No information on other DMARDs *Previous medication*: NSAIDs ≥ 1 month Corticosteroids ≥ 1 month
Result	Hydroxychloroquine achieved a significant decrease in total cholesterol in both dosage groups and also of triglycerides, VLDL and the LDL/HDL ratio in the higher dosage
Patients	19 female patients fulfilling the ACR criteria, with a disease flare • Stable Doses of NSAIDs • Corticosteroids ≥ 1 month
Authors	Kavanaugh A, Adams-Huet B, Jain R, Denke M, McFarlin J
Publication	*J Clin Rheumatol*. 1997 Feb;3(1):3–8
Follow-up	3 months
Note	*Change of*:

	Placebo	400 mg HCQ	800 mg HCQ
Total cholesterol	-6.1	-11.6	-13.4
Triglycerides	+13.6	-9.6	-18.9
VLDL cholesterol	+1.7	-2.0	-4.5
LDL cholesterol	-5.1	-8.9	-11.7
HDL cholesterol	-2.6	+0.7	+2.7
Non-HDL cholesterol	-3.4	-10.9	+16.2
TC/HDL ratio	-0.1	-0.3	-0.8
LDL/HDL ratio	-0.1	-0.2	-0.6

No differences in SLAM scores, C3 and C4 concentrations, antidouble-strand DNA titers, ESR and CRP, physician's or patients visual analogue scale

(continued)

Adverse events		Placebo	400-mg HCQ	800-mg HCQ
	No adverse events	n = 3	n = 0	n = 1
	Headache	n = 1	n = 0	n = 0
	Pleuritic chest pain	n = 1	n = 0	n = 0
	Gastrointestinal symptoms (nausea, abdominal cramping, diarrhea, anorexia)	n = 1	n = 3	n = 3
	Visual disturbance	n = 0	n = 0	n = 2
	Pruritus	n = 0	n = 0	n = 1
	Blurring of vision	n = 0	n = 0	n = 1
	Electrooculography "borderline normal"	n = 0	n = 0	n = 1
	Dizziness	n = 0	n = 1	n = 0
	Fatigue	n = 0	n = 1	n = 0

Trial	A long-term study of Hydroxychloroquine withdrawal on exacerbations in systemic lupus erythematosus The Canadian Hydroxychloroquine Study Group
Substance	**Hydroxychloroquine sulfate 100–400 mg/day** (HCQ, n = 25) **Placebo** (n = 22), dusted with 1 mg of HCQ to give the same unfavorable taste *Concomitant medication*: Prednisone ≤ 10 mg/day
Result	Hydroxychloroquine reduced the major flare rate
Patients	47 patients with clinically stable SLE, fulfilling the ACR criteria • In remission or with minimal disease activity • Treated with 100–400 mg hydroxychloroquine for minimum • 6 months, discontinued at trial entry
Authors	Tsakonas E, Joseph L, Esdaile JM, Choquette D, Senécal JL,Cividino A, Danoff D, Osterland CK, Yeadon C, Smith CD
Publication	*Lupus*. 1998;7(2):80–85
Follow-up	42 months
Note	*Outcome parameters*:

Outcome parameters:

	HCQ	Placebo
Major flare	28%	50%

Secondary flare subtype:

	HCQ	Placebo
Nephritis	4%	14%
Vasculitis	8%	14%
Other	16%	23%
Hospitalization	12%	18%

Trial	Hydroxychloroquine (HCQ), in lupus pregnancy: double-blind and placebo-controlled study
Substance	**Hydroxychloroquine** (HCQ, n = 10) **Placebo** (n = 10) *Concomitant medication*: ASA 100 mg/day was permitted Prednisone was permitted
Result	Hydroxychloroquine was beneficial during lupus pregnancy. SLEPDAI scores and prednisone dosages decreased
Patients	20 consecutive pregnant patients fulfilling the ACR criteria for SLE or • Biopsy-proven discoid Lupus erythematosus for more than 1 year • No CNS involvement
Authors	Levy RA, Vilela VS, Cataldo MJ, Ramos RC, Duarte JL, Tura BR, Albuquerque EM, Jesús NR
Publication	*Lupus*. 2001;10(6):401–404
Note	*Outcome parameters*:

	HCQ	Placebo
Flair	n = 1 (hemolytic anemia, polyserositis and anti-dsDNA antibody)	n = 3 (*skin rashes, arthritis and uveitis*)
Fetal death	n = 0	n = 1
Toxemia during pregnancy	n = 0	n = 3
Early delivery	n = 0	n = 1

SLEPDAI scores (0–3):

	HCQ	Placebo
Study entry	n = 5	n = 8
Delivery	n = 10	n = 5

SLEPDAI scores (4–11):

	HCQ	Placebo
Study entry	n = 5	n = 2
Delivery	n = 0	n = 3

SLEPDAI scores (> 12):

	HCQ	Placebo
Study entry	n = 0	n = 0
Delivery	n = 0	n = 2

Prednisolone doses HCQ treated patients lower than placebo treated patients

Delivery age and Apgar scores were higher in the HCQ group

Neonatal examination did not reveal congenital abnormalities

Examination of children (1.5, 3 years) revealed no differences (height, weight, auditory capacities, cognitive development, ophthalmoscopic examination)

Adverse events	No retinal effects

Trial	Hydroxychloroquine use predicts complete renal remission within 12 months among patients treated with Mycophenolate mofetil therapy for membranous lupus nephritis
Substance	**Hydroxychloroquine (HCQ) 400 mg/day** (n = 11) **No hydroxychloroquine** (n = 18) *Concomitant medication*: Mycophenolate mofetil 2 g/day (increased to 3 g/day if well-tolerated) Prednisone was adjusted to control extrarenal manifestations ACE and angiotensin inhibitors were permitted *Previous medication*: Mycophenolate mofetil ≥ 3 months
Result	Hydroxychloroquine had a benefit for renal remission when mycophenolate mofetil was used as the initial therapy for membranous lupus nephritis
Patients	SLE diagnosed by a rheumatology staff member (n = 29) • 96% fulfilling the ACR criteria • With membranous lupus nephritis or proliferative lupus nephritis
Authors	Kasitanon N, Fine DM, Haas M, Magder LS, Petri M
Publication	*Lupus*. 2006;15(6):366–370
Follow-up	12 months
Note	MMF was discontinued n = 6 (treatment failure)

Outcome parameters:

	All patients	HCQ	No HCQ
Renal remission	38%	64%	22%
Partial remission	7%	–	–
Protein excretion (g)	–	1.52	2.27

Adverse events		All patients
	Death	n = 1

Trial	The BILAG multicenter open randomized controlled trial comparing ciclosporin versus azathioprine in patients with severe SLE
Substance	**Ciclosporin 1.0 mg/kg/day** (n = 42) Increased at 2 weekly intervals by 0.5 mg/kg/day, aiming for a dose of 2.5 mg/kg/day The maximum permissible dose was 3.5 mg/kg/day **Azathioprine 0.5 mg/kg/day** (n = 47) Increased by 0.5 mg/kg/day at 2 weekly intervals to a that a maintenance dose of 2 mg/kg/day The maximum permissible dose was 2.5 mg/kg/day *Concomitant medication*: Prednisolone 15–20 mg, oral, dose at study entry *Previous medication*: Prednisolone at stable dose for ≥ 4 weeks
Result	Both drugs were effective corticosteroid-sparing agents. Ciclosporin was not more effective
Patients	89 patients with SLE requiring a change or initiation of a corticosteroid-sparing agent and who were taking ≥ 15 mg of prednisolone/day • Required the addition of a new corticosteroid-sparing agent • Requirement for ≥ 15 mg prednisolone/day
Authors	Griffiths B, Emery P, Ryan V, Isenberg D, Akil M, Thompson R, Maddison P, Griffiths ID, Lorenzi A, Miles S, Situnayake D, Teh LS, Plant M, Hallengren C, Nived O, Sturfelt G, Chakravarty K, Tait T, Gordon C
Publication	*Rheumatology (Oxford)*. 2010 Apr;49(4):723–32
Follow-up	12 month
Note	*Treatment effect (intention to treat)*:

	Ciclosporin	Azathioprine
Absolute mean change in prednisolone	9.0	10.7
Prednisolone mean daily dose at 12 months (mg)	9.96	8.22
Cumulative prednisolone dose/number of days in study, mg	13.2	11.8
Mean BILAG score at 12 months	5.8	4.7
SLICC (with new damage), n (%)	5	7
SF36 Mean physical component score at 12 months	30.5	32.5
SF36 Mean mental component score at 12 months	45.7	42.6

Treatment effect (per protocol):

	Ciclosporin	Azathioprine
Absolute mean change in prednisolone	10.0	12.3
Prednisolone mean daily dose at 12 months (mg)	8.3	6.0
Cumulative prednisolone dose/number of days in study, mg	11.1	10.1
Mean BILAG score at 12 months	5.2	4.6
SLICC (with new damage), n (%)	2	6
SF36 Mean physical component score at 12 months	30.8	33.9
SF36 Mean mental component score at 12 months	45.7	42.8

(continued) →

Adverse events		Ciclosporin (%)	Azathioprine (%)
	Fatigue	6.4	9.5
	Infection	6.4	2.4
	Abdominal pain	12.8	11.9
	Back pain	6.4	11.9
	Chest pain	8.5	11.9
	Hypertension	48.9	14.3
	Vasculitis	6.4	4.8
	Raynaud´s phenomenon	14.9	7.1
	Anorexia	2.1	9.5
	Diarrhea	6.4	7.1
	Dyspepsia	17.0	7.1
	Nausea	14.9	21.4
	Vomiting	2.1	9.5
	Raised liver function tests	12.8	21.4
	Jaundice	0.0	7.1
	Anemia	38.3	21.4
	Leukopenia	19.1	50
	Thrombocytopenia	0.0	7.1
	Arthralgia	30.0	33.3
	Arthritis	19.1	19.0
	Headache	31.9	23.8
	Depression	17.0	9.5
	Tremor	6.4	4.8
	Dyspnea	2.1	16.7
	Pleurisy	17.0	16.7
	Respiratory tract infection	40.4	47.6
	Upper respiratory tract infection	42.6	21.4
	Lower respiratory tract infection	0.0	7.1
	Acne	0.0	7.1
	Alopecia	12.8	16.7
	Herpes zoster	0.0	4.8
	Herpes simplex	4.3	7.1
	Rash	19.1	28.6
	Lupus rash	12.8	9.5
	Malar rash	23.4	7.1
	Mouth ulcers	2.1	14.3
	Gum hypertrophy	6.4	0.0
	Hirsutism	23.4	2.4
	Raised creatinine	12.8	2.4
	Proteinuria	8.5	4.8
	Urinary tract infection	17.0	26.2
	Hypercholesterolemia	6.4	4.8
	Hyperuricemia	6.4	0.0
	Hypoalbuminemia	6.4	2.4

Trial	Randomized, controlled trial of prednisone, cyclophosphamide, and cyclosporine in lupus membranous nephropathy
Substance	**Prednisolone 40 mg/m²** every other day alone (n = 15) **Cyclophosphamide (Cyc) i. v., every other month (6 doses) 0.5–1.0 g/m²** (n = 15) **Ciclosporin (CsA) 200 mg/m²/day** for 11 months (n = 12) *Concomitant therapy:* Prednisolone 40 mg/m²/day for 8 weeks, then taper 5 mg/week to 10 mg/m² every other day until end of protocol at 1 year
Result	Ciclosporin and cyclophosphamide were more effective in the induction of remissions than prednisone alone, with more relapses of nephrotic syndrome after completion of ciclosporin
Patients	42 patients with lupus membranous nephropathy • Renal biopsy that showed typical lupus membranous nephropathy by light and electron microscopy • ≥ 2 g/day proteinuria
Authors	Austin HA 3 rd, Illei GG, Braun MJ, Balow JE
Publication	*J Am Soc Nephrol.* 2009 Apr;20(4):901–11
Follow-up	12 months

Note	*End of follow-up*:			
		Prednisone	Cyc	CsA
	Remission	27%	60%	83%
	Change of creatinine (mg/dL)	+0.2	+0.1	+0.15

Adverse events		Prednisone	IV CYC	CsA	Extended Cyc
	Diabetes	n = 1	n = 0	n = 2	n = 0
	Infections (total)	n = 0	n = 0	n = 0	n = 0
	Pneumonia	n = 1	n = 0	n = 2	n = 1
	Herpes zoster	n = 0	n = 2	n = 0	n = 0
	Other infections	n = 3	n = 8	n = 5	n = 8
	Leukopenia[b]	n = 0	n = 2	n = 0	n = 0
	Amenorrhea	n = 0	n = 1	n = 0	n = 1
	Increased blood pressure	n = 0	n = 0	n = 9	n = 0
	Nausea/anorexia	n = 0	n = 3	n = 2	n = 0
	Paresthesias/tremor	n = 0	n = 0	n = 4	n = 0
	Gingival hyperplasia/ increased facial hair	n = 0	n = 0	n = 8	n = 0
	Osteoporosis/ avascular necrosis	n = 4	n = 3	n = 2	n = 0
	Basal cell skin cancer	n = 0	n = 1	n = 0	n = 0

Trial	A randomized pilot trial comparing cyclosporine and azathioprine for maintenance therapy in diffuse lupus nephritis over 4 years
Substance	*Induction/Flare treatment*: **Methylprednisolone i. v. pulse** every 24 h for 3 consecutive days (0.5 g ≤ 50 kg; 1 g each for patients > 50 kg) Prednisone 1 mg/kg/day Tapered to 0.7 mg/kg/day for 10 days Tapered to 0.5 mg/kg/day Cyclophosphamide 1–2 mg/kg oral/day for 3 months. *Study Treatments*: **Ciclosporin 4 mg/kg/day** (n = 36) **Azathioprine 2 mg/kg/day** (n = 33) Optional reduction to 1.5 mg/kg/day after 1 month
Result	For patients with diffuse proliferative lupus nephritis, azathioprine or cyclosporine combined with corticosteroids demonstrated equal efficacy in the prevention of flares
Patients	69 patients with SLE • Lupus nephritis class IV, Vc, or Vd nephritis • ≥ 5 erythrocytes/high power field • Proteinuria ≥ 1 g/day • Creatinine levels ≥ 2 g/day and ≤ 4 mg/dL
Authors	Moroni G, Doria A, Mosca M, Alberighi OD, Ferraccioli G, Todesco S, Manno C, Altieri P, Ferrara R, Greco S, Ponticelli C
Publication	*Clin J Am Soc Nephrol*. 2006 Sep;1(5):925–932
Follow-up	4 years

(continued)

Note	Flare rates:		
		Ciclosporin	Azathioprine
	SLE flares	n = 7	n = 8
	Nephritic flare	n = 1	n = 1
	Proteinuric flares	n = 4	n = 6
	Change of:		
		Ciclosporin	Azathioprine
	Change of creatinine clearance (24 months, mL/min)	-9.9	+5.8
	Change of creatinine clearance (4 years, mL/min)	-12.5	-0.1
	Change of mean proteinuria levels (24 months, 42 g/day)	-2.	-1.67
	Change of mean proteinuria levels (4 years)	-2.57	-1.87
	Steroid dose:		
		Ciclosporin	Azathioprine
	Baseline (mg/day)	24.2	22.9
	30 days (mg/day)	21.7	23.1
	60 days (mg/day)	17.2	18.9
	6 months (mg/day)	12.9	12.6
	12 months (mg/day)	8.8	8.9
	24 months (mg/day)	7.5	7.2
	Cumulative (mg)	7,667	7,377
Adverse events		Ciclosporin	Azathioprine
	No. of patients	n = 36	n = 33
	Leukopenia	11.1%	30.3%
	Anemia	13.9%	15.2%
	Hypertension	19.4%	15.2%
	Hypercholesterolemia	5.6%	12.1%
	Gum hyperplasia	5.6%	0%
	Hypertrichosis	5.6%	0%
	Diabetes	0%	3.0%
	Hyperkalemia	2.8%	0%
	Hypertensive crisis	2.8%	0%
	Infections	19.4%	42.4%
	Arthralgias	38.9%	9.1%
	Gastrointestinal disorders	30.6%	9.1%

Trial	Cyclosporine-A plus steroids versus steroids alone in the 12-month treatment of systemic lupus erythematosus
Substance	*Prior to randomization*: **1 g boluses of 6-methylprednisolone** for 3 days *Ciclosporin arm (CsA+PDN, n = 10)*: **Ciclosporin-A < 5 mg/kg/day** plus, gradually reduced until withdrawal after 12 months Prednisone 0.5–1 mg/kg /day Tapered by 5 mg/day every 2 weeks following clinical remission *Prednisone arm (PDN, n = 9)*: **0.5–1 mg/kg prednisone/day** (n = 9) *Previous medication*: Chloroquine Methylprednisolone boluses and subsequently 0.2–0.3 mg/kg steroids/day during the previous 6 months
Result	Ciclosporin-A represents was useful in sparing corticosteroid in the maintenance of clinical remission in patients with an early-stage, active systemic lupus erythematosus
Patients	18 patients with very severe SLE or at first diagnosis fulfilling the ACR criteria
Authors	Dammacco F, Della Casa Alberighi O, Ferraccioli G, Racanelli V, Casatta L, Bartoli E.
Publication	*Int J Clin Lab Res*. 2000;30(2):67–73.
Follow-up	24 months

(continued)

Note	Clinical outcome:		
		CsA+PDN	PDN
	Cumulative mean dose of prednisone (mg/kg)	179.4	231.8
	Change of:		
		CsA+PDN	PDN
	Change of SLE-DAI	-16.3	-11.6
	Change of ESR (mm/h)	-46	-28
	Change of C3 complement	+26	+7
	Change of C4 complement	+7	+26
Adverse events		CsA+PDN	PDN
	Mucocutaneous alterations (hypertrichosis, striae rubrae)	n = 0	n = 4
	Gastrointestinal disturbances (nausea)	n = 0	n = 1
	Neurological disturbances (headache, insomnia, depression)	n = 0	n = 3
	Hypertension (episodes)	n = 4	n = 3
	Infections bacterial	n = 1	n = 0
	Infections viral	n = 0	n = 0
	Infections mycotic	n = 1	n = 0
	Increased liver enzyme levels	n = 2	n = 0
	Thrombocytopenia	n = 1	n = 0
	Increased serum creatinine	n = 1	n = 0
	Increased blood urea nitrogen	n = 1	n = 1
	Renal failure	n = 1	n = 1
	Pulmonary edema	n = 1	n = 1 (death)
	Metabolic disorders (Cushing-like, thyroid goiter)	n = 1	n = 2
	Weight increase > 10% of body weight	n = 3	n = 3

CYCLOFA-LUNE-Trial	Cyclosporine A or intravenous cyclophosphamide for lupus nephritis: the Cyclofa-Lune study CYCLOFA-LUNE: Cyclosporine A or intravenous cyclophosphamide for lupus nephritis
Substance	*Ciclosporin A arm (n = 19)*: **Ciclosporin 4–5 mg/kg/day** for 9 months Followed by gradually decreasing doses of cyclosporine (3.75–1.25 mg/kg/day) within the next 9 months *Cyclophosphamide arm (n = 21)*: **Cyclophosphamide 8 boluses i. v. (10 mg/kg)** within 9 months in subsequently prolonged intervals (2 × 3, 4 × 4, 2 × 6 weeks) Followed by four or five oral cyclophosphamide boluses (10 mg/day in 6–8-week intervals) *Concomitant medication*: Methylprednisolone, oral, 0.8 mg/kg/day Tapered to 0.2 mg/kg/day within 8 weeks *In the case of insufficient control of renal or extrarenal disease activity*: 1–3 i. v. methylprednisolone pulses (15 mg/kg) or Transient 30–50% increase in the dose of peroral methylprednisolone *Previous medication*: No previous cyclosporine A or i. v. cyclophosphamide No high dose glucocorticoids ≤ 3 months, Serum creatinine (≥ 140 mmol/L)
Result	Cyclosporine A was as effective as cyclophosphamide in inducing and maintaining renal remission and response and in preserving renal function
Patients	40 patients with newly diagnosed lupus nephritis • Proliferative glomerulonephritis Class III (focal) or IV (diffuse) ≥ 2 *of the following*: • Abnormal proteinuria (> 500 mg/24 h) • Abnormal microscopic hematuria • C3 hypocomplementemia
Authors	Zavada J, Pesickova S, Rysava R, Olejarova M, Horák P, Hrncír Z, Rychlík I, Havrda M, Vítova J, Lukác J, Rovensky J, Tegzova D, Böhmova J, Zadrazil J, Hána J, Dostál C, Tesar V
Publication	*Lupus*. 2010 Oct;19(11):1281–1289
Follow-up	18 months

(continued) ➔

Note

Outcome parameters (9 months):

	Cyclophosphamide (%)	Ciclosporin A (%)
Remission	24	26
Response	52	43
Stable/improved serum creatinine	86	47
50% decrease in urinary protein	62	84
Urinary protein < 0.3	38	68
Inactive urinary sediment	57	79
Normal/improved C3	86	79
Treatment failure	33	16
Serum creatinine (increase > 50 mmol/L)	5	0
Urinary protein > 3.5 g/24 h	9	0
Persistent nephritic activity	19	16

Outcome parameters (18 months):

	Cyclophosphamide (%)	Ciclosporin A (%)
Remission	14	37
Response	38	58
Stable/improved serum creatinine	57	58
50% decrease in urinary protein	52	74
Urinary protein < 0.3	38	74
Inactive urinary sediment	67	79
Normal/improved C3	76	84
Treatment failure	29	16
Serum creatinine (increase > 50 mmol/L)	10	5
Urinary protein > 3.5 g/24 h	10	5
Persistent nephritic activity	19	5

Change of (9 months):

	Cyclophosphamide	Ciclosporin A
Serum creatinine (mmol/L)	-8.3	+7.5
Estimated GFR (mL/min/1.73 m^2)	+7.6	-11.6
Urinary protein excretion/24 h (g/L)	-2.73	-2.3
Hematuria (present/absent)	76% → 45%	74% → 22%
Estimated GFR < 60 mL/min/1.73 m^2 (present/absent)	14% → 0%	5% → 22%
Proteinuria > 0.5 g/day (present/absent)	90% → 55%	79% → 6%
Proteinuria > 3.5 g/day (present/absent)	29% → 10%	32% → 0%

Change of (18 months):

	Cyclophosphamide	Ciclosporin A
Serum creatinine (mmol/L)	+0.2	+6.0
Estimated GFR (mL/min/1.73 m^2)	+1.3	-7.0
Urinary protein excretion/24 h (g/L)	-2.39	-2.09
Hematuria (present/absent)	76% → 41%	74% → 22%
Estimated GFR < 60 mL/min/1.73 m^2 (present/absent)	14% → 12%	5% → 11%
Proteinuria > 0.5 g/day (present/absent)	90% → 35%	79% → 17%
Proteinuria > 3.5 g/day (present/absent)	29% → 12%	32% → 6%

(continued) ➜

Adverse events		Cyclophosphamide (%)	Cyclosporine A (%)
	Deaths	0	0
	Leukopenia	20	11
	Hair loss	5	0
	Increased facial hair	0	5
	Increased blood pressure	29	53
	Amenorrhea	5	0
	Transient increase in serum creatinine	0	16
	Generalized seizure	0	5
	Herpes Zoster infection	10	5
	Urinary tract infection	5	5
	Sepsis	5	0
	Perianal abscess	0	5
	Transient ischemic attack	0	5

Trial	A double-blind controlled trial comparing Cyclophosphamide, Azathioprine and placebo in the treatment of lupus glomerulonephritis
Substance	**Azathioprine 3 mg/kg/day** (increased to 4 mg/kg after 4 weeks, Aza, n = 13) **Cyclophosphamide 3 mg/kg/day** (increased to 4 mg/kg after 4 weeks, Cyc, n = 10) **Placebo** (n = 15) *Concomitant medication*: Prednisolone < 0.5 mg/kg/day (maximum 30 mg/day)
Result	Cyclophosphamide was better than azathioprine and placebo, leading to an improvement of proteinuria, hematuria, and serum C3 in patients with systemic lupus associated glomerulonephritis
Patients	38 patients with glomerulonephritis • Steroid dose ≤ 0.5 mg/kg/day prednisolone • Hematuria ≥ 20/mL • ≥ 20 white blood cells/mL or proteinuria ≥ 1 g/24 h or high dsDNA antibodies+low complement factors • Renal biopsy proven diffuse glomerulonephritis
Authors	Steinberg AD, Decker JL
Publication	*Arthritis Rheum*. 1974 Nov-Dec; 17(6):923–937
Follow-up	6 months
Note	*Outcome parameters*:

	Cyc	Aza	Placebo
Creatinine Clearance	+5.9	-1.15	-1.27
Proteinuria	-0.79	-0.47	+0.54
Red cells (urine sediment, No./hpf)	-9.3	-1.0	+2.3
Granular and cellular casts (urine sediment, grade)	-1.02	-0.22	-0.09

Trial	Methylprednisolone and cyclophosphamide, alone or in combination, in patients with lupus nephritis. A randomized, controlled trial
Substance	*Initial therapy:*
	Methylprednisolone arm (n = 27):
	1 g/m² methylprednisolone for 3 days i. v.
	Followed by 12 monthly 1 g/m² pulse
	Methylprednisolone for ≥ 12 months
	Cyclophosphamide arm (n = 27):
	6 × 1 g/m² cyclophosphamide/month
	Followed by 1 g/m² cyclophosphamide every 3 months for ≥ 2 years
	Combination arm (n = 28):
	Methylprednisolone plus cyclophosphamide
	After 1 year:
	If inadequate improvement, restart of therapy
	Concomitant medication:
	≤ 0.5 mg/kg prednisone/day
	Tapered by 5 mg every other day each week to minimum
	0.25 mg/kg every other day
	Previous medication:
	No cytotoxic drug treatment ≤ 6 weeks before study entry
	No cyclophosphamide for more than 10 weeks
	No pulse or oral corticosteroids > 0.5 mg/kg/day
Result	Monthly bolus therapy with cyclophosphamide was more effective than methylprednisolone bolus therapy. There was a trend toward greater efficacy with combination therapy
Patients	82 patients with proliferative lupus nephritis
	• Glomerulonephritis ≥ 10 or more erythrocytes per high power field
	• Erythrocyte or leukocyte casts
	• Histologic evidence of active proliferative lupus glomerulonephritis
	• No cytotoxic drugs ≤ 6 weeks for longer than 2 weeks
	• No pulse therapy with corticosteroids during the 6 weeks before study entry
	• No oral corticosteroids (or equivalent) ≥ 0.5 mg/kg/day
Authors	Gourley MF, Austin HA 3 rd, Scott D, Yarboro CH, Vaughan EM, Muir J, Boumpas DT, Klippel JH, Balow JE, Steinberg AD
Publication	*Ann Intern Med.* 1996 Oct 1;125(7):549–557
Follow-up	72 months

(continued) ➜

Note	Outcome parameters:			
		Combination	Cyclophosphamide	Methyl-prednisolone
	Renal remission	n = 17	n = 13	7
	Serum creatinine doubled	0	1	4
	Developed end stage renal disease	0	1	3
Adverse events		Combination (%)	Cyclophosphamide (%)	Methyl-prednisolone (%)
	Amenorrhea	57	52	10
	Cervical dysplasia	7.1	11	0
	Avascular necrosis	18	11	22
	Herpes zoster	21	15	3.7
	Infection	32	26	7.4
	Newly diagnosed avascular necrosis	18	11	22
	Pulmonary infection	7.1	11	3.7
	Gastrointestinal infection	3.6	3.7	0
	Cardiovascular infection	3.6	0	0
	Neutropenic fever	3.6	3.7	0
	Death	3.6	7.4	0

Trial	Treatment of membranous lupus nephritis with nephrotic syndrome by sequential immunosuppression	
Substance	**Prednisolone 0.8 mg/kg/day** plus	
	Cyclophosphamide 2–2.5 mg/kg/day for 6 months	
	Then azathioprine 2 mg/kg/day for 6 months, then further reduction	
	Prednisolone dosage tapered to 10 mg/day at 6 months, then further reduction	
	Concomitant medication:	
	No information provided	
	Previous medication:	
	No information provided	
Result	Sequential immunosuppression with prednisolone and cyclophosphamide was effective in 90% of patients with pure membranous lupus nephropathy	
Patients	20 patients with SLE	
	• Pure membranous lupus nephropathy	
	• WHO Class Va and Vb	
Authors	Chan TM, Li FK, Hao WK, Chan KW, Lui SL, Tang S, Lai KN	
Publication	*Lupus*. 1999;8(7):545–551	
Follow-up	73.5±48.9 months	
Note	*Outcome parameters (within 12 months)*:	
	Complete remission	55%
	Partial remission	35%
	Proteinuria (g/24 h)	6.2 → 2
	Failed to respond	n = 2
	Relapse	n = 8
	Renal function remained stable during follow-up	
Adverse events	Herpes zoster	40%
	Hair loss	30%
	Minor respiratory or urinary tract infections	25%
	Mild leukopenia	15%
	Transient amenorrhea	14.3%
	Pulmonary tuberculosis	n = 4
	Hyperlipidemia	n = 8

Trial	Combination therapy with pulse Cyclophosphamide plus pulse methylprednisolone improves long-term renal outcome without adding toxicity in patients with lupus nephritis
Substance	*Study protocol*:
	Methylprednisolone 12 boluses (1 g/m², n = 27) continued up to 36 months
	Cyclophosphamide 6 boluses (Cyc, 1 g/m², n = 27), followed by 1×/3 months for 24 months
	Methylprednisolone plus cyclophosphamide (n = 28)
	Concomitant medication:
	0.5 mg/kg prednisone/day
	Tapered by 5 mg every other day each week to minimum 0.25 mg/kg every other day
	Extrarenal flares:
	Prednisone 1 mg/kg/day for 2 weeks
	After study protocol:
	Therapy was dictated by the clinical needs
Result	Treatment of lupus nephritis with pulse cyclophosphamide was more effective than pulse methylprednisolone alone in this long term study. The combination of pulse cyclophosphamide and methylprednisolone appeared to provide additional benefit over pulse cyclophosphamide alone
Patients	82 patients with proliferative lupus nephritis glomerulonephritis
	• ≥ 10 or more erythrocytes per high power field erythrocyte or leukocyte casts
	• Histologic evidence of active proliferative lupus glomerulonephritis
	• No cytotoxic drugs ≤ 6 weeks for longer than 2 weeks
	• No pulse therapy with corticosteroids during the 6 weeks before study entry
	• No oral corticosteroids (or equivalent) ≥ 0.5 mg/kg/day
Authors	Illei GG, Austin HA, Crane M, Collins L, Gourley MF, Yarboro CH, Vaughan EM, Kuroiwa T, Danning CL, Steinberg AD, Klippel JH, Balow, JE, Boumpas DT
Publication	*Ann Intern Med.* 2001 Aug 21;135(4):248–257
Follow-up	120 months

(continued)

Note	Outcome parameters (end of study):			
		Cyc	Cyc+methyl-prednisolone	Methyl-prednisolone
	50% increase of creatinine concentration	n = 2	n = 2	n = 5
	Doubling of creatinine concentration	n = 1	n = 0	n = 4
	End stage renal disease	n = 1	n = 0	n = 3
	Outcome parameters (end of follow-up):			
		Cyc	Cyc+methyl-prednisolone	Methyl-prednisolone
	50% increase of creatinine concentration	n = 8	n = 1	n = 9
	Doubling of creatinine concentration	n = 5	n = 0	n = 6
	End stage renal disease	n = 2	n = 0	n = 4
	Patient without treatment failure	n = 7	n = 12	n = 6
Adverse events		Cyc	Cyc+methyl-prednisolone	Methyl-prednisolone
	Hypertension	n = 10	n = 10	–
	Ischemic heart disease	n = 1	n = 4	–
	Hyperlipoproteinemia	n = 7	n = 8	–
	Valvular heart disease	n = 9	n = 7	–
	Premature menopauses	n = 9	n = 10	–
	Herpes zoster infections	n = 7	n = 9	n = 2
	Death	n = 5	n = 5	n = 1
	Avascular necrosis	n = 7	n = 8	n = 6
	Osteoporosis	n = 5	n = 5	n = 3
	Premature menorrhea	n = 12	n = 12	n = 7
	Age of premature menorrhea (years)	n = 33	n = 37	n = 35
	Infections (during protocol)	n = 4	n = 6	n = 1
	Infections (during follow-up)	n = 5	n = 3	n = 1

Euro-Lupus Nephritis trial	Immunosuppressive therapy in lupus nephritis: the Euro-Lupus Nephritis trial, a randomized trial of low dose versus high dose intravenous Cyclophosphamide
Substance	**Cyclophosphamide 0.5 g/m²** i. v. (Cyc, n = 45), 6 monthly pulses and 2 quarterly pulses Doses increased according to the white blood cell count nadir **Cyclophosphamide low dose i. v. (500 mg every 2 weeks**, 6 pulses, n = 44) *Concomitant therapy*: **Methylprednisolone 3 daily pulses 750 mg** i. v. followed by oral 0.5 mg/kg prednisolone/day for 4 weeks Prednisolone was tapered by 2.5 mg every 2 weeks *Maintenance therapy*: **Azathioprine (Aza, 2 mg/kg/day)** started 2 weeks after the last Cyc application, continued at least until month 30 after study inclusion *Benign renal flares*: ≤ 15 mg of prednisolone/day for a 2-week plus hydroxychloroquine (6 mg/kg/day) ± NSAIDs *Severe renal flairs*: Renal impairment: > serum creatinine increase > 33% Increase in proteinuria: albuminemia ≥ 3.5 g/dL and proteinuria ≥ 3 g *Severe systemic disease*: central nervous system disease, thrombocytopenia (< 100,000 platelets/μL), hemolytic anemia, lupus pneumonitis, lupus, myocarditis, extensive skin vasculitis, or serositis not responding to low dose glucocorticoid and/or NSAID treatment Both severe flares: 0.5–1 mg prednisolone/kg/day of for 1 month Promptly tapered to the patient's preflare dosage 2 × i. v. pulses 750 mg methylprednisolone within a 1-week period allowed
Result	Low dose and high dose i. v. cyclophosphamide regimen, followed by azathioprine in SLE patients with proliferative lupus nephritis achieved comparable clinical results
Patients	90 SLE patients with biopsy proven proliferative lupus glomerulonephritis (WHO class III, IV, Vc, or Vd) • Proteinuria ≤ 500 mg/24 h • Not pretreated with Cyc or Aza • No prednisolone ≤ 15 mg/day
Authors	Houssiau FA, Vasconcelos C, D'Cruz D, Sebastiani GD, Garrido Ed Ede R, Danieli MG, Abramovicz D, Blockmans D, Mathieu A, Direskeneli H, Galeazzi M, Gül A, Levy Y, Petera P, Popovic R, Petrovic R, Sinico RA, Cattaneo R, Font J, Depresseux G, Cosyns JP, Cervera R
Publication	*Arthritis Rheum.* 2002 Aug;46(8):2121–2131
Follow-up	60 months

(continued)

Note	Outcome parameters:		
		High dose cyclophosphamide (%)	Low dose cyclophosphamide (%)
	Renal flare	27	29
	Treatment failure	20	16
	Renal remission	54	71
Adverse events		High dose cyclophosphamide	Low dose cyclophosphamide
	Death	n = 0	n = 2
	End stage renal disease	n = 2	n = 1
	Doubling of creatinine level	n = 1	n = 3
	Severe infections	n = 10	n = 5
	Pneumonia	n = 4	n = 3
	Other bacterial infections	n = 5	n = 1
	CMV	n = 3	n = 1
	VZV	n = 5	n = 2
	Mucocutaneous infections	n = 5	n = 4
	Lower urinary tract	n = 2	n = 5
	Upper resp. tract	n = 2	n = 1
	Ear nose throat	n = 1	n = 0
	Leucopenia	n = 5	n = 5
	Toxic anemia	n = 0	n = 1
	Bone marrow aplasia	n = 0	n = 1
	Menopause	n = 2	n = 2
	Transient amenorrhea	n = 1	n = 1
	Azathioprine induced hepatitis	n = 0	n = 3
	Ischemic heart disease	n = 1	n = 2
	Deep venous thrombosis	n = 2	n = 0
	Diabetes	n = 1	n = 1
	Avascular osteonecrosis	n = 1	n = 0
	Tendon rupture	n = 0	n = 1

Trial	Therapy with intermittent pulse Cyclophosphamide for pulmonary hypertension associated with systemic lupus erythematosus
Substance	**Cyclophosphamide 6 monthly i. v. (IVCYC, 0.5 g/m²/month**, n = 16) **Enalapril Oral** (10 mg/day, n = 18) *Concomitant medication*: Prednisone in stable doses < 15 mg/day Antimalarials Anti-inflammatory drugs Antibiotics in the case of infections Ondansetron was used for treatment of nausea and vomiting No prednisone doses > 15 mg/day, beta-blockers, or calcium channel blockers trial
Result	Cyclophosphamide was more effective than enalapril in mild and moderate pulmonary hypertension associated with SLE
Patients	34 patients fulfilling the ACR criteria for SLE • Prednisone doses of < 15 mg/day • Doppler echocardiography: • SPAP > 30 mmHg with exercise or • SPAP > 25 mmHg at rest
Authors	Gonzalez-Lopez L, Cardona-Muñoz EG, Celis A, García-de la Torre I, Orozco-Barocio G, Salazar-Paramo M, Garcia-Gonzalez C, Garcia-Gonzalez A, Sanchez-Ortiz A, Trujillo-Hernandez B, Gamez-Nava JI
Publication	*Lupus.* 2004;13(2):105–112
Follow-up	34 patients with SLE who had systolic pulmonary artery pressure (SPAP), > 30 mmHg by Doppler echocardiography

(continued) ➔

Note	*Outcome parameters (patients who finished the trial)*:		
		Cyclophosphamide	Enalapril
	SPAP > 30 mmHg at baseline	12/15	12/18
	SPAP ≥ 35 mmHg at baseline	11/11	3/9
	Outcome parameters (intent to treat):		
		Cyclophosphamide	Enalapril
	SPAP > 30 mmHg at baseline	12/16	12/18
	SPAP ≥ 35 mmHg at baseline	11/12	3/9
	Change of:		
		Cyclophosphamide	Enalapril
	SPAP (mmHg)	-15	-7
	SPAP (Patients with initial SPAP ≥ 35 mmHg)	-15	-10
Adverse events		Cyclophosphamide (%)	Enalapril (%)
	Withdrawals	6	0
	Side effects (total)	94	67
	Infections total by group	87	55
	Mild infections	81	55
	Severe infections	6	0
	Nausea or vomiting	81	6
	Arterial hypotension	0	44
	Leucopenia	6	0

Trial	EULAR randomized controlled trial of pulse Cyclophosphamide and methylprednisolone versus continuous Cyclophosphamide and prednisolone followed by Azathioprine and prednisolone in lupus nephritis
Substance	*Intermittent pulse therapy protocol*: **Cyclophosphamide (Cyc,) 4×10 mg/kg** pulses (3 weekly, maximum 1 g, n = 16) 2×5 mg/kg Cyc p. o. for 2 days in 4 weekly intervals for 9 months After week 58 6 weekly intervals for 12 months Dose modification for neutrophil nadir, cytopenia, renal impairment Methylprednisolone pulses i. v. 6.6 mg/kg (maximum 1 g) Then orally at the same dose split together with oral Cyc
	Concomitant medication: Low dose orally 3 mg/kg prednisolone/day Reducing by 0.1 mg/kg/day with each pulse Maintenance dose of 0.05 mg/kg/day, or 0.1 mg/kg/day Metoclopramide or ondansetron were recommended as antiemetics 3×oral mesna at 25% of the Cyc dose in mg at 0, 4, and 18 h after Cyc
	Continuous therapy protocol: **Cyc continuous (2 mg/kg day, n = 13)** After 3 months change to azathioprine (1.5 mg/kg/day), for 2 years Dose modification for neutrophil nadir, cytopenia, renal impairment
	Concomitant medication: Starting at 0.85 mg/kg prednisolone/day (maximum 60 mg) Tapering: and reducing according to protocol (see paper)
Result	There was no difference in efficacy and side effects between the two regimens. Infectious complications were common
Patients	32 SLE patients • Biopsy proven proliferative glomerulonephritis caused by SLE • No Cyc or Aza treatment within the preceding 3 weeks • No pure membranous or pure mesangial proliferative glomerulonephritis • No previous treatment with cyclophosphamide for more than 3 months
Authors	Yee CS, Gordon C, Dostal C, Petera P, Dadoniene J, Griffiths B, Rozman B, Isenberg DA, Sturfelt G, Nived O, Turney JH, Venalis A, Adu D, Smolen JS, Emery P
Publication	*Ann Rheum Dis.* 2004 May;63(5):525–529
Follow-up	104 weeks

(continued) ➜

Note	Outcome parameters:		
		Continuous cyclophosphamide (%)	Pulse cyclophosphamide (%)
	Doubled serum creatinine	6.3	0
	Dialysis	12.5	0
Adverse events		Continuous cyclophosphamide (%)	Pulse cyclophosphamide (%)
	Neutropenia	18.8	7.7
	Infections	25	38.5
	Nausea/vomiting	6.3	23.1
	Hemorrhagic cystitis	6.3	0
	Malignancy	0	7.7
	Permanent amenorrhea	6.3	7.7
	Withdrawn from therapy	43.8	53.8
	Death	6.3	15.4

Trial	Controlled clinical trial of i. v. cyclophosphamide versus i. v. methylprednisolone in severe neurological manifestations in systemic lupus erythematosus
Substance	*Induction treatment*: **Methylprednisolone 1 g i. v./day** for 3 days *Followed by*: **Cyclophosphamide monthly 0.75 g/m²** i. v. for 1 year (n = 19) Then every 3 months, or **Methylprednisolone monthly 1 g** i. v. for 3 months (n = 13) Then bimonthly for 6 months Then every 3 months for 1 year *Concomitant therapy*: Oral 1 mg/kg prednisone/day started on the fourth day (maximum 3 months) Tapered according to disease activity/remission
Result	Cyclophosphamide was more effective than methylprednisolone in the treatment of acute, severe neurological manifestations of systemic lupus erythematosus
Patients	32 patients fulfilling the ACR criteria for SLE • With severe neuropsychiatric manifestations such as seizures, optic neuritis, peripheral or cranial neuropathy, coma, brainstem disease, or transverse myelitis • Not antiphospholipid antibody associated manifestations. No pure psychiatric manifestations
Authors	Barile-Fabris L, Ariza-Andraca R, Olguín-Ortega L, Jara LJ, Fraga-Mouret A, Miranda-Limón JM, Fuentes de la Mata J, Clark P, Vargas F, Alocer-Varela J
Publication	*Ann Rheum Dis*. 2005 Apr;64(4):620–625
Follow-up	18 months

(continued) ➔

Note	Outcome parameters:		
		Cyclophosphamide	Methylprednisolone
	Response rate	n = 18/19	n = 7/13
	Disappearance of epileptogenic foci of seizures	n = 5/5	n = 2/5
	Improved visual function after optic neuritis	n = 4/4	n = 0/2
	Improvement of peripheral neuropathy	n = 3/4	n = 1/3
	Improvement of coma	n = 1/1	n = 1/1
	Improvement of brainstem disease	n = 1/1	n = 0/0
	Change of (after 12 months):		
		Cyclophosphamide	Methylprednisolone
	Leucocytes (cells × 106/ L)	+0.1	- 4.5
	Lymphocytes (cells × 106/L)	+10.8	+10.9
	SLEDAI	-9	-10
	SLICC	-0.16	-0.02
	Prednisone (mg/day)	-48.8	-29.4
Adverse events		Cyclophosphamide	Methylprednisolone
	Urinary tract infections	n = 10	n = 8
	Respiratory infections	n = 6	n = 4
	Oropharyngeal candidiasis	n = 2	n = 0
	Herpes zoster	n = 2	n = 0
	Systemic hypertension	n = 0	n = 1
	Hyperglycemia	n = 0	n = 1
	Pancreatitis	n = 0	n = 1
	Death	n = 3	n = 1

The Dutch Lupus Nephritis group-trial	Azathioprine/methylprednisolone versus Cyclophosphamide in proliferative lupus nephritis. A randomized controlled trial	
Substance	*Cyclophosphamide pulses (750 mg/m², 6 pulses every 4 weeks)*: Followed by seven pulses every 12 weeks Plus oral 1 mg/kg prednisone/day (n = 50) Tapered to 10 mg/day after 6 months *Azathioprine (2 mg/kg/day in 2 years)*: Plus methylprednisolone i. v. pulses of (3 × 3 pulses of 1,000 mg) Plus prednisone 20 mg/day for 5 months (n = 37) Tapered to 10 mg/day after 6 months	
Result	Cyclophosphamide was superior to azathioprine with regard to renal relapses and less herpes zoster virus infections. No differences in serum creatinine or proteinuria between the two groups	
Patients	87 patients with proliferative lupus nephritis • Creatinine clearance (Cockcroft-Gault > 25 mL/min) • Biopsy-proven proliferative lupus nephritis • WHO-class IV or Vd lupus nephritis • No membranous lupus nephritis WHO-class Va or Vb 56 renal impairment (56%, clearance < 70 mL/min)	
Authors	Grootscholten C, Ligtenberg G, Hagen EC, van den Wall Bake AW, de Glas-Vos JW, Bijl M, Assmann KJ, Bruijn JA, Weening JJ, van Houwelingen HC, Derksen RH, Berden JH; Dutch Working Party on Systemic Lupus Erythematosus	
Publication	*Kidney Int.* 2006 Aug;70(4):732–742	
Note	*Outcome parameters*:	

	Cyclophosphamide	Azathioprine
Primary treatment failure	n = 0	n = 1
Renal relapse	n = 2	n = 10
Renal relapse rate (relapse/100 patient years)	1.1	7.1
Reaching study end point (doubling of serum creatinine)	n = 2	n = 6
Therapy switch	n = 1	n = 3
End-stage renal disease	n = 0	n = 1
Death	n = 2	n = 3
Became pregnant during follow-up	n = 9	n = 5
Pregnancies during follow-up	n = 10	n = 10
Unwillingly childless	n = 3	n = 1
Became postmenopausal during follow-up	n = 6	n = 3
Premature ovarian failure	n = 2	n = 2
Creatinine (µmol/L)	80	86
Proteinuria (g/24 h)	0.2	0.4
Cumulative steroid dose (g)	11	20

Adverse events	Cyclophosphamide	Azathioprine
Infection rate/100 patient years	18	37

Euro-Lupus Nephritis Trial	The 10-year follow-up data of the Euro-Lupus Nephritis Trial comparing low dose and high dose intravenous cyclophosphamide
Substance	**Cyclophosphamide 0.5 g/m² i. v.** (Cyc, n = 45), 6 monthly pulses and 2 quarterly pulses Doses increased according to the white blood cell count nadir Cyclophosphamide low dose i. v. (500 mg every 2 weeks, 6 pulses, n = 44) *Concomitant therapy:* Methylprednisolone three daily pulses 750 mg of i. v. Followed by oral 0.5 mg/kg prednisolone/day for 4 weeks Prednisolone was tapered by 2.5 mg every 2 weeks *Maintenance therapy:* **Azathioprine 2 mg/kg/day** started 2 weeks after the last Cyc application Continued at least until month 30 after study inclusion *Benign renal flares:* Prednisolone ≤ 15 mg of /day for a 2-week plus hydroxychloroquine (6 mg/kg/day) ± NSAIDs *Severe renal flairs:* Renal impairment: > serum creatinine increase > 33% Increase in proteinuria: albuminemia ≥ 3.5 g/dL and proteinuria ≥ 3 g *Severe systemic disease:* Central nervous system disease, Thrombocytopenia (< 100,000 platelets/μL), hemolytic anemia, lupus pneumonitis, lupus, myocarditis, extensive skin vasculitis, or serositis not responding to low dose glucocorticoid and/or NSAID treatment Both severe flares: 0.5–1 mg prednisolone/kg/day of for 1 month Promptly tapered to the patient's preflare dosage 2 × i. v. pulses 750 mg methylprednisolone within a 1-week period allowed
Result	Low dose intravenous cyclophosphamide regimen followed by azathioprine-the "Euro-Lupus regimen"-achieved good clinical results in the very long term
Patients	90 SLE patients with biopsy proven proliferative lupus glomerulonephritis • (WHO class III, IV, Vc, or Vd) • Proteinuria ≤ 500 mg/24 h • Not pre-treated with Cyc or Aza • No Prednisolone ≤ 15 mg/day
Authors	Houssiau FA, Vasconcelos C, D'Cruz D, Sebastiani GD, de Ramon Garrido E, Danieli MG, Abramovicz D, Blockmans D, Cauli A, Direskeneli H, Galeazzi M, Gül A, Levy Y, Petera P, Popovic R, Petrovic R, Sinico RA, Cattaneo R, Font J, Depresseux G, Cosyns JP, Cervera R
Publication	*Ann Rheum Dis.* 2010 Jan;69(1):61–64
Follow-up	10 years

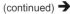
(continued) ➜

Note	End of follow-up:		
		Low dose cyclophosphamide	High dose cyclophosphamide
	Death	11%	4%
	Sustained doubling of serum creatinine	14%	11%
	End-stage renal disease	5%	9%
	Lost during follow-up	n = 3	n = 3
Adverse events		Low dose cyclophosphamide	High dose cyclophosphamide
	Cardiac or arterial event	n = 3	n = 4
	Cancer	n = 6	n = 1
	Lost during follow-up	n = 3	n = 3
	Pregnancies	n = 10	n = 9

Trial	High dose cyclophosphamide versus monthly intravenous cyclophosphamide for systemic lupus erythematosus: a prospective randomized trial
Substance	*Traditional i. v. cyclophosphamide (n = 27)*: **Cyclophosphamide i. v. 750 mg/m²/month** for 6 months Followed by quarterly i. v. cyclophosphamide for 2 years *High dose cyclophosphamide (n = 21)*: **Cyclophosphamide i. v. 50 mg/kg/day** for 4 days
Result	There were no differences comparing monthly cyclophosphamide and high dose cyclophosphamide. Nonresponders to monthly cyclophosphamide could sometimes be rescued with high dose cyclophosphamide
Patients	51 patients fulfilling the ACR criteria for SLE • Moderate-to-severe activity: • 1 × BILAG A • Combination therapy with both hydroxychloroquine and quinacrine as well as immunosuppression had to have failed for SLE patients with cutaneous lupus • No musculoskeletal lupus • Lupus nephritis n = 22
Authors	Petri M, Brodsky RA, Jones RJ, Gladstone D, Fillius M, Magder LS
Publication	*Arthritis Rheum.* 2010 May;62(5):1487–1493
Follow-up	30 months

(continued)

Note	Induction response at 6 months:		
		High dose (%)	Traditional (%)
	Overall complete response	52	35
	Overall partial response	19	15
	Overall no response	29	50
	Renal complete response	10	8
	Renal partial response	30	33
	Renal no response	60	58
	Neurologic complete response	100	71
	Neurologic partial response	0	0
	Neurologic no response	0	29
	Other complete response	75	43
	Other partial response	25	0
	Other no response	0	57

	Induction response at 30 months:			
		High dose (%)	Traditional (%)	Crossover (%)
	Overall complete response	48	65	50
	Overall partial response	19	10	17
	Overall no response	33	25	33
	Renal complete response	20	64	100
	Renal partial response	20	18	0
	Renal no response	60	18	0
	Neurologic complete response	86	100	50
	Neurologic partial response	0	0	0
	Neurologic no response	14	0	50
	Other complete response	50	25	33
	Other partial response	50	0	33
	Other no response	0	75	33

Adverse events		High dose	Traditional
	Hospitalizations	n = 29	n = 29
	Serious infections	n = 11	n = 15
	Death	n = 2	n = 1
	Premature ovarian failure	30%	43%

Trial	Comparison of high and low dose of cyclophosphamide in lupus nephritis patients: a long-term randomized controlled trial
Substance	*Group I (n = 73)* **6 × 10 mg/kg cyclophosphamide monthly** i. v. Then every 2 months for 12 months *Group II (n = 44)* **6 × 5 mg/kg cyclophosphamide monthly** i. v. Then every 2 months for 36 months *Concomitant medication*: 1 mg/kg prednisolone/day for 4 weeks Tapered to 0.2 mg/kg/day *Maintenance therapy*: 200 mg hydroxychloroquine 1 mg/kg azathioprine
Result	Low dose cyclophosphamide therapy is sufficiently effective for WHO class IV lupus nephritis patients with lower side-effects compared with standard dose
Patients	117 biopsy-proven, de novo lupus nephritis • WHO class IV
Authors	Mitwalli AH, Al Wakeel JS, Hurraib S, Aisha A, Al Suwaida A, Alam A, Hammad D, Sulimani F, Memon NA, Askar A, Al Tuwaijri A, Qudsi A
Publication	*Saudi Kidney Dis Transpl.* 2011;22(5):935–940
Follow-up	36 months

(continued)

Note	Clinical outcome:		
		Group I	Group II
	Complete remission	34.2%	25%
	End-stage renal disease	13.7%	20.4%
	Change of:		
		Group I	Group II
	Urinary protein	-1.23	-1.37
	Creatinine clearance	-17.1	-3.5
	Serum creatinine	+140.8	+89.6
Adverse events		Group I (%)	Group II (%)
	Amenorrhea	34.6	13.6
	Abortion	1.4	0
	Infections	31.3	13.6
	Pneumonia	1.3	2.27
	Meningitis	1.3	0
	Pleural effusions	1.3	2.27
	Bronchiectasis	1.3	0
	Cerebritis	1.3	0
	Herpes	4.1	0
	Upper respiratory tract infection	8.2	4.5
	Urinary tract infection	4.1	2.27
	Vaginal infection	8.4	2.27
	Miscellaneous	20.3	11.35
	Digital infarction	1.4	0
	Hypothyroidism	1.3	2.27
	Thrombopenia	2.7	2.27
	Pulmonary hemorrhage	1.3	0
	Tuberculosis	2.7	2.27
	Diabetes	4.1	2.27
	Leukopenia	2.7	0
	Vasculitis	4.1	2.27
	Neoplasm	5.4	0
	Hospitalization	9.5	2.27

Trial	The effects of cyclophosphamide and mycophenolate on end-stage renal disease and death of lupus nephritis
Substance	*Cyclophosphamide (Cyc, n = 51)* **0.5 g/m² cyclophosphamide/month** 1 mg/kg of oral steroids, tapered according to clinical response over 6–12 months *Mycophenolate (MMF, n = 20)* **2 × 1–1.5 g/day mycophenolate mofetil**
Result	The results of this retrospective study showed advantages of intravenous cyclophosphamide over mycophenolate in averting end stage renal disease and death
Patients	71 SLE patients • Presence of lupus nephritis in renal biopsy or • Proteinuria of ≥ 0.5 g/g • Proteinuria of ≥ 500 mg/ 24-h urine collection. • No former immunosuppressive therapy other than Cyc and MMF
Authors	Koo H, Kim Y, Lee S, Kim D, Oh KH, Joo K, Kim Y, Ahn C, Han J, Kim S, Chin H
Publication	*Lupus.* 2011;20(13):1442–1449
Follow-up	144 months

Note	*Clinical outcome:*		
		Mycophenolate (%)	Cyclophosphamide (%)
	Complete Remission	47.4	38.7
	Partial remission	5.3	18.4
	No response	47.4	42.9
Adverse events		Mycophenolate (%)	Cyclophosphamide (%)
	Total	25.0	29.4
	Avascular necrosis	5.0	5.9
	Cerebrovascular disease	5.0	3.9
	Infection	15.0	19.6

Trial	Benefits of Leflunomide in systemic lupus erythematosus: a pilot observational study
Substance	Leflunomide 100 mg/day loading dose for 3 days Followed by **leflunomide 20 mg/day** (n = 18) *Concomitant medication*: No information on concomitant DMARDs and corticosteroids
Result	Leflunomide was efficacious and safe in this cohort of SLE patients after 2–3 months of therapy
Patients	18 SLE patients from a single private rheumatology practice • With non organ threatening signs and symptoms
Authors	Remer CF, Weisman MH, Wallace DJ
Publication	*Lupus*. 2001;10(7):480–483
Follow-up	6 months
Note	*Change of*:

Note		
	SLEDAI	−2.1
	ESR (mm/h)	−9
	Anti-ds DNA (IU/mL)	−13.7
	Complement C3 (mg/dL)	−2.1

Adverse events	Diarrhea	n = 7
		n = 2 discontinued
	Rash	n = 1 after discontinuation of leflunomide

Trial	Double-blind, randomized, placebo-controlled pilot study of Leflunomide in systemic lupus erythematosus
Substance	**Leflunomide 20 mg/day** after a loading dose of 100 mg/day for 3 days (n = 6) **Placebo** (n = 6) *Concomitant medication*: Prednisolone 20 mg/day Tapered by 5 mg every 4 weeks until 10 mg/day Tapered by 2.5 mg every 4 weeks until 5 mg/day Hydroxychloroquine and NSAIDs were allowed to continue safe contraceptive methods
Result	Leflunomide was more effective than placebo in treating SLE patients with mild to moderate disease activity. It was safe and well tolerated
Patients	12 patients with SLE • With mild to moderate disease activity (SLEDAI of ≥ 6) • < 0.5 mg/kg prednisolone/day • No life-threatening disease requiring addition of immunosuppressants such as cyclophosphamide or azathioprine
Authors	Tam LS, Li EK, Wong CK, Lam CW, Szeto CC
Publication	*Lupus.* 2004;13(8):601–604
Follow-up	24 weeks

Note	*Change of*:		
		Leflunomide	Placebo
	SLEDAI	−11.0	−4.5
	The changes in proteinuria, complement C3 levels, anti ds-DNA binding and prednisolone dosage were similar between the two groups		

Adverse events		Leflunomide	Placebo
	Transient elevation in ALT > 5×	n = 1	n = 0
	Hypertension	n = 2	n = 0
	Diarrhea	n = 0	n = 0

Trial	Methotrexate in patients with moderate systemic lupus erythematosus (exclusion of renal and central nervous system disease)
Substance	**Methotrexate (MTX) p. o. 15 mg/week** over 6 months *Concomitant medication*: Prednisolone was continued Antimalarial drugs were discontinued 100 mg indomethacin/day was permitted No other anti-inflammatory drugs
Result	Treatment with methotrexate reduced disease activity and the dose of corticosteroids
Patients	22 patients fulfilling the ACR criteria for SLE • Refractory cutaneous rashes • Active vasculitis of the skin • Active pleurisy • Active arthritis • No active lupus nephritis • No central nervous system involvement • Prednisolone > 7.5 mg/day ≥ 6 months without achieving remission
Authors	Gansauge S, Breitbart A, Rinaldi N, Schwarz-Eywill M
Publication	*Ann Rheum Dis*. 1997 June;56(6):382–385
Follow-up	6 months
Note	*Outcome parameters*:

	Start	End
SLEDAI	12.2	4
Prednisolone dose (mg)	17.4	8.8
ESR (mm/h)	46	32

Disappearance of symptoms:

Arthritis	n = 10 of 12
Dermatitis	n = 8 of 10
Pleuritis	n = 3 of 4
Vasculitis of the skin	n = 6 of 9
Disease activity completely suppressed	n = 16 (SLEDAI score = 2)
Disease activity considerable reduced	n = 4 (SLEDAI score 3–6)

Adverse events	General malaise	n = 4
	Increased in liver enzymes	n = 2
	MTX had to be stopped	n = 0

SMILE-trial	Double-blind, randomized, placebo controlled clinical trial of Methotrexate in systemic lupus erythematosus SMILE: Study of methotrexate in lupus erythematosus
Substance	**Methotrexate (MTX) 15 mg/week** (< 50 kg body weight) or **Methotrexate 20 mg/week** (> 50 kg body weight, n = 20) **Placebo** (n = 21) *Concomitant medication*: Prednisone < 0.5 mg/kg/day Safe contraception *Previous medication*: No antimalarials or immunosuppressives ≤ 4 months
Result	Methotrexate treatment led to a control of cutaneous and articular activity of SLE. Prednisone could be reduced
Patients	41 patients fulfilling the ACR criteria for SLE • Arthralgia ≥ 3 joints ≥ 1 week • Active discoid lesions, molar rash, pleuritis, pericarditis, vasculitis, proteinuria, or urinary casts
Authors	Carneiro JR, Sato EI
Publication	*J Rheumatol.* 1999 June;26(6):1275–1279
Follow-up	6 months

Note	*Outcome parameters (end of the follow-up)*:		
		Placebo	Methotrexate
	Articular complaints	n = 16	n = 1
	Cutaneous lesions	n = 16	n = 3
	Prednisone dose decreased by 50%	n = 1	n = 13

SLEDAI scores were higher in placebo treated patients

VAS scores for pain were higher in the placebo group than in the MTX group

Adverse events		Placebo	Methotrexate
	Nausea	n = 0	n = 6
	Weakness	n = 0	n = 5
	Diarrhea	n = 0	n = 5
	Oral ulcers	n = 0	n = 6
	Dyspepsia	n = 0	n = 9
	Increased AST	n = 0	n = 10
	Increased ALT	n = 0	n = 8
	Increased gGT	n = 0	n = 6
	Increased AP	n = 0	n = 3
	Increased bilirubin	n = 0	n = 4
	Urticaria	n = 0	n = 1
	Infection	n = 0	n = 4
	Tuberculosis	n = 0	n = 1
	Increase of serum creatinine	n = 1	n = 0

Trial	Steroid-sparing effects of methotrexate in systemic lupus erythematosus: a double-blind, randomized, placebo-controlled trial
Substance	**Methotrexate 7.5 mg/week**, increased monthly by 2.5 mg to ≤ 20 mg/day (MTX, n = 41) **Placebo** (n = 45) *Concomitant medication*: Folic acid 2.5 mg/day Anticonception Stable on NSAIDs, prednisolone, antimalarials ≥ 4 weeks
Result	Methotrexate was more efficient in lowering daily prednisolone and slightly decreasing disease activity in moderately active SLE than placebo
Patients	86 patients with SLE • SLAM-R ≥ 8 • SLICC-DI/ACR ≤ 15
Authors	Fortin PR, Abrahamowicz M, Ferland D, Lacaille D, Smith CD, Zummer M; Canadian Network For Improved Outcomes in Systemic Lupus
Publication	*Arthritis Rheum.* 2008 Dec 15;59(12):1796–1804
Follow-up	12 months

Note	*Outcome parameters*:	MTX (%)	Placebo (%)
	No prednisolone at baseline and 12 months	44	37
	Prednisolone at baseline but not 12 months	5	2
	No prednisolone at baseline but taken at 12 months	2	13
	Prednisolone decreased from baseline	24	13
	Same dose	12	16
	Dose increased	12	18

Adverse events		MTX (%)	Placebo (%)
	Total	78.1	73.3
	Cardiovascular	0	0
	Central nervous system	7.3	4.4
	Ear, nose, throat, larynx	2.4	0
	Endocrine/metabolic	2.4	0
	Gastrointestinal	56.1	33.3
	Genitourinary	2.4	0
	Hematologic	26.8	22.2
	Infection	4.9	2.2
	Mucocutaneous	31.7	46.7
	Musculoskeletal	2.4	2.2
	Psychological	9.8	0
	Renal	0	0
	Respiratory	0	0

Trial	Long-term study of Mycophenolate mofetil as continuous induction and maintenance treatment for diffuse proliferative lupus nephritis
Substance	*Mycophenolate (n = 32)*: **Mycophenolate mofetil 2 × 1,000 mg/day** for 6 months Followed by 2 × 500 mg mycophenolate mofetil/day for 6 months Drug was then discontinued Followed by 1–1.5 mg/kg azathioprine/day *Cyclophosphamide-Azathioprine (n = 31)*: **Cyclophosphamide 2.5 mg/kg/day** p. o. for 6 months Followed by azathioprine 1.5–2 mg/kg/day for 6 months Followed by azathioprine 1.0–1.5 mg/kg/day for 6 months *Concomitant medication*: Plus prednisolone 0.8 mg/kg/day Tapered to 10 mg/day at approximately 6 months Tapered to 7.5 mg/day 9 months Tapered to 7.5 mg/day 12 months *Cellular or fibrocellular crescents affecting > 50% of the glomeruli*: Methylprednisolone 500 mg/day i. v. for 3 days at the initiation of treatment Intravenous Ig or plasmapheresis was not used
Result	Mycophenolate mofetil and prednisolone was an effective continuous induction and maintenance treatment for diffuse proliferative lupus nephritis in Chinese patients

Patients	62 patients with diffuse proliferative lupus nephritis (WHO class IV)
	  • Urinary protein excretion of ≥ 1 g/24 h
	  • Serum albumin concentration < 35 g/L

Authors	Chan TM, Tse KC, Tang CS, Mok MY, Li FK; Hong Kong Nephrology Study Group
Publication	*J Am Soc Nephrol*. 2005 Apr;16(4):1076–1084
Follow-up	24 months

(continued)

Note	Outcome parameters:		
		Mycophenolate mofetil	Cyclophosphamide/ Azathioprine
	Doubling of baseline creatinine during follow-up	6.3%	10%
	Complete remission	72.7%	74.2%
	Partial remission	24.2%	22.6%
	Time to reach complete remission (weeks)	15.3	19.7
	Doubling of baseline creatinine	n = 2	n = 3
	End stage renal failure	not depicted	n = 2
	Renal impairment	n = 4	n = 3
	Disease relapse	n = 11	n = 9
	Time of relapse (weeks)	20.2	32.7
Adverse events		Mycophenolate mofetil	Cyclophosphamide/ Azathioprine
	Leucopenia	0%	25.8%
	Gastrointestinal	9.1%	3.2%
	Severe hair loss	0%	29%
	Amenorrhea	n = 1 of 28	n = 9 of 25
	Withdrawal as a result of side effects	3%	9.7%
	Death	0%	6.5%
	Infections	12.5%	40%
	Infection requiring hospitalization	6.3%	30%
	VZV	6.3%	16.7%
	Progressive renal impairment	12.5%	10%

ALMS-trial	Mycophenolate mofetil as induction and Maintenance therapy for lupus nephritis: rationale and protocol for the randomized, controlled Aspreva Lupus Management Study (ALMS) ALMS: Aspreva Lupus Management Study
Substance	*First phase*: *Mycophenolate (MMF, n = 179)*: Week 1: **2 × 500 mg mycophenolate mofetil/day** Week 2: 2 × 1´000 mg mycophenolate mofetil/day Week 3–24: 2 × 1´500 mg mycophenolate mofetil/day *Cyclophosphamide i. v. (Cyc, n = 179)*: Week 1–4: **0.75 g cyclophosphamide/m²** Week 4–24: 0.5–1 g cyclophosphamide/m² *Re-randomization of responders* (week 24, *n = 278*): *MMF-arm (n = 139)*: **2 × 1´000 mg mycophenolate mofetil/day** If prior Cyc arm 1 week 2 × 500 mg MMF/day *Aza-arm*: **Start azathioprine (2 g/kg/day**, n = 139) *Concomitant therapy*: Corticosteroids ≤ 60 mg/day Tapering of prednisolone by 10 mg/day every 2 weeks until 40 mg/day. Then tapered by 5 mg/day every 3 weeks until 10 mg/day Reductions below 10 mg/day are allowed after 4 weeks of stable response No MMF, Cyc, nitrogen mustard, chlorambucil, vincristine, procarbazine, etoposide, Aza, CsA, MTX ≤ 12 months No i. v. corticosteroids, plasmapheresis, i. v. immunoglobulin ≤ 2 weeks No infliximab, adalimumab, etanercept, efalizumab, alefacept ≤ 6 months No rituximab within 12 months No enteric-coated corticosteroids during the study No allopurinol within 4 weeks No cholestyramine or other agents No NSAIDs or cyclo-oxygenase-2 inhibitors No phenobarbital at high dose
Result	Mycophenolate mofetil as an induction therapy was comparably effective in controlling lupus nephritis as i. v. cyclophosphamide. For maintenance therapy mycophenolate mofetil was comparably effective in controlling lupus nephritis as azathioprine

(continued) ➜

Patients	358 patients fulfilling the ACR criteria for SLE (n = 278 after second randomization) • Biopsy-demonstrated lupus nephritis (Class III-V) *Active nephritis*: • Proteinuria $\geq$ 1,000 mg/24 h • Serum creatinine > 1.3 mg/dL • Active urinary sediment in patients with class IV-S or IV-G disease • Plus significant proteinuria ($\geq$ 2,000 mg/24 h) • Elevated serum creatinine levels (> 1.3 mg/dL) in patients with Class III or V disease			
Authors	Sinclair A, Appel G, Dooley MA, Ginzler E, Isenberg D, Jayne D, Wofsy D, Solomons N			
Publication	*Lupus*. 2007;16(12):972–980			
Follow-up	24 months			
Note	*Outcome parameters*:			
		Cyc	MMF	Aza
	Response rate first phase	70%	85%	–
	Flares after randomization	–	40.7%	59.5%

Trial	Sequential therapies for proliferative lupus nephritis
Substance	*Introduction therapy (n = 59)*: Cyclophosphamide (Cyc) 0.5–1 g/m² i. v. boli followed by corticosteroids *Maintenance therapy*: **Mycophenolate mofetil 500–3,000 mg/day** (MMF, n = 20) **Azathioprine 1–3 mg/kg/day** (Aza, n =19) **Cyclophosphamide 0.5–1 mg/sqm** (n = 20) every 3 months Combined with mesna (hemorrhagic cystitis) and granisetron hydrochloride (nausea/vomiting) *Concomitant medication*: Prednisone 0.5 mg/kg (or equivalent) for 1–3 years Maintenance immunosuppressive therapy was stopped *Prior randomization*: ≤ 7 intravenous cyclophosphamide prior randomization ≤ 8 weeks azathioprine prior randomization
Result	Induction therapy with intravenous cyclophosphamide followed by maintenance therapy with mycophenolate mofetil or azathioprine was more efficacious and safer than long-term therapy with intravenous cyclophosphamide in lupus nephritis
Patients	59 patients fulfilling the ACR criteria for SLE • Biopsy: type III/IV/Vb lupus nephritis • No creatinine clearance ≤ 20 mL/min
Authors	Contreras G, Pardo V, Leclercq B, Lenz O, Tozman E, O'Nan P, Roth D
Publication	*N Engl J Med*. 2004 Mar 4;350(10):971–980
Follow-up	72 months

(continued) ➔

Note	Outcome parameters:			
		Aza	MMF	Cyc
	Death during follow-up	n = 0	n = 1	n = 4
	Chronic renal failure	n = 1	n = 1 (after 2 weeks of therapy)	n = 3
	Cumulative rate of renal survival	80%	95%	74%
	Relapse rate	n = 6	n = 3	n = 8
	Relapse with increase in the serum creatinine	n = 2	n = 1	n = 3
Adverse events		Aza (%)	MMF (%)	Cyc (%)
	Amenorrhea	8	6	32
	Pneumonia	2	2	15
	Total infections	29	32	77
	Major infections	2	2	25
	Sepsis with bacteremia	0	0	8
	Meningitis	0	0	3
	Upper respiratory tract infections	22	14	32
	Urinary tract infections	2	10	3
	Herpes zoster infection	4	6	17
	Leucopenia	6	2	10
	Nausea	7	14	65
	Vomiting	4	10	55
	Diarrhea	9	12	12

ALMS-Trial	Nonrenal disease activity following mycophenolate mofetil or intravenous cyclophosphamide as induction treatment for lupus nephritis: findings in a multicenter, prospective, randomized, open-label, parallel-group clinical trial
	ALMS Aspreva Lupus Management Study
Substance	*First phase*:
	Mycophenolate (MMF, n = 179):
	Week 1: **2 × 500 mg mycophenolate mofetil/day**
	Week 2: 2 × 1´000 mg mycophenolate mofetil/day
	Week 3–24: 2 × 1´500 mg mycophenolate mofetil/day
	Cyclophosphamide i. v. (Cyc, n = 179):
	Week 1–4: **0.75 g cyclophosphamide/m^2**
	Week 4–24: 0.5–1 g cyclophosphamide/m^2
	Re-randomization of responders (week 24, n = 278):
	MMF-arm (n = 139):
	2 × 1´000 mg mycophenolate mofetil/day
	If prior Cyc arm 1 week 2 × 500 mg MMF/day
	Aza-arm:
	Start **azathioprine (2 g/kg/day**, n = 139)
	Concomitant therapy:
	Corticosteroids ≤ 60 mg/day
	Tapering of prednisolone by 10 mg/day every 2 weeks until 40 mg/day. Then tapered by 5 mg/day every 3 weeks until 10 mg/day
	Reductions below 10 mg/day are allowed after 4 weeks of stable response
	No MMF, Cyc, nitrogen mustard, chlorambucil, vincristine, procarbazine, etoposide, Aza, CsA, MTX ≤ 12 months
	No i. v. corticosteroids, plasmapheresis, i. v. immunoglobulin ≤ 2 weeks
	No infliximab, adalimumab, etanercept, efalizumab, alefacept ≤ 6 months
	No rituximab within 12 months
	No enteric-coated corticosteroids during the study
	No allopurinol within 4 weeks
	No cholestyramine or other agents
	No NSAIDs or cyclooxygenase-2 inhibitors
	No phenobarbital at high dose
Result	There was no clear difference in efficacy between mycophenolate mofetil and intravenous cyclophosphamide in ameliorating either the renal or nonrenal manifestations

(continued) ➜

Patients	358 patients fulfilling the ACR criteria for SLE (n = 278 after second randomization)
	• Biopsy-demonstrated LN (Class III–V)
	Active nephritis:
	• Proteinuria ≥ 1´000 mg/24 h
	• Serum creatinine > 1.3 mg/dL
	• Active urinary sediment in patients with class IV-S or IV-G disease+Significant proteinuria (≥ 2,000 mg/24 h)
	• Elevated serum creatinine levels (> 1.3 mg/dL) in patients with Class III or V disease
Authors	Ginzler EM, Wofsy D, Isenberg D, Gordon C, Lisk L, Dooley MA; ALMS Group
Publication	*Arthritis Rheum.* 2010 Jan;62(1):211–221
Follow-up	24 weeks
Note	*Change of (week 24):*

	MMF	CYC
Withdrawals	18.9%	15.7%
BILAG improvement, general	100%	93.5%
BILAG improvement, mucocutaneous	84%	93%
BILAG improvement, musculoskeletal	91%	96%
BILAG improvement, hematologic	60%	67%
SELENA–SLEDAI	−7.0	−7.3

Trial	Is mycophenolate mofetil superior to pulse intravenous cyclophosphamide for induction therapy of proliferative lupus nephritis in Egyptian patients?
Substance	**Mycophenolate 2 × 1 g/day** for 6 months (MMF, n = 24) **Cyclophosphamide i. v. 0.5–1 g/m²** monthly for 6 months (Cyc, n = 23) *Concomitant medication*: Prednisolone 60 mg/day for 4–6 weeks Then 40 mg/day for 2 weeks Tapered by 5 mg/day every 2 weeks until 20 mg/day Then 2.5 mg/day every 2 weeks until 12.5 mg/day. Then by 2.5 mg/day reduction every 4 weeks until a maintenance dose of between 5 and 10 mg/day
Result	In this 24-week trial, mycophenolate and intravenous cyclophosphamide combined with corticosteroids demonstrated equal efficacy in inducing remission of proliferative lupus nephritis.
Patients	47 patients fulfilling the ACR criteria for SLE • With newly diagnosed active proliferative lupus nephritis class III or IV • No glomerular filtration rate < 30 mL • No serum creatinine on repeated testing > 200 µmol/L
Authors	El-Shafey EM, Abdou SH, Shareef MM
Publication	*Clin Exp Nephrol.* 2010 Jun;14(3):214–221
Follow-up	24 weeks

(continued)

Note	Response criteria:		
		MMF	Cyc
	Responders with renal biopsy Class III(A)/IV-S, G(A)	14/24	12/23
	Complete remission	6/24	5/23
	Partial remission	8/24	7/23
	Nonresponders	10	11/23
	ESR (mm/h)	22.55	30.84
	Creatinine (µmol/L)	81.68	92.95
	eGFR (mL/min)	103.15	89.05
	Proteinuria (g/day)	0.68	0.72
	Urine red blood cells per HPF	12.25	14.26
	Change of:		
		MMF	Cyc
	Change in SLAM score	−22.1	−17.84
	Change in anti-dsDNA antibody titer (Au/mL)	−92.5	−71.79
	Change in C3 concentration (mg/dL)	54.9	41.84
	Change in C4 concentration (mg/dL)	10.23	11.31
	Change in sIL-2R (pg/mL)	−4357.4	−3950.3
Adverse events		MMF (%)	Cyc (%)
	Severe infections	8.33	8.69
	Necrotizing fasciitis	0	4.34
	Pneumonia	8.33	4.34
	Oral vaginal candida	8.33	13.04
	Tinea of skin	4.17	17.39
	Herpes zoster	8.33	13.04
	UTI, bronchitis, pharyngitis	12.5	17.39
	Upper GI symptoms	16.67	21.74
	Diarrhea	20.83	8.69
	Rectal bleeding	0	4.34
	Leucopenia < 3.5 × 10⁹/L	16.67	13.04
	Anemia unrelated to SLE	4.17	4.34
	Menstrual irregularities	4.17	8.69

MAINTAIN-Trial	Azathioprine versus mycophenolate mofetil for long-term immunosuppression in lupus nephritis: results from the MAINTAIN Nephritis Trial MAINTAIN: To maintain a response		
Substance	*Corticosteroid tapering*: **Methylprednisolone 750 mg/day** for 3 first days Followed by prednisolone equivalent 0.5 m /kg/day for 4 weeks Tapered by 2.5 mg prednisolone/day every 2 weeks to 7.5 mg/day at week 24 Tapered to 5 mg/day at week 52 From week 76 onward, tapering of glucocorticosteriods and their stop if possible was strongly advised *Intravenous cyclophosphamide pulses*: 6 fortnightly cyclophosphamide intravenous pulses of 500 mg *After week 12*: **Azathioprine 2 mg/kg/day** (Aza, n = 52) **Mycophenolate 2 g/day** (MMF, n = 53) *Concomitant medication*: Contraception Angiotensin-converting enzyme inhibitors in all patients with nephrotic-range proteinuria ($\geq$ 3 g/day) *Previous medication*: No glucocorticoids > 15 mg equivalent prednisolone/day $\leq$ 1 month No treatment with Cyc, Aza, MMF, or ciclosporin A $\leq$ 1 year		
Result	Fewer renal flares were observed in patients receiving mycophenolate mofetil		
Patients	105 patients fulfilling the ACR criteria for SLE • With proliferative lupus nephritis • Proteinuria $\geq$ 500 mg/24 h • Biopsy-proven proliferative WHO class III, IV, Vc, or Vd lupus glomerulonephritis • No non-lupus related renal disease		
Authors	Houssiau FA, D'Cruz D, Sangle S, Remy P, Vasconcelos C, Petrovic R, Fiehn C, de Ramon Garrido E, Gilboe IM, Tektonidou M, Blockmans D, Ravelingien I, le Guern V, Depresseux G, Guillevin L, Cervera R; MAINTAIN Nephritis Trial Group		
Publication	*Ann Rheum Dis.* 2010 Dec;69(12):2083–2089		
Follow-up	48 months		
Note		Azathioprine	Mycophenolate
	Renal flares	25%	19%
	Recurrence/development of nephrotic syndrome	n = 8	n = 6
	$\geq$ 50% reduction of 24 h proteinuria	n = 48	n = 50

(continued)

Adverse events	Azathioprine	Mycophenolate
Death due to SLE	n = 0	n = 1
Death due to legionellosis 0 1	n = 0	n = 1
Doubling of serum creatinine	n = 4	n = 3
End-stage renal failure	n = 1	n = 1
Benign infection	n = 14	n = 21
Herpes zoster	n = 5	n = 4
Herpes simplex	n = 0	n = 2
Cytomegalovirus	n = 2	n = 2
Chickenpox	n = 1	n = 0
Salmonella sepsis	n = 2	n = 0
Upper urinary tract infection	n = 0	n = 2
Sepsis of unknown origin	n = 1	n = 0
Streptococcus pneumonia	n = 0	n = 1
Leucopenia	n = 11	n = 2
Leucopenia and anemia	n = 1	n = 0
Anemia	n = 2	n = 0
Renal hematoma	n = 1	n = 1
Psoas bleeding	n = 0	n = 1
Nausea/diarrhea	n = 8	n = 8
Hepatitis	n = 2	n = 1
Depression	n = 4	n = 3
Psychosis	n = 1	n = 0
Headaches	n = 2	n = 1
Antimalarial retinopathy	n = 1	n = 0
Drug-induced rash	n = 2	n = 2
Alopecia	n = 1	n = 2
Transient amenorrhea	n = 1	n = 2
Gynecological bleeding	n = 1	n = 1
Cushing	n = 1	n = 3
Diabetes mellitus	n = 1	n = 0
Angina pectoris	n = 1	n = 0
Cerebrovascular accident	n = 1	n = 0
Renal vein thrombosis	n = 1	n = 0
Subclavian vein thrombosis	n = 1	n = 0
Avascular osteonecrosis	n = 1	n = 0
Osteopenia	n = 1	n = 0
Rib fractures	n = 1	n = 0
Cervix carcinoma	n = 2	n = 0

Trial	Long-term follow-up after tapering mycophenolate mofetil during maintenance treatment for proliferative lupus nephritis
Substance	*Induction of remission (all)*: **Cyclophosphamide 5–7 monthly pulses i. v. 1 g/m²** Plus i. v. 1 g methylprednisolone *Maintenance treatment*: Group 1: **Mycophenolate 2 g/day** (MMF, n = 22) MMF dose **tapered after a median of 22 months** via 1.5 g/day–1.0 g/day–0.5 g/day, discontinued based on the physician's clinical assessment (n = 18) Group 2: MMF dose **tapered after a median of 17 months** to 1.0 g/day–0.5 g/day and discontinued based on the physician's clinical assessment (n = 26) *Concomitant medication*: Methylprednisolone oral 0.5–1 mg/kg/day for 1 month
Result	Tapering mycophenolate 1.5 years after induction of remission had no increased risk of disease flare in proliferative lupus nephritis in this retrospective study. Patients reducing mycophenolate within 18 months after remission had a higher risk of relapse compared to those taking a stable dose
Patients	44 patients with SLE • With biopsy-proven proliferative lupus nephritis
Authors	Laskari K, Tzioufas AG, Antoniou A, Moutsopoulos HM
Publication	*J Rheumatol.* 2011 Jul;38(7):1304–1308
Follow-up	60 months

(continued)

Note	Relapse rate:		
		Group 1	Group 2
	At 12 or 18 months	n = 1	n = 0
	At 24 months	n = 2	n = 0
	At 36 months	n = 5	n = 3
	At 48 months	n = 6	n = 9
	At 60 months	n = 6	n = 10
	Last minute	n = 6	n = 10
Adverse events		Group 1	Group 2
	Herpes zoster virus infections	n = 3	n = 0
	Salmonella species gastroenteritis	n = 1	n = 0
	Diarrhea that remitted after tapering of MMF	n = 2	n = 0
	Hypercholesterolemia	n = 2	n = 5
	Human papilloma virus	n = 1	n = 0
	Epstein-Barr virus infection	n = 1	n = 0
	Chlamydia-related myocarditis	n = 0	n = 1
	Ulcerative gastritis	n = 0	n = 1
	Gastrointestinal discomfort that resolved after reducing MMF from 3 to 2 g/day	n = 0	n = 1
	Alopecia	n = 0	n = 1

Trial	Tacrolimus for induction therapy of diffuse proliferative lupus nephritis: an open-labeled pilot study
Substance	**Tacrolimus p. o. 0.1 mg/kg/day** for 2 months Followed by 0.06 mg/kg/day *Concomitant medication*: Prednisolone 0.6 mg/kg /day for 6 weeks Tapered by 5 mg/week until a dose of ≤ 10 mg/day Maintained throughout the study period Antimalarials at the discretion of attending physicians No angiotensin-converting enzyme (ACE) inhibitors Other antihypertensive agents could be used No NSAIDs No prior treatment with CsA or tacrolimus
Result	Tacrolimus was safe and effective as an induction treatment of SLE-diffuse proliferative glomerulonephritis
Patients	Nine consecutive SLE patients • Biopsy-proven diffuse proliferative glomerulonephritis (WHO class IV) • Serum creatinine < 200 μmol/L
Authors	Mok CC, Tong KH, To CH, Siu YP, Au TC
Publication	*Kidney Int*. 2005 Aug;68(2):813–817
Follow-up	6 months

(continued) ➔

Note	*Change of:*	
	Daily proteinuria (g)	−3.28
	Nephrotic syndrome	−67%
	Serum albumin (g/L)	+8.8
	Serum complement C3 (mg/dL)	+0.28
	Serum creatinine (μmol/L)	−8.6
	Creatinine clearance (mL/min)	-0.5
	Hemoglobin (g/dL)	+1.9
	SLEDAI scores	−9.1
	Complete response	67%
	Partial response	22%
	Seroconversion of dsDNA antibodies	33%
Adverse events	Herpes zoster	0%
	Major infection (hospitalization)	0%
	Amenorrhea > 2 months	0%
	Alopecia	22%
	Transient hyperglycemia	22%
	Nausea, vomiting	0%
	Diarrhea	0%
	Hemorrhagic cystitis	0%
	Cervical dysplasia	0%
	New onset hypertension	0%
	Neurotoxicity (e.g., tremor)	11%
	Hypertrichosis	0%
	Gingivitis/gum hypertrophy	0%
	Increase in serum creatinine by 30%	11%

Trial	Tacrolimus for the treatment of systemic lupus erythematosus with pure class V nephritis
Substance	**Tacrolimus 0.1–0.2 mg/kg/day** for 6 months (n = 18) *Control group (n = 19)*: **Azathioprine** (n = 26), or **Cyclophosphamide** p. o. (n = 25), doses for both decided by clinician *Concomitant therapy*: Prednisolone 30 mg/day Tapered by 5 mg every 2 weeks until 20 mg/day Tapered by 5 mg every 4 weeks until 10 mg/day Tapered by 2.5 mg every 4 weeks until 5 mg/day Angiotensin-converting enzyme inhibitor or angiotensin receptor blocker Additional antihypertensive therapy if needed *Maintenance therapy*: After 6 months tacrolimus was stopped Azathioprine 1.5 mg/kg/day
Result	Tacrolimus, as compared to standard immunosuppressive treatment, was a safe and effective treatment of pure class V lupus nephritis
Patients	69 patients meeting the ACR criteria for SLE • Biopsy: pure class V (membranous) nephritis • Secondary to nephropathy secondary to SLE • With nephrotic syndrome: • Proteinuria (> 3 g/day) • Serum albumin < 30 g/dL • ± active urinary sediments
Authors	Szeto CC, Kwan BC, Lai FM, Tam LS, Li EK, Chow KM, Gang W, Li PK
Publication	*Rheumatology (Oxford)*. 2008 Nov;47(11):1678–1681
Follow-up	12 months

(continued) ➔

Note	Outcome parameters (after 12 weeks):		
		Tacrolimus	Control patients
	Complete remission	27.8%	15.8%
	Partial remission	50%	47.4%
	New lupus flares	n = 4	n = 11
	SLEDAI	no differences	
	Outcome parameters (after 24 weeks):		
		Tacrolimus	Control patients
	Complete remission	38.9%	36.8%
	Partial remission	44.4%	57.9%
	Change of (after 12 weeks):		
		Tacrolimus	Control patients
	Proteinuria	-76.2%	-47.1%
Adverse events		Tacrolimus	Control patients
	Infection	n =3 (gastroenteritis, oral herpes, urinary tract infection)	n =2 (gastroenteritis, herpes zoster)
	Elevated liver enzymes	n = 1	n = 1
	Dyspepsia	n = 8	n = 0
	Tremor	n = 2	n = 0
	Angioedema	n = 1	n = 0

Trial	Efficacy and safety of tacrolimus for lupus nephritis: a placebo-controlled double-blind multicenter study
Substance	**Tacrolimus 3 mg/day** (n = 28) **Placebo** (n = 35) *Concomitant medication*: Other immunosuppressants were not permitted Potassium-sparing diuretics were not permitted bosentan hydrate was not permitted Glucocorticoid pulse therapy was not permitted Plasma exchange, hemodialysis, and surgical procedures were not permitted *Previous medication*: ≥ 10 mg prednisolone/day (or equivalent)
Result	In patients on glucocorticoid therapy for lupus nephritis, addition of tacrolimus to basal therapy achieved significant improvement compared with placebo
Patients	Patients meeting the ACR criteria for SLE • With clinical signs of persistent nephritis: • Proteinuria ≥ 0.5 g/day and/or • Urinary red blood cell (RBC) count ≥ 21/hpf • Anti-double-stranded (ds)-DNA antibody ≥ 10 IU/mL • Serum complement (C3) < 84 mg/dL • LNDAI ≥ 3
Authors	Miyasaka N, Kawai S, Hashimoto H
Publication	*Mod Rheumatol.* 2009;19(6):606–615
Follow-up	28 weeks
Note	*Changes in the lupus nephritis activity index*:

Changes in the lupus nephritis activity index:

	Tacrolimus	Placebo
% Change	-32.9	2.3
Absolute change	-1.8	0.0

Normalization of:

	Tacrolimus	Placebo
Daily urinary protein excretion	n = 27	n = 33
Urinary RBC count	n = 12	n = 15
Anti-ds-DNA antibody	n = 14	n = 19
Complement (C3)	n = 21	n = 33
Maintenance of-normal serum creatinine	n = 24	n = 29

(continued)

Adverse events	Tacrolimus (%)	Placebo (%)
Acute myocardial infarction	7.1	0
Hypertension	7.1	80.6
Nausea	14.3	0
Stomatitis	0	5.7
Headache	0	8.6
Migraine	7.1	0
Weight gain	0	5.7
Blood creatinine increased	7.1	11.4
Creatinine clearance decreased	7.1	0
Blood uric acid increased	0	8.6
Urine b_2 microglobulin increased	10.7	17.1
NAG increased	25.0	17.1
Blood glucose increased	14.3	0
Glycosylated hemoglobin increased	7.1	0
Urine glucose positive	10.7	0
Hemoglobin decreased	0	5.7
White blood cell count increased	7.1	0
AST increased	7.1	0
Blood LDH increased	7.1	0
c-GTP increased	0	5.7
Blood albumin decreased	0	5.7
Blood urea increased	7.1	5.7
b_2 microglobulin increased	0	11.4
Blood amylase increased	0	8.6
Blood cholesterol increased	7.1	8.6
Blood triglycerides increased	0	5.7
All infections	57.1	57.1
Serious infections	7.1	2.9

Trial	Short-term outcomes of induction therapy with tacrolimus versus cyclophosphamide for active lupus nephritis: A multicenter randomized clinical trial
Substance	**Tacrolimus 0.05 mg/kg/day**, titrated to achieve a trough blood concentration of 5–10 ng/mL (n = 42) **Cyclophosphamide 750 mg/m² i. v.**, then adjusted to 500–1,000 mg/m², every 4 weeks, total of 6 pulse treatments (n = 39) *Concomitant medication:* Prednisone 1 mg/kg/day (maximum, 60 mg/day) Tapered by 10 mg/day every 2 weeks to 40 mg/day Followed by a decrease of 5 mg/day every 2 weeks until 10 mg/day 10 mg/day was maintained to the end of 6 months. Angiotensin-converting enzyme inhibitors and/or angiotensin receptor blockers at stable doses Statins and/or fibric acid derivatives were required Contraception *Previous medication:* No mycophenolate mofetil ≤ 1 month No cyclophosphamide ≤ 1 month No cyclosporine ≤ 1 month No methotrexate ≤ 1 month No other immunosuppressive agents ≤ 1 month
Result	In conjunction with prednisone, induction therapy with tacrolimus was as efficacious as intravenous cyclophosphamide and prednisone in producing complete remission of lupus nephritis and had a more favorable safety profile
Patients	81 patients, diagnosis according to the ACR criteria for SLE • Biopsy-proven lupus nephritis Class III, IV-S, or IV-G, (A) or (A/C), or Class V *Active nephritis:* • Proteinuria ≥ 1 g/24 h • Increased serum creatinine level (≥ 1.3 mg/dL) • Active urinary sediment (any of ≥ 5 red blood cells/high power field, ≥ 5 white blood cells/high power field, or red blood cell casts in the absence of infection or other causes) • No cerebral lupus
Authors	Chen W, Tang X, Liu Q, Chen W, Fu P, Liu F, Liao Y, Yang Z, Zhang J, Chen J, Lou T, Fu J, Kong Y, Liu Z, Fan A, Rao S, Li Z, Yu X
Publication	*Am J Kidney Dis.* 2011 Feb;57(2):235–244
Follow-up	6 months

(continued) ➔

Note	Patients achieving complete remission:		
		Tacrolimus	Cyclophosphamide i. v.
	Partial remission	n = 16	n = 17
	No. of patients failing to meet complete remission	n = 17	n = 19
	Proteinuria ≥ 0.3 g/24 h	n = 17/17	n = 19/19
	Serum albumin < 3.5 g/dL	n = 4/17	n = 4/19
	Serum creatinine ≥ 1.47 mg/dL or ≥ 115% of baseline	n = 1/17	n = 1/19
	No. of patients failing to meet complete or partial remission	n = 1	n = 2
	Proteinuria ≥ 3.0 g/24 h or decrease < 50% from baseline	n = 1/1	n = 2/2
	Serum albumin ≥ 3.0 g/dL	n = 0/1	n = 0/2
	Serum creatinine ≥120% of baseline	n = 1/1	n = 1/2
	Adjusted mean after 1 months:		
		Tacrolimus	Cyclophosphamide i. v.
	Proteinuria (g/24 h)	0.01	0.23
	Serum albumin (g/dL)	0.54	0.50
	Serum creatinine (mg/dL)	-0.04	-0.08
	MDRD Study eGFR (mL/min)	1.84	1.88
	Serum C3 (mg/dL)	1.85	1.82
	Adjusted mean after 6 months:		
		Tacrolimus	Cyclophosphamide i. v.
	Proteinuria (g/24 h)	-0.33	-0.28
	Serum albumin (g/dL)	0.62	0.60
	Serum creatinine (mg/dL)	-0.05	-0.10
	MDRD Study eGFR (mL/min)	1.91	1.97
	Serum C3 (mg/dL)	-0.04	-0.10
Adverse events		Tacrolimus	Cyclophosphamide i. v.
	No. of patients with infections	n = 5	n = 4
	No. of infectious episodes	n = 12	n = 7
	Upper respiratory tract	n = 3	n = 2
	Pulmonary	n = 1	n = 1
	Urinary tract	n = 3	n = 2
	Herpes zoster	n = 5	n = 2
	Leukopenia	n = 0	n = 5
	Gastrointestinal symptoms	n = 4	n = 10
	Hair loss	n = 0	n = 3
	Liver function disorder	n = 3	n = 4
	Amenorrhea	n = 0	n = 2
	Hyperglycemia	n = 7	n = 6
	Transient increase in serum creatinine	n = 3	n = 1
	Death	n = 0	n = 1

Trial	The efficacy and safety of abatacept in patients with non–life-threatening manifestations of systemic lupus erythematosus: results of a 12-month, multicenter, exploratory, Phase IIb, randomized, double-blind, placebo-controlled trial
Substance	**Abatacept 10 mg/kg day** 0–15–29, and then every 4 weeks (n = 61) **Placebo** (n = 57) *Concomitant medication:* Prednisone 30 mg/day (or equivalent) for 1 month Dosage was tapered NSAIDs were permitted if given at a stable dose ≥ 1 months Azathioprine were permitted if given at a stable dose ≥ 1 months MMF was permitted if given at a stable dose ≥ 1 months Chloroquine was permitted if given at a stable dose ≥ 1 months Hydroxychloroquine were permitted if given at a stable dose ≥ 1 months MTX was permitted if given at a stable dose ≥ 1 month Angiotensin-converting enzyme inhibitors or angiotensin receptor–blocking agents and statins at a stable dose ≥ 1 months
Result	Effects of abatacept were seen in post-hoc analyses with respect to new BILAG-A flares, physician-assessed flares and patient reported outcomes, especially in the polyarthritis group, in patients with non–life-threatening manifestations of SLE. There was an increased rate of severe adverse events
Patients	118 patients meeting the ACR criteria for SLE 1 of the following primary manifestations: • Active polyarthritis • Active discoid lesions • Active pleuritis and/or pericarditis • Disease activity was defined according to the British Isles Lupus Activity Group (BILAG) index • ≥ 1 BILAG A or ≥ 2 BILAG B
Authors	Merrill JT, Burgos-Vargas R, Westhovens R, Chalmers A, D'Cruz D, Wallace DJ, Bae SC, Sigal L, Becker JC, Kelly S, Raghupathi K, Li T, Peng Y, Kinaszczuk M, Nash P
Publication	*Arthritis Rheum.* 2010 Oct;62(10):3077–3087
Follow-up	12 months
Note	

	Abatacept (%)	Placebo (%)
New BILAG A/B flares	79.7	82.5
BILAG A flare	40.7	54.4
Physician-assessed flare	63.6	82.5

(continued) ➔

Adverse events		Abatacept (%)	Placebo (%)
	Total	90.9	91.5
	Serious adverse events	19.8	6.8
	Musculoskeletal and connective tissue disorders	5.0	1.7
	General disorders and administration site conditions	3.3	0
	Infections and infestations	2.5	1.7
	Renal and urinary disorders	2.5	0
	Gastrointestinal disorders	1.7	1.7
	Nervous system disorders	1.7	1.7
	Psychiatric disorder	1.7	1.7
	Cardiac disorders	1.7	0
	Immune system disorders	1.7	0
	Injury, poisoning, and procedural complications	1.7	0
	Respiratory, thoracic, and mediastinal disorders	1.7	0
	Blood and lymphatic system disorders	0.8	0
	Metabolism and nutrition disorders	0.8	0
	Skin and subcutaneous tissue disorders	0	1.7
	Vascular disorders	0	1.7

Trial	Biologic activity and safety of belimumab, a neutralizing anti-B-lymphocyte stimulator (BLyS) monoclonal antibody: a phase I trial in patients with systemic lupus erythematosus BLISS-Belimumab in Subjects With Systemic Lupus Erythematosus
Substance	**Placebo** (n = 13) **Belimumab 1.0 mg/kg** (n = 15) **Belimumab 4.0 mg/kg** (n = 14) **Belimumab 10.0 mg/kg** (n = 14) **Belimumab 20.0 mg/kg** (n = 14) As a single infusion or two infusions 21 days apart
Result	Belimumab was well-tolerated and reduced peripheral B-cell levels in this phase-I trial
Patients	70 patients with mild-to-moderate SLE
Authors	Furie R, Stohl W, Ginzler EM, Becker M, Mishra N, Chatham W, Merrill JT, Weinstein A, McCune WJ, Zhong J, Cai W, Freimuth W; Belimumab Study Group
Publication	*Arthritis Res Ther.* 2008;10(5):R109
Follow-up	84–105 days
Note	*Outcome measures:*

	Placebo	Belimumab
SELENA SLEDAI score scoring 0	33%	37%

(continued) ➔

Adverse events		Placebo	1 mg/kg belimumab	4 mg/kg belimumab	10 mg/kg belimumab	20 mg/kg belimumab
	Arthralgia	n = 4	n = 3	n = 2	n = 7	n = 3
	Headache	n = 1	n = 3	n = 3	n = 4	n = 2
	Rash	n = 0	n = 4	n = 2	n = 2	n = 4
	Diarrhea	n = 0	n = 5	n = 1	n = 1	n = 3
	Nausea	n = 4	n = 2	n = 3	n = 2	n = 3
	Fatigue	n = 0	n = 1	n = 2	n = 3	n = 1
	Back pain	n = 1	n = 0	n = 2	n = 1	n = 3
	Joint swelling	n = 2	n = 0	n = 1	n = 0	n = 4
	Synovitis	n = 1	n = 2	n = 0	n = 3	n = 0
	Depression	n = 0	n = 3	n = 0	n = 0	n = 0
	Infections and infestations	n = 8	n = 4	n = 8	n = 4	n = 5
	Upper respiratory tract infection	n = 2	n = 0	n = 3	n = 1	n = 3
	Thrombocytopenia	n = 0	n = 0	n = 1	n = 0	n = 0
	Pancreatitis	n = 0	n = 0	n = 0	n = 0	n = 1
	Cellulitis staphylococcal	n = 0	n = 0	n = 0	n = 1	n = 0
	Sepsis	n = 1	n = 0	n = 0	n = 0	n = 0
	Aspartate aminotransferase increased	n = 0	n = 0	n = 0	n = 0	n = 1
	Blood creatinine increased	n = 0	n = 0	n = 0	n = 0	n = 1
	Neutrophil count decreased	n = 0	n = 0	n = 0	n = 2	n = 0
	Dehydration	n = 0	n = 0	n = 0	n = 0	n = 1
	Pain in extremity	n = 0	n = 0	n = 1	n = 0	n = 0
	Headache	n = 0	n = 0	n = 0	n = 1	n = 0
	Sinus headache	n = 0	n = 1	n = 0	n = 0	n = 0
	Angioneurotic edema	n = 0	n = 0	n = 1	n = 0	n = 0
	Urticaria	n = 0	n = 0	n = 0	n = 0	n = 1
	Activated partial thromboplastin time (grade 3)	n = 0	n = 1	n = 1	n = 0	n = 1
	Creatinine (grade 3)	n = 0	n = 0	n = 0	n = 0	n = 1
	Hemoglobin (grade 3)	n = 0	n = 0	n = 0	n = 0	n = 0
	Hyperglycemia (grade 3)	n = 0	n = 1	n = 0	n = 0	n = 0
	Neutropenia (grade 3)	n = 0	n = 1	n = 1	n = 2	n = 0
	Thrombocytopenia (grade 4)	n = 0	n = 0	n = 1	n = 0	n = 0
	Proteinuria (grade 3)	n = 0	n = 0	n = 0	n = 1	n = 1
	Proteinuria (grade 4)	n = 0	n = 0	n = 0	n = 0	n = 1
	Prothrombin time (grade 3)	n = 3	n = 1	n = 0	n = 0	n = 0
	Prothrombin time (grade 4)	n = 2	n = 0	n = 0	n = 0	n = 0

Trial	A Phase II, randomized, double-blind, placebo-controlled, dose-ranging study of belimumab in patients with active systemic lupus erythematosus
Substance	**Placebo** (n = 113) **Belimumab 1 mg/kg** (n = 114) **Belimumab 4 mg/kg** (n = 111) **Belimumab 10 mg/kg** (n = 111) on days 0, 14, 28, and then every 28 days for 52 weeks plus SOC *Concomitant medication*: Standard of care Prednisone 5–40 mg/day Antimalarials or immunosuppressives ≥ 60 days *Previous medication*: No cyclosporine, intravenous immunoglobulin biologics, cyclophosphamide, or doses of prednisone > 100 mg/day < 6 months
Result	Belimumab was biologically active and well tolerated in this Phase-II trial. There were effects of belimumab on the time to flare. In serologically active patients, belimumab demonstrated improvement in disease activity and of patient reported outcomes, as compared to placebo
Patients	Patients fulfilling the ACR criteria for SLE, and • SELENA-SLEDAI score ≥ 4 • Positive antinuclear antibodies • Positive anti-dsDNA, anti-Smith, anti-RNP, anti-Ro, anti-La, or anti-cardiolipin • No active lupus nephritis • No central nervous system disease
Authors	Wallace DJ, Stohl W, Furie RA, Lisse JR, McKay JD, Merrill JT, Petri MA, Ginzler EM, Chatham WW, McCune WJ, Fernandez V, Chevrier MR, Zhong ZJ, Freimuth WW
Publication	*Arthritis Rheum*. 2009 Sep 15;61(9):1168–1178
Follow-up	52 weeks

(continued)

Note

Outcome parameters (all patients):

	Placebo	1 mg/kg Belimumab	4 mg/kg Belimumab	10 mg/kg Belimumab
Time to first flare from weeks 24–52	108	154	135	152
SLE flare from weeks 24–52, %	72.8	67.7	66.4	63.9
% Increase prednisolone to > 7.5 mg/day	12.3	12.2	6.6	2.7
Delete ≥ 1 DMARD	5.3	5.3	5.4	2.7
No change DMARD therapy	83.2	90.3	85.6	91.9
Add ≥ 1 DMARD	11.5	4.4	9.0	5.4
New 1A or 1B BILAG, %	35.4	33.3	28.8	26.1
Time to first flare over week 52	83	68	61	70

Outcome parameters (serological active patients):

	Placebo	1 mg/kg Belimumab	4 mg/kg Belimumab	10 mg/kg Belimumab
Time to first flare from weeks 24–52	111	170	167	126
SLE flare from weeks 24–52, %	71.4	64.2	62.7	65.2
% Increase prednisolone to > 7.5 mg/day	12.8	14.6	8.0	2.3
Delete ≥ 1 DMARD	4.7	5.1	2.5	1.3
No change DMARD therapy	81.4	88.5	86.1	91.0
Add ≥ 1 DMARD	14.0	6.4	11.4	7.7
New 1A or 1B BILAG, %	39.5	35.9	26.6	25.6
Time to first flare over week 52	84	68	77	84

Change of (all patients):

	Placebo	1 mg/kg Belimumab	4 mg/kg Belimumab	10 mg/kg Belimumab
SELENA-SLEDAI at week 24	-17.2	-23.3	-11.3	-23.7
SELENA-SLEDAI at week 52	-20.6	-29.7	-23.9	-27.9
Modified SELENA-SLEDAI at week 52	-23.9	-37.1	-34.7	-32.6
PGA at week 52	-13.8	-28.3	-30.6	-33.0
SF-36 PCS at week 52	1.4	2.7	1.7	3.4
% Prednisone reduction	27.1	20.0	31.4	44.7
Prednisone dose reduction mg/day Days 309–337	-1.7	+0.4	-2.6	-6.4
Prednisone dose reduction mg/day Days 337–364	-2.1	+0.3	-2.4	-6.4

Change of (serological active patients):

	Placebo	1 mg/kg Belimumab	4 mg/kg Belimumab	10 mg/kg Belimumab
SELENA-SLEDAI at week 24	-15.6	-25.5	-6.8	-30.0
SELENA-SLEDAI at week 52	-14.2	-34.3	-19.3	-33.0
Modified SELENA-SLEDAI at week 52	-17.8	-44.4	-33.0	-40.1
PGA at week 52	-10.7	-30.1	-34.2	-33.7
SF-36 PCS at week 52	1.2	3.6	1.9	3.5
% Prednisone reduction	30.8	23.3	37.9	50.0
Prednisone dose reduction mg/day Days 309–337	-3.1	+0.3	-2.6	-7.8
Prednisone dose reduction mg/day Days 337–364	-3.4	+0.4	-2.7	-7.8

(continued) ➜

Adverse events		Placebo (%)	1 mg/kg Belimumab (%)	4 mg/kg Belimumab (%)	10 mg/kg Belimumab (%)
	≥ 1 AE	97.3	97.4	96.4	97.3
	≥ 1 serious AE	19.5	18.4	13.5	16.2
	Infections and infestations	72.6	74.6	79.3	73.0
	≥ 1 serious infection AE	3.5	6.1	6.3	2.7
	≥ 1 severe infection AE	2.7	7.0	5.4	3.6
	Musculoskeletal and connective tissue disorders	70.8	64.9	64.0	68.5
	Skin and subcutaneous tissue disorders	50.4	63.2	58.6	49.6
	Gastrointestinal disorders	55.8	55.3	54.1	57.7
	Nervous system disorders	46.9	43.9	51.4	54.1
	General disorders and administration site conditions	54.9	41.2	57.7	48.7
	Respiratory, thoracic, and mediastinal disorders	46.0	44.7	34.2	44.1
	Arthralgia	37.2	36.0	33.3	36.9
	Upper respiratory tract infection	29.2	31.6	32.4	26.1
	Headache	23.9	25.4	27.9	31.5
	Fatigue	31.0	23.7	29.7	24.3
	Nausea	23.9	27.2	19.8	29.7
	Diarrhea	16.8	16.7	20.7	15.3
	Arthritis	16.8	14.0	18.9	16.2
	Urinary tract infection	15.9	14.0	17.1	18.0

BLISS-52-Trial	Efficacy and safety of belimumab in patients with active systemic lupus erythematosus: a randomized, placebo-controlled, Phase III trial BLISS-Belimumab in Subjects With Systemic Lupus Erythematosus
Substance	**Placebo** (n = 288) **Belimumab 1 mg/kg** (n = 289) **Belimumab 10 mg/kg** (n = 290) on days 0, 14, and 28, and then every 28 days until 48 weeks *Concomitant medication*: No changes of immunosuppressive drugs after 16 weeks No changes of antimalarial drugs after 24 weeks Changes for prednisone dose was not restricted in the first 24 weeks, thereafter return to 25% or 5 mg greater than baseline dose Addition of a new immunosuppressive or biological drug at any time was prohibited New antimalarial drug after 4 months was prohibited New angiotensin-converting-enzyme inhibitors after 4 months was prohibited New statins after 6 months were prohibited *Previous medication*: And a stable treatment regimen with fixed doses of prednisone (0–40 mg/day), or Nonsteroidal antiinflammatory, antimalarial, or immunosuppressive drugs ≥ 30 days No previous B-lymphocyte-targeted drug No intravenous cyclophosphamide ≤ 6 months of enrolment No i. v. immunoglobulin Ig or prednisone (> 100 mg/day) ≤ 3 months
Result	Belimumab was more effective than placebo in reducing disease activity and carticosteroid use, without clear dose dependency and with adequate safety, in this phase-III trial of serologically and clinically active disease
Patients	867 patients fulfilling the ACR criteria for SLE With active disease: • SELENA-SLEDAI score ≥ 6 • Positive ANA (titer ≥ 1:80) or anti-dsDNA antibody (≥ 30 IU/mL) • No active lupus nephritis or CNS lupus
Authors	Navarra SV, Guzmán RM, Gallacher AE, Hall S, Levy RA, Jimenez RE, Li EK, Thomas M, Kim HY, León MG, Tanasescu C, Nasonov E, Lan JL, Pineda L, Zhong ZJ, Freimuth W, Petri MA; BLISS-52 Study Group
Publication	*Lancet.* 2011 Feb 26;377(9767):721–31
Follow-up	52 weeks

(continued)

Note		Belimumab 1 mg	Belimumab 10 mg	Placebo
	SRI response rate	51%	58%	44%
	Reduction ≥ 4 points in SELENA-SLEDAI	53%	58%	46%
	No worsening with BILAG	78%	81%	73%
	No worsening with PGA (total)	79%	80%	69%
	No worsening with PGA (Asia-Pacific)	38%	50%	39%
	No worsening with PGA (Latin America)	59%	61%	49%
	No worsening with PGA (Eastern Europe)	62%	74%	36%
	Time to first flare during 52 weeks (days)	126	119	84
	Patients with flare	70%	71%	80%
	SFI, severe	18%	14%	23%
	New BILAG 1A or 2B	27%	19%	30%
	New BILAG 1A PGA score	19%	10%	20%
	Change of PGA at week 24	-0.39	-0.50	-0.35
	Improvement (decrease ≥ 0·3) at week 52 Steroid-sparing activity	59%	64%	49%
	Prednisone dose reduced by ≥ 25% to ≤ 7·5 mg/day during weeks 40–52	21%	19%	12%
	Prednisone dose reduced by ≥ 50% at week 52	23%	28%	18%
	Prednisone dose increased to > 7·5 mg/day at week 52 from ≤ 7·5 mg/day	30%	20%	36%
	Patients with sustained reduction (≥ 12 weeks) in prednisone dose from a baseline of > 7·5 mg/day	24%	28%	15%
	Health-related quality of life (SF-36 PCS score, absolute change from baseline) Week 24	3.39	3.34	3.26
	Health-related quality of life (SF-36 PCS score, absolute change from baseline) Week 52	4.17	4.19	2.84
	Median (IQR) change in C3 concentration from baseline at week 52	2.74%	5.59%	-3.03%
	Return of low C3 concentrations to normal	23%	34%	14%
	Median (IQR) change in C4 concentrations from baseline at week 52	21.83%	30.38%	0%
	Return of low C4 concentrations to normal	36%	43%	19%
	Return of hypergammaglobulinemia to normal	50%	49%	19%
	Median (IQR) change in anti-dsDNA concentrations from baseline to week 52	-35.13%	-37.57%	-12.26%
	Anti-dsDNA positive to negative at week 52	13%	17%	6%

(continued)

Adverse events	Belimumab 1 mg (%)	Belimumab 10 mg (%)	Placebo (%)
Adverse event ($n \geq 1$)	92	92	92
Serious adverse event ($n \geq 1$)	16	14	13
Severe adverse event ($n \geq 1$)	13	11	12
Discontinuations due to adverse events	6	5	7
Deaths	< 1	1	1
Malignant neoplasm	0	0	0
Infections(all)	68	67	64
Serious infection ($n \geq 1$)	8	4	6
Severe infection ($n \geq 1$)	3	2	3
Admission to hospital due to infections	7	4	6
Opportunistic infections	0	< 1	0
Headache	20	23	26
Upper respiratory tract infection	14	12	16
Arthralgia	7	11	12
Urinary tract infection	10	9	9
Influenza	8	11	9
Diarrhea	10	10	7
Nasopharyngitis	10	7	8
Hypertension	9	6	10
Nausea	6	8	11
Infusion reactions (all)	16	17	17
Infusion reactions requiring medical intervention	7	9	8
Severe infusion reactions	1	1	< 1
White blood cells ($< 2 \times 10^9$ L)	1	4	3
Neutrophils ($< 1 \times 10^9$ L)	4	4	4
Lymphocytes ($< 5 \times 10^8$ L)	28	26	25
Hemoglobin (≤ 80 g/L)	4	2	5
Prothrombin time (17.25 s)	6	6	4
Proteinuria (> 2 g/24 h)	16	14	18
Hypogammaglobulinemia (< 4 g/L)	0	< 1	0
Change of IgG	-14.1	-15.6	-3.6
Change of IgA	-16.8	-16.0	-2.7
Change of IgM	-28.5	-30.0	-3.2
Pregnancy	1	4	2
Spontaneous abortion or still-birth	33	46	60

BLISS-76-Trial	A phase III, randomized, placebo-controlled study of belimumab, a monoclonal antibody that inhibits B lymphocyte stimulator, in patients with systemic lupus erythematosus BLISS: Belimumab in Subjects With Systemic Lupus Erythematosus
Substance	**Placebo** (n = 275) **Belimumab 1 mg/kg** (n = 271) **Belimumab 10 mg/kg** (n = 273) Intravenously on days 0, 14, and 28 and then every 28 days for 72 weeks *Concomitant medication*: No new immunosuppressive drugs New antimalarial drug and dosage increases of concomitant immunosuppressives or antimalarial drugs were permitted until week 16 Corticosteroids at any dose through week 24; thereafter dose within 25% or 5 mg or greater than baseline dose *Previous medication*: Stable prednisone (or equivalent) (7.5–40 mg/day) or stable antimalarial drugs Stable nonsteroidal antiinflammatory drugs Stable immunosuppressive therapies No B cell–targeted agent No i. v. cyclophosphamide ≤ 6 months No tumor necrosis factor inhibitor, anakinra, IVIG, prednisone ≥ 100 mg/day, or plasmapheresis ≤ 3 months
Result	Belimumab at 10 mg/kg, plus standard therapy unambiguosly reduced SLE disease activity and severe flares in week 52, but not anymore in week 76, in this phase-III trial of serologically and clinically active SLE, and was generally well-tolerated
Patients	819 patients fulfilling the ACR criteria for SLE • Antinuclear antibody ≥ 1:80 • Anti-dsDNA antibody ≥ 30 IU/mL • SELENA-SLEDAI scores ≥ 6 • No serious intercurrent illness • No severe active lupus nephritis • No severe central nervous system manifestations
Authors	Furie R, Petri M, Zamani O, Cervera R, Wallace DJ, Tegzová D, Sanchez-Guerrero J, Schwarting A, Merrill JT, Chatham WW, Stohl W, Ginzler EM, Hough DR, Zhong ZJ, Freimuth W, van Vollenhoven RF; BLISS-76 Study Group
Publication	*Arthritis Rheum.* 2011 Dec;63(12):3918–3930
Follow-up	76 weeks

(continued) ➜

Note | *Outcome parameters:*

	Placebo (%)	Belimumab 1 mg/kg (%)	Belimumab 10 mg/kg (%)
Responder Index (SRI) response rate	32.4	39.1	38.5
SPI response after 52 weeks	33.8	40.6	43.2
Durability of week 52 SRI response ≥ 1 month	35.6	38.8	41.0
Durability of week 52 SRI response ≥ 2 months	30.2	37.3	38.2
Durability of week 52 SRI response ≥ 3 months	28.7	36.5	38.1
Durability of week 52 SRI response ≥ 4 months	28.7	36.3	38.1
Durability of week 52 SRI response ≥ 5 months	28.4	33.6	35.4
Durability of week 52 SRI response ≥ 6 months	25.1	30.5	34.1
≥ 6-point reduction in SELENA	20.4	26.9	28.9
Percent change from baseline in SELENA–SLEDAI	-27.8	-36.1	-37.0
Patients with corticosteroid dose reduced to ≤ 7.5 mg/day	17.5	27.7	25.8
Patients with corticosteroid dose increase to ≤ 7.5 mg/day	18.1	13.5	11.8
Increase in corticosteroid use	20.7	14.7	11.8
Flare rate	26.5	18.5	20.5
Median percent change in anti-dsDNA	-9.7	-43.3	-49.5
Median percent change in C4	16.7	38.5	51.9
Median percent change in CD20pos B cells	0	-55.7	-54.8
Median change in short-lived plasma B cells	-7.7	-17.9	-42.9
≥ 4-point reduction in SELENA–SLEDAI	35.3	40.6	46.5
No worsening by BILAG	65.5	74.9	69.2
No worsening by PGA	62.9	72.7	69.6
SRI modified by SELENA–SLEDAI ≥ 5 points (week 52)	20.4	31.0	32.6
SRI modified by SELENA–SLEDAI ≥ 6 points (week 52)	18.9	28.8	30.8
SRI modified by SELENA–SLEDAI ≥ 7 points (week 52)	13.4	19.4	21.3

(continued)

SRI modified by SELENA–SLEDAI ≥ 8 points (week 52)	13.3	18.5	21.4
SRI modified by SELENA–SLEDAI ≥ 9 points (week 52)	8.2	14.0	15.4
SRI modified by SELENA–SLEDAI ≥ 10 points (week 52)	8.6	13.9	15.4
SRI response rate at week 76	32.4	39.1	38.5
≥ 4-point reduction in SELENA–SLEDAI score§	33.8	42.1	41.4
No worsening by BILAG	58.9	69.0	63.4
No worsening by PGA	58.2	65.7	63.0
SRI modified by SELENA–SLEDAI ≥ 5 points (week 76)	21.8	28.4	30.8
SRI modified by SELENA–SLEDAI ≥ 6 points (week 76)	20.4	26.9	29.9
SRI modified by SELENA–SLEDAI ≥ 7 points (week 76)	13.9	21.7	21.8
SRI modified by SELENA–SLEDAI ≥ 8 points (week 76)	12.9	19.9	21.9
SRI modified by SELENA–SLEDAI ≥ 9 points (week 76)	4.8	14.7	15.4
SRI modified by SELENA–SLEDAI ≥ 10 points (week 76)	5.0	14.6	14.0

(continued)

Adverse events		Placebo (%)	Belimumab 1 mg/kg (%)	Belimumab 10 mg/kg (%)
	Patients with ≥ 1 AE	92.0	93.4	92.7
	≥ 1 serious AE	19.6	23.2	22.3
	≥ 1 severe AE	18.9	18.8	19.8
	Discontinuations due to AEs	8.4	6.6	8.4
	Deaths	0	0.7	0.4
	Malignant neoplasms	0.4	1.5	0.7
	Malignancy solid organs	0.4	1.1	0.4
	Nonmelanoma skin	0	0.4	0.4
	Infections all	69.1	74.5	74.0
	≥ 1 serious infection AE	5.8	7.0	7.3
	≥ 1 severe infection AE	4.0	3.0	2.6
	Opportunistic infection	0	0	0.4
	Upper respiratory tract infection	21.1	19.6	19.8
	Headache	13.8	20.7	16.1
	Urinary tract infection	15.6	18.5	16.1
	Arthralgia	15.6	15.9	15.0
	Nausea	9.8	15.9	16.8
	Diarrhea	10.2	12.9	12.1
	Nasopharyngitis	8.7	10.7	15.8
	Sinusitis	10.2	7.7	11.4
	Back pain	7.6	9.6	9.9
	Fatigue	9.1	10.0	7.7
	Pyrexia	7.6	8.5	10.6
	Bronchitis	7.6	7.0	11.7
	Insomnia	4.7	10.0	6.2
	Infusion reactions (all)	9.8	15.5	13.6
	Infusion reactions requiring medical intervention	3.3	5.9	6.2
	Severe infusion reactions	0.4	0.4	1.1
	WBC count $< 2 \times 10^9/L$	4.4	4.1	4.0
	Neutrophil count $< 1 \times 10^9/L$	7.3	6.7	5.9
	Lymphocyte count $< 5 \times 10^8/L$	29.1	29.2	27.9
	Hemoglobin ≤ 80 g/L	5.5	2.6	1.8
	Prothrombin time	11.6	13.6	11.2
	Proteinuria (> 2 g/24 h)	7.7	7.1	10.4
	Hypogammaglobulinemia (< 4 g/L)	0.4	0.4	0.4
	Change of IgG	-0.8	-15.1	-16.4
	Change of IgA	-2.1	-18.0	-20.4
	Change of IgM	-3.8	-31.8	-35.0
	Pregnancy (all)	n = 0	n = 3	n = 2
	Live birth without congenital anomaly	n = 0	n = 2	n = 1

Trial	Safety and efficacy of tumor necrosis factor alpha blockade in systemic lupus erythematosus: an open-label study
Substance	**Infliximab 300 mg** i. v. ($\approx$ 5 mg/kg), at weeks 0, 2, 6, and 10 Plus azathioprine or methotrexate *Concomitant medication*: Azathioprine, methotrexate, chloroquine continued at stable doses Prednisone was continued at stable doses
Result	Infliximab had a therapeutic effect in patients with low or moderate disease activity with respect to kidney and joint disease. Severe adverse events or adverse events related to an increase in SLE activity were not observed
Patients	6 patients fulfilling the ACR criteria for SLE • Low-to-moderate disease activity, for at least 3 months prior to inclusion • In case of renal disease: patients unresponsive to cytotoxic therapy
Authors	Aringer M, Graninger WB, Steiner G, Smolen JS
Publication	*Arthritis Rheum*. 2004 Oct;50(10):3161–3169
Follow-up	52 weeks
Note	*Outcome parameters*: No significant serum titer changes of dsDNA antibodies None of the patients experienced an increased disease activity Joint swelling stopped in all three patients with active arthritis In all 4 patients with nephritis proteinuria decreased

		Baseline	End of follow-up
	Systemic Lupus Erythematosus Index Score (SIS)	10	6
	SLEDAI	9	5
	Creatinine clearance rate (mL/min)	79	100

Adverse events	Febrile episode	n = 1
	Urinary tract infection	n = 3
	Increase of anti dsDNA level	n = 4
	Increase of anti cardiolipin antibodies	n = 4

Trial	Efficacy and safety of Infliximab in active SLE: a pilot study	
Substance	Control group with standard care (n = 18) **Infliximab 3 mg/kg** i. v. at 0, 2, 6 weeks and then every 8 weeks (n = 9) *Concomitant medication*: INH Prophylaxis in case of positive TBC testing Corticosteroids were continued DMARds were continued	
Result	Several clinical and serological parameters improved, the safety profile was good	
Patients	27 patients with active SLE satisfying the ACR criteria for SLE	
Authors	Uppal SS, Hayat SJ, Raghupathy R	
Publication	*Lupus*. 2009 Jul;18(8):690–697	
Follow-up	24 weeks	
Note	*Outcome parameters*:	

		Infliximab	Control
	Requirement of glucosteroid pulses	0.4	0.4

Change of (after 6 months):

	Infliximab	Control
SLEDAI	-27.75	-13.33
SLICC	0.0	+0.1
VAS Fatigue	-35.0	-15.0
Glucosteroid dose (mg)	-38.75	+4
SF36-Physical	+10.9	+3.36
SF36-Role physical	+16.92	+5.63
SF36-Bodily pain	+17.56	+15.15
SF36-General	+8.74	+0.93
SF36-Vitality	+6.6	+2.13
SF36-Social	+16.26	+10.31
SF36-Role emotional	+14.76	+8.42
SF36-Mental	+14.08	+4.1
SF36-Physical component	+13.22	+6.13
SF36-Mental component	+12.26	+5.79
SF36-Total	+25.48	+11.92
24 h urine protein (g)	-1.23	-2.22
Total ds DNA (IU/mL)	-5.4	-25.81
Complement C3 (g/L)	+0.41	+0.39
Complement C4 (g/L)	+0.11	+0.07

Adverse events		Infliximab	Control
	Infections/patient	0.4	0.5
	Admissions/patient	0.6	1.2
	Fever and chills	n = 1	n = 0
	Chest pain and dyspnea	n = 1	n = 0
	Hypostension, headache and vomiting	n = 1	n = 0
	Intense Pruritus/urticarial rash	n = 1	n = 0

Trial	A multicenter Phase I/II trial of Rituximab for refractory systemic lupus erythematosus
Substance	**Rituximab 4 infusions of 500 mg** every week (n = 5) **Rituximab 2 infusions of 1′000 mg** every other week (n = 10) *Concomitant medication*: No corticosteroid boli No DMARDs
Result	Rituximab therapy was safe for the treatment of active SLE patients
Patients	15 patients who met the ACR criteria for SLE • With active and refractory disease • Flares according to BILAG score: • 1 × BILAG A or 2 × BILAG B • Moderate to severe flare, although they were treated with ≥ 30.4 mg/kg/day prednisolone
Authors	Tanaka Y, Yamamoto K, Takeuchi T, Nishimoto N, Miyasaka N, Sumida T, Shima Y, Takada K, Matsumoto I, Saito K, Koike T
Publication	*Mod Rheumatol.* 2007;17(3):191–197
Follow-up	28 weeks

Note: *Outcome parameters (change from BILAG B)*:

	Baseline	Improvement	No change	Worsened
General	n = 4	n = 3	n = 1	n = 0
Mucocutaneous	n = 9	n = 3	n = 6	n = 0
Nervous system baseline	n = 2	n = 2	n = 0	n = 0
Musculoskeletal	n = 2	n = 1	n = 1	n = 1
Cardiovascular/ respiratory	n = 0	n = 0	n = 0	n = 0
Vasculitis	n = 2	n = 0	n = 2	n = 0
Renal	n = 4	n = 1	n = 3	n = 0
Hematological	n = 2	n = 1	n = 1	n = 3

Outcome parameters (change from BILAG A):

	Baseline	Improvement	No change	Worsened
General	n = 1	n = 0	n = 1	n = 0
Mucocutaneous	n = 0	n = 0	n = 0	n = 0
Nervous system baseline	n = 3	n = 3	n = 0	n = 0
Musculoskeletal	n = 0	n = 0	n = 0	n = 0
Cardiovascular/ respiratory	n = 1	n = 0	n = 1	n = 0
Vasculitis	n = 0	n = 0	n = 0	n = 0
Renal	n = 2	n = 2	n = 0	n = 0
Hematological	n = 1	n = 1	n = 0	n = 0

(continued)

Adverse events		Grade 1 (n = 16)	Grade 2 (n = 27)	Grade 3 (n = 3)
	Infection	n = 5	n = 21	n = 3
	Redness of foot pad	n = 1	n = 0	n = 0
	Flush	n = 1	n = 0	n = 0
	Muscle weakness of hands	n = 1	n = 0	n = 0
	Tremor	n = 1	n = 0	n = 0
	Tachycardia	n = 1	n = 0	n = 0
	Edema of feet	n = 1	n = 0	n = 0
	Subcutaneous nodule	n = 1	n = 0	n = 0
	Hypertension	n = 1	n = 0	n = 0
	Headache	n = 1	n = 0	n = 0
	Sore throat	n = 1	n = 0	n = 0
	Paresthesia	n = 1	n = 0	n = 0
	Diarrhea	n = 0	n = 1	n = 0
	Skin eruption	n = 0	n = 1	n = 0
	Muscular	n = 0	n = 1	n = 0
	Pain of lower limbs	n = 0	n = 1	n = 0
	Abdominal pain	n = 0	n = 1	n = 0
	Keratosis of foot pad	n = 0	n = 1	n = 0
	Sleeping disturbance	n = 0	n = 1	n = 0

Trial	Efficacy of Rituximab (anti-CD20), for refractory systemic lupus erythematosus involving the central nervous system
Substance	Patient 1–5 and 10: **Rituximab 375 mg/m² 1×/week for 2 weeks** Patient 9: **Rituximab 375 mg/m² 1×** Patients 6, 7: Rituximab 500 mg 1x for 4 weeks Patient 8: **Rituximab 1´000 mg once biweekly for 4 weeks** *Concomitant therapy:* Moderate doses of corticosteroids (15–40 mg/day) No precise information on concomitant DMARD usage
Result	Rituximab rapidly improved refractory neuropsychiatric SLE, as evident by resolution of various clinical signs and symptoms and improvement of radiographic findings

Patients	10 patients with refractory neuropsychiatric SLE
	 • Despite intensive treatment
	  1. Presence of a highly active disease
	  2. CNS lesions resistant to conventional treatment (intravenous cyclophosphamide pulse, ciclosporin)

Authors	Tokunaga M, Saito K, Kawabata D, Imura Y, Fujii T, Nakayamada S, Tsujimura S, Nawata M, Iwata S, Azuma T, Mimori T, Tanaka Y
Publication	*Ann Rheum Dis.* 2007 Apr;66(4):470–475
Follow-up	3 months
Note	*Outcome parameters:*	
	SLEDAI scores reduced at day 28	n = 10
	These effects lasted for 1 year in five patients:	
	Complete recovery	n = 4
	Improvement of psychosis	n = 1
	Improvement of depression	n = 2
	Improvement of consciousness	n = 1
	Resolution of headache	n = 1
	Resolution of paresthesia	n = 1
	Reduction of paresis	n = 1
Adverse events	Pneumonia	n = 2
	Herpes zoster	n = 1
	Chickenpox	n = 1
	Intractable infection of decubitus ulceration	n = 1
	All infections were successfully controlled with antibiotics	

Trial	Treatment of refractory SLE with Rituximab plus Cyclophosphamide: clinical effects, serological changes, and predictors of response
Substance	**Rituximab 375 mg/m²** once weekly for 4 weeks, First and last infusion combined with cyclophosphamide 0.5 g/m² *Concomitant medication*: Methylprednisolone 250 mg i. v. together with cyclophosphamide Followed by oral glucocorticoids (0.5 mg/kg/day) for 4 weeks Glucocorticoids were rapidly tapered down to the lowest possible dose *Previous medication*: All patients were pretreated with DMARDs
Result	The majority of patients improved following rituximab plus cyclophosphamide
Patients	16 patients meeting the ACR criteria for SLE • 1 × BILAG A or 2 × BILAG B in any organ system • Not responding to conventional immunosuppressive treatment including cyclophosphamide
Authors	Jónsdóttir T, Gunnarsson I, Risselada A, Henriksson EW, Klareskog L, van Vollenhoven RF
Publication	*Ann Rheum Dis*. 2008 Mar;67(3):330–334 (Epub Sep7, 2007)
Follow-up	6 months
Note	*Outcome parameters*:	
	50% reduction in SLEDAI	n = 13
	Response according to BILAG	n = 15
	Remission defined as SLEDAI < 3	n = 9
	Relapse	n = 7
	Time to relapse (median)	18 months, range 10–40

EXPLORER trial	Efficacy and safety of rituximab in moderately-to-severely active systemic lupus erythematosus: The randomized, double-blind, phase ii/iii systemic lupus erythematosus evaluation of rituximab trial
	EXPLORER: The Exploratory Phase II/III SLE Evaluation of Rituximab
Substance	**Rituximab 1´000 mg** (RTX) on days 1, 15, 168, and 182 (n = 169) **Placebo** (n = 88)
	Concomitant medication:
	Acetaminophen together with RTX
	Diphenhydramine together with RTX
	Methylprednisolone 100 mg together with RTX
	Azathioprine 100–250 mg/day, mycophenolate mofetil 1–4 g/day, methotrexate 7.5–27.5 mg/week were continued at stable doses
	Oral prednisone 0.5 mg/kg, 0.75 mg/kg, or 1 mg/kg based on the BILAG score at entry and the amount of steroids already Steroids were tapered after day 16 (aim ≤ 10 mg/day over 10 weeks, ≤ 5 mg/day by week 52)
Result	Placebo and rituximab treatment of patients with moderately to severely active SLE on aggressive background treatment did not clearly differ with regard to clinical response in the outcome parameters used in this study
Patients	257 patients fulfilling the ACR criteria for SLE
	• 1 BILAG A score or ≥ 2 BILAG B scores despite treatment with one the immunosuppressives listed under "substance"
	• No central nervous system manifestations
	• No organ threatening disease or active condition requiring cyclophosphamide or a calcineurin inhibitor
	• Despite background immunosuppressant therapy
Authors	Merrill JT, Neuwelt CM, Wallace DJ, Shanahan JC, Latinis KM, Oates JC, Utset TO, Gordon C, Isenberg DA, Hsieh HJ, Zhang D, Brunetta PG
Publication	*Arthritis Rheum.* 2010 Jan;62(1):222–233
Follow-up	52 weeks

(continued)

Note	Outcome parameters:		
		Placebo (%)	Rituximab (%)
	No clinical response	71.6	70.4
	Partial clinical response	12.5	17.2
	Major clinical response	15.9	12.4
	Anti-dsDNA antibody (median decrease)	76	55
	Complement C3 (median increase)	129	114
	Complement C4 (median increase)	173	115
	Subgroup analysis among Hispanic patients:		
		Placebo (%)	Rituximab (%)
	Partial clinical response	9.4	13.8
	Major clinical response	6.3	20
	Change of:		
		Placebo	Rituximab
	Area under the curve minus baseline of the BILAG score	-5.9	-5.8
Adverse events		Placebo (%)	Rituximab (%)
	Cardiac disorder	5.7	3
	Infections and infestations	17	9.5
	Gastrointestinal disorders	8	4.7
	General disorder	5.7	4.1
	Musculoskeletal and connect tissue disorders	5.7	5.3
	Neutropenia	0	3.6
	Any study drug-related treatment emergent SAE	9.1	7.7
	Any infusion-related AE	38.6	43.8
	Any infusion-related AE, first infusion	29.5	27.2
	Any infusion-related AE , second infusion	16.5	17.6
	Any infusion-related AE, third infusion	10	16.3
	Any infusion-related AE, fourth infusion	5.9	18.5
	Any infusion-related SAE	17	9.5
	Any treatment-emergent infection related SAE	17	9.5
	Lower respiratory tract and lungs	4.5	3
	Bacterial	4.5	2.4
	Abdominal and gastrointestinal	4.5	1.2
	Sepsis, bacteremia, viremia, and fungemia infections	3.4	1.2
	Death	1.1	2.4

Trial	Is combination rituximab with cyclophosphamide better than rituximab alone in the treatment of lupus nephritis?
Substance	*Rituximab (n = 9)*:
	Day 1: methylprednisolone 250 mg i. v. plus **rituximab 1´000 mg**
	Day 2 to Day 5: prednisolone 30 mg /day
	Then prednisolone 0.5 mg/kg/day for 4 weeks
	Then a reduction of 5 mg every 2 weeks to 5 mg/day
	Combination rituximab with cyclophosphamide (n = 10):
	Day 1: methylprednisolone i. v. 250 mg plus
	Rituximab 1´000 mg plus 750 mg cyclophosphamide i. v.
	Day 2–5: prednisolone 30 mg/day
	Then prednisolone 0.5 mg/kg/day for 4 weeks
	Then a reduction of 5 mg every 2 weeks to 5 mg/day
	Premedication:
	Chlorpheniramine 10 mg i. v.
	Paracetamol 1 g
	Concomitant medication:
	Other immunosuppressive drugs were stopped ≥ 8 weeks
	Hydroxychloroquine was permitted
	Oral prednisolone was permitted
	Statins were permitted
	Angiotensin-converting enzymes inhibitors were started
Result	Rituximab monotherapy was effective as induction therapy in lupus nephritis with no additional improvement by cyclophosphamide
Patients	19 patients meeting the ACR criteria for SLE
	• With proliferative lupus nephritis
	• Proven by renal biopsies according to the classification of the World
	• Health Organization as proliferative glomerulonephritis Class III (focal) or intravenous (IV) (diffuse)
	• Clinical activity 56/24
	• Urinary protein excretion of ≥ 1.5 g/24 h
	• Serum albumin concentration of ≤ 35 g/L
	• No renal failure requiring dialysis
Authors	Li EK, Tam LS, Zhu TY, Li M, Kwok CL, Li TK, Leung YY, Wong KC, Szeto CC
Publication	*Rheumatology (Oxford)*. 2009 Aug;48(8):892–898
Follow-up	48 weeks

(continued) ➜

Note	At week 48:		
	Complete response	n = 4	
	Partial response	n = 11	
	Remained the same or stable	n = 3	
	Worsened	n = 2	
	Differences between the two groups	none	
	Significant improvement in activity indices in renal biopsies	n = 9	
	Effective B-cell depletion	n = 18	
	Differences in the proportion of patients with complete depletion	none	
Adverse events		RTX	RTX+Cyc
	Infections (total)	n = 7	n = 5
	Respiratory infections	n = 5	n = 7
	Urinary tract infections	n = 2	n = 2
	Gastroenteritis	n = 1	n = 2
	Septicemia	n = 1	n = 0
	Herpes zoster	n = 1	n = 0
	Abscess	n = 0	n = 1
	Cramps	n = 4	n = 0
	Ankle swelling	n = 3	n = 4
	Insomnia	n = 0	n = 2
	Pruritis	n = 0	n = 2
	Dyspepsia	n = 0	n = 2
	Urticaria	n = 0	n = 2
	Chest pain	n = 0	n = 1
	Abdominal distension	n = 0	n = 1
	Depression	n = 1	n = 0
	Malaise	n = 0	n = 1

Trial	The administration of low doses of rituximab followed by hydroxychloroquine, prednisone and low doses of mycophenolate mofetil is an effective therapy in Latin American patients with active systemic lupus erythematosus
Substance	**Rituximab 2 × 500 mg** i. v., 2 weeks apart
	Concomitant medication:
	Mythylprednisolone 500 mg i. v. before RTX-infusion
	Then prednisone, initial doses 15–60 mg/day
	Tapered according to clinical response
	Mycophenolate mofetil 500 mg/day (patients with nonrenal SLE)
	Mycophenolate mofetil 2 × 500 mg/day (patients with lupus nephritis)
	Hydroxychloroquine 400 mg/day, tapered to 200 mg/day after 6 months
Result	Low doses of rituximab with concomitant hydroxychloroquine, prednisone and low doses of mycophenolate were an effective therapy in this open study
Patients	46 patients fulfilling the ACR criteria for SLE
	• With mildly to very severely active disease
Authors	Galarza-Maldonado C, Kourilovitch MR, Molineros JE, Cardiel MH, Zurita L, Soroka NF, Yagur VY, Doukh N, Cervera R
Publication	*Autoimmun Rev.* 2010 Dec;10(2):108–111
Follow-up	24 months
Note	*MEX-SLEDAI score*:

	Baseline (%)	3 months (%)	6 months (%)	12 months (%)	18 months (%)	24 months (%)
Remission (0–1)	0	19.6	34.8	41.3	45.7	50
Mild (2–5)	4.3	2.2	4.3	4.3	4.3	6.5
Moderate (6–9)	19.6	58.7	58.7	45.7	45.7	39.2
Severe (10–13)	34.8	15.2	0	6.5	0	0
Very severe (≥ 14)	41.3	4.3	2.2	2.2	4.3	4.3

Adverse events		
Hypotension	n = 4
Tachycardia	n = 1
Skin rash	n = 1
Acute bronchitis	n = 1
Sinusitis	n = 1
Herpes zoster	n = 1
Malignancies	n = 0

Trial	Tocilizumab in systemic lupus erythematosus: data on safety, preliminary efficacy, and impact on circulating plasma cells from an open-label phase I dosage-escalation study
Substance	**Tocilizumab 2 mg/kg/2 weeks** (n = 4) **Tocilizumab 4 mg/kg/2 weeks** (n = 6) **Tocilizumab 8 mg/kg/2 weeks** (n = 6) *Concomitant medication*: Prednisone (or equivalent) ≤ 0.3 mg/kg/day Gradual tapering to 0.15 mg/kg/day Temporary increases in prednisone ≤ 0.5 mg/kg/day were permitted Hydroxychloroquine was permitted Nonsteroidal antiinflammatory drugs were permitted Angiotensin-converting enzyme inhibitors were permitted Angiotensin receptorn antagonists were permitted *Previous medication*: Prednisone at a stable dosage of ≤ 0.3 mg/kg/day for at least 2 weeks before the first dose No cyclophosphamide No pulse methylprednisolone or IVIG within 4 weeks
Result	There was improvement of disease activity in a considerable number of patients in this open study of active SLE. The safety profile was adequate, with 2 cases of marked neutropenia in the group receiving the highest dose

Patients	16 patients fulfilling the ACR criteria for SLE
	  • With mild-to-moderate disease activity as defined by 1 of the following criteria sets:
	
	Criteria set 1:
	  • Chronic glomerulonephritis, with an inadequate response to ≥ 6 months of adequate immunosuppressive therapy
	
	Plus the following four features:
	  • > 30% increase in serum creatinine levels as compared with the lowest level achieved during treatment
	  • Proteinuria at levels ≤ 1.5 times the value at baseline
	  • ≤ 2+ cellular casts in the urinary sediment
	  • Extrarenal disease activity not exceeding a score of 10 on the nonrenal components of the Safety of Estrogens in Lupus Erythematosus National Assessment (SELENA) version of the Systemic Lupus
	  • Erythematosus Disease Activity Index (SLEDAI)
	
	Criteria set 2:
	  • Moderately active extrarenal lupus
	  • Extrarenal SELENA–SLEDAI score in the range of 3–10
	  • The SELENA–SLEDAI score must have been stable for at least 2 weeks prior to screening.
	
	Plus ≥ 1 of the following 4:
	  • Serum anti-dsDNA antibody level ≥ 30 IU
	  • IgG anticardiolipin antibody level ≥ 20 IgG phospholipid units/mL
	  • CRP ≥ 0.8 mg/dL, or
	  • ESR ≥ 25 mm/h in men and ≥ 42 mm/h in women

(continued) ➔

Authors	Illei GG, Shirota Y, Yarboro CH, Daruwalla J, Tackey E, Takada K, Fleisher T, Balow JE, Lipsky PE	
Publication	*Arthritis Rheum.* 2010 Feb;62(2):542–552	
Follow-up	8 weeks	
Note	Disease activity showed decrease of ≥ 4 points SLEDAI	n = 8
	Arthritis improved	n = 7
	Change of:	
		4/8 mg/kg Toci
	Levels of anti-double-stranded DNA antibodies	-47%
	IgG level	-7.8%
Adverse events	Urinary tract infection	n = 3
	Folliculitis	n = 1
	Upper respiratory tract infection	n = 5
	Otitis media	n = 1
	Sinusitis	n = 1
	Herpes zoster keratitis	n = 1
	Oral candidiasis	n = 1
	Labial herpes simplex	n = 1
	Acute pyelonephritis	n = 1
	Fungal vaginosis	n = 1
	Severe neutropenia	n = 2
	CTC grade 3 neutropenia	n = 2
	Decreases in the absolute neutrophil count	38% (4 mg) 56% (8 mg)

Antiphospholipid Syndrome

Aspirin

Trial	Does aspirin have a role in improving pregnancy outcome for women with the antiphospholipid syndrome? A randomized controlled trial
Substance	**75 mg aspirin/day** (n = 20) **Placebo** (n = 20) *Concomitant medication*: No NSAIDs No corticosteroids No heparin
Result	Low dose aspirin treatment of women with antiphospholipid syndrome and recurrent miscarriages had no benefit
Patients	50 women • ≥ 3 miscarriages • Antiphospholipid antibodies: (≥ 5 U IgG, ≥ 5 U IgM anti-phospholipid antibodies, or pos. lupus anticoagulant) • No SLE
Authors	Pattison NS, Chamley LW, Birdsall M, Zanderigo AM, Liddell HS, McDougall J
Publication	*Am J Obstet Gynecol.* 2000;183(4):1008–1012

(continued) ➔

R. Müller, J. von Kempis, *Clinical Trials in Rheumatology,*
DOI 10.1007/978-1-4471-2870-0_5, © Springer-Verlag London 2013

Note	*Pregnancy complications*:		
		Placebo (%)	ASS (%)
	Bleeding (any in pregnancy)	35	45
	Hypertension or preeclampsia	18	19
	Preterm birth	0	13
	Cesarean delivery	29	31
	Outcome:		
		Placebo (%)	ASS (%)
	Live birth	85	80
	Neonatal outcome:		
		Placebo	ASS
	Birth weight	3´367 g	3´038 g
	Small for gestational age	24%	6%
	Neonatal admission	12%	13%
	Congenital anomalies	6%	6%

APLASA-Trial	Aspirin for primary thrombosis prevention in the antiphospholipid syndrome: a randomized, double-blind, placebo-controlled trial in asymptomatic antiphospholipid antibody-positive individuals APLASA: Antiphospholipid Antibody Acetylsalicylic Acid
Substance	**Aspirin 81 mg/day** (n = 48) **Placebo** (n = 50) *Concomitant medication*: No warfarin No prior aspirin
Result	Asymptomatic, persistently antiphospholipid-antibody-positive individuals did not benefit from low dose aspirin for primary thrombosis prophylaxis
Patients	98 patients, with or without systemic autoimmune diseases, and ≥ 1 *of the following*: • Positive lupus anticoagulant test • On ≥ 2 occasions, at least 6 weeks apart, and/or • Positive cardiolipin IgG/IgM/IgA • ≥ 20 units on ≥ 2 occasions ≥ 6 weeks apart • No thrombosis or pulmonary embolism or transient ischemic attack • No history of bleeding ≤ 5 years • No thrombocytopenia ($< 30 \times 10^9$ cells/L)
Authors	Erkan D, Harrison MJ, Levy R, Peterson M, Petri M, Sammaritano L, Unalp-Arida A, Vilela V, Yazici Y, Lockshin MD
Publication	*Arthritis Rheum*. 2007;56(7):2382–2391
Follow-up	3 years

Note		Aspirin	Placebo
	Incidence rate of acute thrombosis (No./100 patient-years)	2.75	0
	Incidence rate of chronic vascular events (No./100 patient-years)	1.83	0.86

Adverse events		Aspirin	Placebo
	Mild gastrointestinal disturbances	n = 5	n = 1
	Minor bleeding events	n = 3	n = 1
	Easy bruising	n = 2	n = 1
	Malignancies	n = 1	n = 1
	Death	n = 1	n = 1

Trial	Randomized controlled trial of aspirin and aspirin plus heparin in pregnant women with recurrent miscarriage associated with phospholipid antibodies (or antiphospholipid antibodies)
Substance	**Aspirin 75 mg/day** after positive pregnancy test (n = 45) *After detection of fetal heart activity* $\Rightarrow$ *Randomization*: Plus 2 × 5´000 U unfractionated heparin/day s. c. (ASS-Hep, n = 45) No additional heparin (ASS, n = 45)
Result	Treatment with aspirin and heparin of women with a history of recurrent miscarriage associated with antiphospholipid antibodies led to a significantly higher rate of live births than that achieved with aspirin alone
Patients	90 women with antiphospholipid syndrome • History of recurrent miscarriage (minimum 3, median 4, range 3–15) Positive results for phospholipid antibodies on minimum two occasions • No SLE patients • No uterine abnormality • No hypersecretion of luteinizing hormone. No multiple pregnancy • No women with partner who had an abnormal karyotype
Authors	Rai R, Cohen H, Dave M, Regan L
Publication	*BMJ.* 1997;314(7076):253–257

(continued) ➔

Note	Outcome parameters:		
		ASS	ASS-Hep
	Gestation age (weeks) at randomization	6.6	6.7
	Live births	n = 19	n = 32
	Miscarriages	n = 26	n = 13
	Live birth:		
		ASS	ASS-Hep
	Gestation age at randomization (weeks)	6.7	6.8
	Gestation age at delivery (weeks)	39.6	38.0
	Deliveries before 37 weeks' gestation	n = 4	n = 8
	Median birth weight (g)	3´080	3´330
	Congenital abnormalities were detected	n = 0	n = 0
	Caesarean section	n = 1 (growth retardation)	n = 0
	Baby with parietal lobe infarction	n = 1	n = 0
	Unsuccessful pregnancies:		
		ASS	ASS-Hep
	Gestation age at randomization (weeks)	6.5	6.4
	Gestation age at miscarriage	8.3	9.4
	No. with loss of pregnancy:		
		ASS	ASS-Hep
	≤ 14 weeks	n = 24	n = 11
	Between 14 and 28 weeks	n = 2	n = 2

Trial	A randomized, double-blind, placebo-controlled trial of heparin and aspirin for women with in vitro fertilization implantation failure and antiphospholipid or antinuclear antibodies
Substance	**Unfractionated heparin subcutaneous 2×5´000 IU/day** **Plus 100 mg aspirin (ASS)/day** (158 transfers of 296 embryos) **Placebo** (neither heparin nor ASS, 142 transfers of 259 embryos)
Result	Heparin and aspirin combination therapy did not improve pregnancy or implantation rates for antiphospholipid or antinuclear antibodies-positive patients with in vitro fertilization implantation failure
Patients	143 women without achieving pregnancy • Positive for antiphospholipid, antinuclear, or beta 2 glycoprotein I autoantibodies • ≥ 10 embryos transferred
Authors	Stern C, Chamley L, Norris H, Hale L, Baker HW
Publication	*Fertil Steril.* 2003;80(2):376–383

Note	*Outcome parameters:*		
		Hep+ASS	Placebo
	Total embryo transfers	n = 296	n = 259
	Fetal hearts detected	n = 20	n = 22
	Number of babies born	n = 18	n = 17
	Live birth rate	6%	7%
	Pos. Pregnancy test	14.6%	17.6%
Adverse events		Hep+ASS (%)	Placebo (%)
	Bruising at the injection site	64	6

HepASA-Trial	Low Molecular Weight Heparin and Aspirin for Recurrent Pregnancy Loss: Results from the Randomized, Controlled HepASA Trial HepASA: Heparin and ASA
Substance	**Low molecular weight heparin 5´000 IU/day** (n = 45) Until 35th week of gestation or delivery **Plus 81 mg ASA/day** (Heparin plus ASA) **Acetylsalicylic acid 81 mg/day** (ASA, n = 43)
Result	Low molecular weight heparin and acetylsalicylic acid had no additional effect as compared to acetylsalicylic acid alone with respect to pregnancy outcome, regardless of the presence of absence of antiphospholipid antibodies
Patients	88 women with confirmed pregnancies • Age 18–44 years • ≥ 2 unexplained consecutive pregnancy losses prior to 32 weeks gestation • ≥ 1 of the following: ANA, antiphospholipid antibodies, or an inherited thrombophilia on two occasions • No SLE • No peptic ulcer disease • No hypersensitivity to ASA or heparin obtained No bone mineral density Z score < −2.5 No previous thromboembolic event requiring ongoing anticoagulant therapy No genetic, anatomic, or hormonal etiology for pregnancy loss No hysterosalpingogram/sonohystogram
Authors	Laskin CA, Spitzer KA, Clark CA, Crowther MR, Ginsberg JS, Hawker GA, Kingdom JC, Barrett J, Gent M
Publication	*J Rheumatol*. 2009;36(2):279–287

(continued) ➔

Note	*Outcome parameters all patients*:		
		Heparin+ASA	ASA
	Pregnancy loss ≤ 14 weeks gestation	15.6%	18.6%
	Pregnancy loss 14–20 weeks gestation	0%	0%
	Ectopic pregnancy	4.4%	0%
	Still birth (20–32 weeks)	2.2%	2.3%
	Live birth	77.8%	79.1%
	Induced delivery	20.0%	18.2%
	Caesarian section	24.4%	31.8%
	Neonatal death	n = 0	n = 1

Pregnancy outcome dependent on the presence or absence of antiphospholipid antibodies:

	aPL pos.		aPL neg.	
	Heparin+ASA	ASA	Heparin+ASA	ASA
Spontaneous abortion	n = 3	n = 5	n = 4	n = 3
Still birth	n = 1	n = 0	n = 0	n = 1
Ectopic pregnancy	n = 1	n = 0	n = 1	n = 0
Neonatal death	n = 0	n = 0	n = 0	n = 1
Live birth	n = 17	n = 15	n = 18	n = 19
Birth weight < tenth percentile	n = 1	n = 0	n = 2	n = 6

Adverse events		Heparin+ASA	ASA
	BMD at the spine (g/cm^2)	−0.05	−0.01

Trial	Efficacy and safety of two doses of low molecular weight heparin (enoxaparin) in pregnant women with a history of recurrent abortion secondary to antiphospholipid syndrome
Substance	**Enoxaparin 40 mg/day** (n = 30) **Enoxaparin 20 mg/day** (n = 30) *Concomitant medication*: Low dose 75 mg aspirin/day
Result	There were no significant differences between both dosages with respect to neonatal outcome or of obstetric and maternal complications during pregnancy or puerperium
Patients	60 pregnant women with a history of recurrent abortion secondary to antiphospholipid syndrome • ≥ 3 consecutive abortions before 10 weeks' gestation • Positive lupus anticoagulant and/or anticardiolipin antibodies on at least two occasions at least 12 weeks apart • No chromosomal abnormalities or uterine abnormalities luteal phase defect, abnormal thyroid function tests hyperprolactinemia, polycystic ovary syndrome systemic lupus erythematosus, previous thromboembolism, peptic ulcer
Authors	Fouda UM, Sayed AM, Ramadan DI, Fouda IM.
Publication	*J Obstet Gynaecol*. 2010;30(8):842–846
Follow-up	Until end of pregnancy
Note	*Pregnancy outcome*:

	Enoxaparin 40 mg (%)	Enoxaparin 20 mg (%)
First trimester loss	20	26.67
Second trimester loss	3.33	3.33
Intrauterine fetal death	0	0
Live birth	76.67	70
Preeclampsia	10	6.67
Intrauterine growth restriction	6.67	3.33
Placenta abruption	0	0
Postpartum bleeding	0	0
Vaginal Delivery	78.26	80.95
Caesarean section	21.74	19.05

Neonatal outcome:

	Enoxaparin 40 mg	Enoxaparin 20 mg
Gestational age at birth (weeks)	38.48	38.76
Birth weight (Kg)	3.104	3.014
Preterm delivery	13.04%	9.52%
Neonatal bleeding	0%	0%
Congenital anomalies	0%	0%

Trial	Antiphospholipid antibodies associated with recurrent pregnancy loss: prospective, multicenter, controlled pilot study comparing treatment with low molecular weight heparin vs. unfractionated heparin
Substance	Low molecular weight heparin (**40 mg enoxaparin/day,** n = 25)
	Until 5 days before scheduled Cesarean section
	2 × 5´000 IE unfractionated heparin (n = 25)
	Both heparin dosages were continued postpartum for 2 weeks
	Concomitant medication:
	Low dose 81 mg aspirin/day until 37 gestational weeks
	Oral 2 × 600 mg calcium
Result	Combination therapy of low dose aspirin and unfractionated heparin or low molecular weight heparin during pregnancy for the prevention of recurrent pregnancy loss in women with antiphospholipid syndrome was equally safe and effective
Patients	50 women
	• ≥3 pregnancy losses before 20th weeks of gestation
	• Positive antiphospholipid antibodies (cardiolipin IgG > 80 units/mL, or phosphatidylserine IgM > 70 units/mL)
	• No other reasons for pregnancy loss (chromosomal, TSH, anatomical, hormonal, infections)
Authors	Noble LS, Kutteh WH, Lashey N, Franklin RD, Herrada J
Publication	*Fertil Steril.* 2005;83(3):684–690
Note	*Outcome parameters*:

	Enoxoparin – ASS	Unfract. heparin – ASS
Life birth	84%	80%
Estimated gestation age (weeks)	37.3	38.1
Birth weight	3´047 g	2´973 g
Vaginal delivery	66.7%	75.0%
Miscarriages	16%	20%
Estimated gestation age at miscarriage	8.7	7.2

(continued) →

Adverse events		Enoxoparin – ASS	Unfract. heparin – ASS
	Major bleeding episodes	n = 0	n = 0
	Deep venous thrombosis, thrombocytopenia, preeclampsia, gestational diabetes, or bone fractures	n = 0	n = 0
	Hematuria	n = 1	n = 0
	Bleeding at injection site	n = 2	n = 0
	Minor bleeding	n = 3	n = 2
	Intrauterine growth retardation	n = 1	n = 1

Trial	Enoxaparin vs. unfractionated heparin in the management of recurrent abortion secondary to antiphospholipid syndrome
Substance	**Unfractionated heparin (UFH, 5'000 units, twice daily)** (n = 30) **Low molecular weight heparin (enoxaparin 40 mg/day)** (n = 30) As soon as pregnancy was diagnosed *Concomitant medication*: Low dose aspirin
Result	Low molecular weight heparin plus low dose aspirin was safe and comparatively effective as an alternative to unfractionated heparin plus low dose aspirin in the management of recurrent abortion secondary to antiphospholipid antibody syndrome
Patients	60 pregnant women • ≥ 3 consecutive spontaneous abortions before 10 weeks of gestation • Positive antiphospholipid antibodies ≥ 40 GPL on ≥ 2 occasions ≥ 12 weeks apart • Body mass index 19–29 • Exlusion of: paternal chromosomal abnormalities; uterine malformation detected by hysterosalpingography or office hysteroscopy; cervical incompetence; luteal-phase defect; abnormal thyroid function tests; hyperprolactinemia; polycystic ovary syndrome; hereditary thrombophilia; systemic lupus erythematosus; previous venous or arterial thrombotic episodes; diabetes mellitus; and sensitivity to aspirin, UFH, or enoxaparin
Authors	Fouda UM, Sayed AM, Abdou AM, Ramadan DI, Fouda IM, Zaki MM
Publication	*Int J Gynaecol Obstet.* 2011 Mar;112(3):211–215
Follow-up	Until end of pregnancy
Note	*Pregnancy outcome*

	UFH	Enoxaparin
First-trimester miscarriage	n = 6	n = 9
Second-trimester miscarriage	n = 0	n = 1
Live birth	n = 24	n = 20

Adverse events	UFH	Enoxaparin
Osteoporotic fractures	n = 0	n = 0
Excessive bleeding episodes	n = 0	n = 0
Thrombocytopenia	n = 0	n = 0
Subcutaneous bruises	n = 3	n = 3
Skin allergy	n = 0	n = 1
Complications among pregnancies progressing beyond 24 weeks	n = 24	n = 20
Preeclampsia	n = 2	n = 1
Intrauterine growth	n = 1	n = 2
Preterm labor	n = 3	n = 2
Intrauterine fetal death	n = 0	n = 0
Neonatal bleeding	n = 0	n = 0
Congenital anomalies	n = 0	n = 0
Admission to neonatal intensive care unit	n = 2	n = 2

Trial	Adjusted prophylactic doses of nadroparin plus low dose aspirin therapy in obstetric antiphospholipid syndrome. A prospective cohort management study
Substance	**Low molecular weight heparin (LMWH) patients** **54–64 kg ≥ 3´800–5´700 U/daily** Patients 65–76 kg ≥ 4´750 and 6´650 U/daily LMWH LMWH was resumed 12 h after delivery and was continued at a dosage of 3´800 (weight ≤ 60 kg) to 4´750 (weight > 60 kg) U/daily for 6 weeks *Concomitant medication*: 100 mg aspirin/daily, stopped 10 days before the expected birth date
Result	Daily doses of low molecular weight heparin together with low dose aspirin treatment of pregnant antiphospholipid syndrome patients with no history of thrombosis led to a high live birth rate and a satisfactory mean gestational age and weight at birth. Major pregnancy/neonatal-associated complications were absent
Patients	33 pregnant women *History of ≥ 1of the following*: • ≥ 1 unexplained deaths of morphologically normal fetuses at or beyond the tenth week of gestation • ≥ 1 premature births of morphologically normal neonates before the 34th week of gestation because of severe preeclampsia–eclampsia or recognized symptoms of placental insufficiency • ≥ 3 unexplained consecutive spontaneous abortions before the tenth week of gestation *Laboratory criteria included*: • Lupus anticoagulant and/or medium/high titers of anticardiolipin antibodies and/or • β2 Glucoprotein antibodies • Detected on two or more occasions at least 12 weeks apart
Authors	Ruffatti A, Gervasi MT, Favaro M, Ruffatti AT, Hoxha A, Punzi L
Publication	*Clin Exp Rheumatol.* 2011 May-Jun;29(3):551–554
Note	*Follow-up*:	
	Life birth	n = 32, 37.4 weeks of gestation
	Pregnancy loss	n = 1, unknown origin eighth week of gestation
	Cesarean delivery	n = 24
	Vaginal birth	n = 8
	Born prematurely	n = 1 due to *placenta previa*
	Birth weight	3´084 g
	Apgar score at 1 min	8.5
	Apgar score at 5 min	9.6
Adverse events	Decreasing platelet counts	n = 2
	Hypothyroidism of the mother	n = 1
	Neonatal Intensive Care Unit due to pneumothorax	n = 1

Trial	Antiphospholipid syndrome in pregnancy: a randomized, controlled trial of treatment
Substance	**Aspirin 75 mg/day** (ASS, n = 47) **Aspirin 75 mg/day plus 5'000 IU heparin/day** (ASS-heparin, n = 51) *Concomitant medication*: No use of steroids during pregnancy No systemic lupus erythematosus requiring medication
Result	Low dose aspirin was effective in pregnant women with antiphospholipid syndrome. The addition of low molecular weight heparin did not significantly improve pregnancy outcome
Patients	98 consecutive women • Pregnant before 12th weeks of gestation • ≥ 3 consecutive pregnancy losses or • ≥ 2 consecutive pregnancy losses with proven fetal death after tenth week of gestation • ≥ 9 U/mL IgG anticardiolipin and/or • ≥ 5 U/mL IgM anticardiolipin • No parental chromosomal abnormality • No uterine anomaly • No previous arterial or venous thrombosis • No complicated by nephritis • No other thrombophilia
Authors	Farquharson RG, Quenby S, Greaves M
Publication	*Obstet Gynecol.* 2002;100(3):408–413

Note: *Outcome parameters*:

	ASS	ASS-heparin
Live Birth	72%	78%
Mean birth weight	3´221 g	3´127 g
Embryo loss	n = 9	n = 3
Fetal loss	n = 4	n = 8

Gestation age at delivery:

	ASS	ASS-heparin
< 30 week	n = 1	n = 1
30–36 week	n = 3	n = 1
> 36 weeks	n = 30	n = 38

Trial	Treatment of antiphospholipid antibody syndrome (APS), in pregnancy: a randomized pilot trial comparing low molecular weight heparin to unfractionated Heparin
Substance	*Dalteparin group* (n = *14*): **Acetylsalicylic acid 81 mg/day,** started preconceptionally **Plus dalteparin 2´500 IE/day** Increased to 5´000 IE/day in the second trimester Increased to 7´500 IE/day in the third trimester *Unfractionated heparin group* (n = *14*): **Unfractionated heparin 2×5'000 IE/day** Increased to 2×10'000 IE/day in the second trimester *Concomitant medication*: No prior heparin treatment
Result	Dalteparin was an effective alternative to unfractionated heparin for the treatment of antiphospholipid antibody syndrome in during pregnancy
Patients	28 pregnant women • ≥ 3 consecutive, unexplained miscarriages • Lupus anticoagulant positive • Anticardiolipin pos (IGM or IgG) • No thrombophilia
Authors	Stephenson MD, Ballem PJ, Tsang P, Purkiss S, Ensworth S, Houlihan E, Ensom MH
Publication	*J Obstet Gynaecol Can.* 2004;26(8):729–734
Note	*Outcome parameters*:

	Dalteparin	Unfractionated heparin
Live Birth 33	n = 9	n = 4
Mean birth weight	3´304 g	3´536 g
Embryonic demise	n = 0	n = 2
Anembryonic demise	n = 4	n = 7

Trial	Treatment of recurrent miscarriage and antiphospholipid syndrome with low dose enoxaparin and aspirin
Substance	**Enoxaparin 20 mg/day** **Plus aspirin 75 mg/day** Treatment started shortly after positive pregnancy test Until the women went into labor or the day before elective delivery
Result	In this open study of 20 mg enoxaparin in combination with 75 mg aspirin treatment of women with recurrent miscarriages and antiphospholipid syndrome a rate of live birth of 80% was observed
Patients	35 women with antiphospholipid syndrome • Confirmed pregnancy • Positive lupus anticoagulant on two occasions • Antiphospholipid antibodies IgG ($\geq$ 8 U/L) IgM ($\geq$ 5 U/L) • $\geq$ 3 consecutive miscarriages before tenth week' gestation or • $\geq$ 1 consecutive miscarriages beyond tenth week' gestation • $\geq$ 1 premature birth of morphological normal neonate before 34th week' gestation because of preeclampsia or eclampsia or placental insufficiency
Authors	Mo D, Saravelos S, Metwally M, Makris M, Li TC
Publication	*Reprod Biomed Online.* 2009;19(2):216–220
Note	*Outcome of 35 pregnancies:*	
	Biochemical pregnancy	3%
	First trimester loss:	
	Biochemical pregnancy	3%
	Ultrasound gestation sac only	6%
	Ultrasound showed gestation sac and fetal pole	9%
	Ultrasound demonstrated fetal heart beats	3%
	Second trimester loss	0%
	Third trimester loss	0%
	Live birth	80%

Trial	Treatment of recurrent miscarriage and antiphospholipid syndrome with low dose enoxaparin and aspirin
Substance	**Enoxaparin low dose 20 mg/day** **Plus aspirin low dose 75 mg/day**
Result	Low dose enoxaparin in conjunction with low dose aspirin treatment produced resulted in a birth rate of 80%
Patients	35 pregnant women with antiphospholipid syndrome • ≥ 3 miscarriage before 20 weeks' gestation • ≥ 1 clinical criterion • ≥ 3 unexplained consecutive spontaneous miscarriages before week 10 of gestation • ≥ 1 unexplained deaths of a morphologically normal fetus at or beyond week 10 of gestation • ≥ 1 premature births of a morphologically normal neonate at or before week 34 of gestation because of severe preeclampsia or eclampsia, or severe placental insufficiency • ≥ 1 laboratory criterion • Lupus anticoagulant on two separate occasions at least 6 weeks • Elevated Ig G (≥ 8.5 unit/L) or Ig M (≥ 5 unit/L) antiphospholipid antibodies (APA) on two separate occasions at least 6 weeks apart.
Authors	Mo D, Saravelos S, Metwally M, Makris M, Li TC
Publication	*Reprod Biomed Online.* 2009 Aug;19(2):216–220
Follow-up	One pregnancy
Note	Miscarriage rate	20%
	Birth rate	80%
	First trimester loss; Ultrasound showed gestation sac only	6%
	First trimester loss; Ultrasound showed gestation sac and fetal pole	9%
	First trimester loss; Ultrasound demonstration of fetal heart beat	3%

Trial	Prednisone and aspirin in women with autoantibodies and unexplained recurrent fetal loss
Substance	**Prednisone 0.8 mg/kg/day** for 4 weeks (maximum 60 mg/day) Followed by 0.5 mg/kg/day after week 4 until delivery (maximum 40 mg/day) **Plus 100 mg aspirin/day** until 36th weeks of gestation (n = 101) **Placebo** (n = 101)
Result	Treatment of women with different autoantibodies — including antiphospholipid-antibodies-autoantibodies and recurrent fetal loss with prednisone and aspirin was not effective in promoting live birth, and it increased the risk of prematurity
Patients	202 pregnant women • ≥ 2 consecutive fetal losses before 32 weeks of gestation ≥ 1 autoantibody: • Antinuclear antibodies n = 83 • Anti-DNA antibodies (single- or double-stranded) n = 37 • Antilymphocyte IgM n = 64 • Anticardiolipin IgG n = 20 • Lupus anticoagulant n = 74 Exclusion criteria: • No chromosomal or anatomical abnormality • No luteal-phase defect • No peptic ulcer disease ≤ 3 years • No systemic lupus erythematosus • No diabetes mellitus
Authors	Laskin CA, Bombardier C, Hannah ME, Mandel FP, Ritchie JW, Farewell V, Farine D, Spitzer K, Fielding L, Soloninka CA, Yeung M
Publication	N Engl J Med. 1997;337(3):148–153

Note — Outcome parameters:

	Treatment	Placebo
Live birth	65%	56%
At term delivery	38%	88%
Before term delivery	62%	12%
Fetal loss	35%	44%
Birth weight < 2,500 g	28%	18%
Male sex	62%	46%
Admission to neonatal intensive care unit	35%	4%
Days in neonatal intensive care unit	4.4	6.0
Sepsis	2%	0%
Congenital anomaly	0%	4%

Adverse events

	Treatment	Placebo
Hypertension	13%	5%
Gestational diabetes mellitus	15%	5%
Cataract	n = 2	n = 0

Trial	Comparative trial of prednisone plus aspirin versus aspirin alone in the treatment of anticardiolipin antibody-positive obstetric patients
Substance	**Prednisone 20 mg/day** (increased or decreased on the basis of observed changes in serial antibody levels, range 10–40 mg/day) **Plus aspirin low dose 81 mg/day** (n = 17) **81 mg/day aspirin alone** (n = 22)
Result	The use of prednisone therapy in conjunction with low dose aspirin did not improve and may have contributed to worse pregnancy outcome in antiphospholipid antibody-positive patients, in comparison with aspirin alone
Patients	39 pregnant women • Positive for anticardiolipin antibodies (IgG > 8 units/mL, IgM > 5 units/mL) or lupus anticoagulant • ≥ 1 fetal abortus before 12th week of gestation or • ≥ 2 unexplained first trimester miscarriages • No anatomical abnormalities • No hormonal abnormalities
Authors	Silver RK, MacGregor SN, Sholl JS, Hobart JM, Neerhof MG, Ragin A
Publication	*Am J Obstet Gynecol.* 1993;169(6):1411–1417

Note	*Outcome parameters*:		
		Prednisone+ASS	ASS
	Gestation age at onset treatment (week)	6.7	8.4
	Perinatal losses	n = 0	n = 0
	Preterm delivery	n = 8/12	n = 3/22
Adverse events		Prednisone+ASS	ASS
	Diabetes	n = 2	n = 0
	Endometritis	n = 3	n = 0
	Wound dehiscence	n = 1	n = 0
	Bilateral lower extremity thrombosis	n = 1	n = 0
	Autoimmune pneumonitis	n = 0	n = 1

Trial	Repeated fetal losses associated with antiphospholipid antibodies: a collaborative randomized trial comparing prednisone with low dose heparin treatment
Substance	**Prednisone 20 mg every 12 h** (n = 8) **Heparin 10´000 IU every 12 h** (n = 12) Dose was reduced by 2´000 IU until PTT was within normal range *Concomitant medication*: Aspirin 80 mg/day (all patients) Start treatment after exclusion ectopic pregnancy Vitamin D 600–800 U Calcium carbonate 4 g No prednisone treatment
Result	Serious maternal morbidity and the frequency of preterm delivery were higher in high risk pregnant women with antiphospholipid antibodies treated with prednisone rather than heparin
Patients	20 patients with antiphospholipid syndrome • Confirmed pregnancy • Lupus anticoagulant or anticardiolipin antibodies ($\geq 2 \times$ positive tests within 6 weeks) • ≥ 2 unexpected unexplained fetal losses on two occasions • No other causes of recurrent miscarriages or fetal death • No diabetes mellitus • No lupus like disorders
Authors	Cowchock FS, Reece EA, Balaban D, Branch DW, Plouffe L
Publication	*Am J Obstet Gynecol.* 1992;166(5):1318–1323
Note	*Outcome parameters*:

	Prednisone	Heparin
Live birth	68%	73%
Preterm delivery	n = 6	n = 2
Premature rupture of membrane	n = 3	n = 0
Mean week of delivery	32nd week	37th week
Minor thrush	n = 2	n = 0
Minor bleeding	n = 0	n = 2
Superficial thrombosis	n = 0	n = 1
Manageable diabetes	n = 3	n = 1
Serious preeclampsia	n = 3	n = 0
Cataract	n = 1	n = 0
Life birth	n = 6	n = 9
Fetal death after 12th week of gestation	n = 2	n = 1

Trial	First trimester low dose prednisolone in refractory antiphospholipid antibody-related pregnancy loss
Substance	**Prednisolone 10 mg/day** *Concomitant medication*: Standard anticoagulation (aspirin or aspirin plus heparin)
Result	The addition of first trimester low dose prednisolone to conventional treatment appeared to be effective in refractory antiphospholipid antibody-related pregnancy loss(es), although complications remain elevated
Patients	18 women with antiphospholipid syndrome, according to the Sapporo criteria
Authors	Bramham K, Thomas M, Nelson-Piercy C, Khamashta M, Hunt BJ
Publication	*Blood*. 2011 Jun 23;117(25):6948–6951
Note	*During/before follow-up*:	
	Life births before low dose prednisolone	n = 4/97 (4%)
	Live births after low dose prednisolone	n = 14/23 (61%)
	First trimester miscarriages	n = 8
	Ectopic pregnancy	n = 1
	Fetal deaths after 10 weeks' gestation	n = 0

Trial	A multicenter, placebo-controlled pilot study of intravenous immune globulin treatment of antiphospholipid syndrome during pregnancy. The Pregnancy Loss Study Group
Substance	**I. v. immune globulin (IVIG, 1 g/kg,** n = 7) **Placebo** (n = 9) For 2 consecutive days/month until 36 weeks of gestation *Concomitant medication*: 7´500 units of unfractionated sodium heparin by s. c./12 h Increased to 10´000 U in the second trimenon plus 81 mg aspirin
Result	Intravenous immune globulin did not improve obstetric or neonatal outcomes beyond those achieved with a heparin and low dose aspirin regimen
Patients	16 women • With a single live conception at ≤ 12 weeks gestation • ≥ 20 U IgG phospholipid-binding anticardiolipin antibodies or • Lupus anticoagulant or ≥ 40 units/mL • History of fetal death (unexplained intrauterine death of a fetus) or • History of unexplained venous or arterial thromboembolism • No thrombocytopenia • No history of a bleeding disorder • No osteoporosis, or a known allergy to immune globulin, heparin, or aspirin • No renal disease • No active systemic lupus erythematosus • No insulin-dependent diabetes mellitus or hypertension
Authors	Branch DW, Peaceman AM, Druzin M, Silver RK, El-Sayed Y, Silver RM, Esplin MS, Spinnato J, Harger J
Publication	Am J Obstet Gynecol. 2000 Jan;182(1 Pt 1):122–7.

(continued)

Note	Outcome parameters:		
		IVIG	Placebo
	Eclampsia	n = 0	n = 0
	Preeclampsia	n = 3	n = 1
	Comparison of neonatal outcomes:		
		IVIG	Placebo
	Neonatal intensive care unit admissions	n = 1	n = 4
	Length of intensive care unit stay (days)	21	20.8
	Length of ventilator requirement (days)	1.0	3.0
	Infant respiratory distress syndrome	n = 0	n = 1
	Pregnancy outcome:		
		IVIG	Placebo
	Gestational age at delivery (week)	34.8	36.7
	Birth weight (g)	2´432.9	2´604.4
	Preterm delivery (gestational age < 37 week)	n = 7	n = 3
	Oligohydramnios	n = 2	n = 2
	Intrauterine growth restriction (birth weight ≤ 10th percentile)	n = 1	n = 3
	Fetal distress	n = 0	n = 3
	Preeclampsia	n = 3	n = 1
Adverse events	No cases heparin-induced thrombocytopenia		
	No bleeding		
	No osteopenic fracture		

Trial	Randomized study of subcutaneous low molecular weight heparin plus aspirin versus intravenous immunoglobulin in the treatment of recurrent fetal loss associated with antiphospholipid antibodies
Substance	*Intravenous immunoglobulin group (IVIG*, n = 21): **Intravenous immunoglobulin 400 mg/kg/day** for 2 days Followed by a single dose every month Stopped after 31st week's gestation: *Low molecular weight heparin group (LMW*, n = 19): **Heparin low molecular weight 5´700 IU/day** **Aspirin low dose 75 mg/day** *Concomitant medication*: No antihypertensive drugs No previous prednisone therapy
Result	Treatment with low molecular weight heparin plus low dose aspirin of pregnant patients with antiphospholipid antibodies was superior to intravenous immunoglobulin treatment
Patients	40 pregnant women • ≥ 3 consecutive abortions before tenth week of gestation • ≥ 2 positive test results for anticardiolipin or lupus anticoagulant (> 40 IU) • No chromosomal or anatomic abnormality • No luteal phase defect • No confirmed peptic ulcer • No diabetes mellitus • No SLE • No previous thromboembolism • No hypertension
Authors	Triolo G, Ferrante A, Ciccia F, Accardo-Palumbo A, Perino A, Castelli A, Giarratano A, Licata G
Publication	*Arthritis Rheum.* 2003;48(3):728–731
Note	*Outcome parameters*:

	IVIG	LMW
Number of pregnancies	n = 21	n = 19
Live births	57%	84%
Duration of pregnancy (weeks)	38.3	38.7
Birth weight	3´246 g	3´298 g
Preterm deliveries	n = 1	n = 0
Infants admitted to neonatal intensive care unit	n = 1	n = 0
Congenital anomalies	n = 0	n = 0
Caesarean deliveries	n = 1	n = 0
First trimester fetal loss	29%	11%
Fetal loss after 13 weeks	n = 2	n = 0
Intrauterine death	n = 1	n = 1

Trial	Low molecular weight heparin versus intravenous immunoglobulin for recurrent abortion associated with antiphospholipid antibody syndrome
Substance	*LMW group* (n = 40): **75 mg aspirin plus 4´500 IU heparin** (adapted to recommended prophylactic factor Xa levels) Aspirin was discontinued at 32 weeks, heparin at 38 weeks *IVIG group* (n = 38): **400 mg/kg i. v. immunoglobulins every 28 days** *Concomitant medication*: 500 mg of calcium daily for heparin treated women
Result	Low molecular weight heparin plus low dose aspirin resulted in a higher live birth rate than IVIG in the treatment of antiphospholipid antibody syndrome in women with recurrent abortion
Patients	85 patients • ≥ 1 unexplained deaths of a morphologically normal fetus ≥ 10th week of gestation • ≥ 1 premature births of a morphologically normal neonate ≤ 34th week of gestation because of severe preeclampsia, eclampsia, or severe placental insufficiency • ≥ 3 or more unexplained consecutive spontaneous abortions ≤ 10th week of gestation *Laboratory criteria*: • Anticardiolipin antibody of IgG and/or IgM isot ≥ 2 occasions ≥ 6 weeks apart • Lupus anticoagulant ≥ 2x, ≥ 6 weeks apart • No factor V Leiden, prothrombin G20210A mutation, protein C and protein S, antithrombin III, factor XII coagulant, activated protein C resistance, plasminogen, and 5,10-methylenetetrahydrofolate reductase (MTHFR 677CNT)
Authors	Dendrinos S, Sakkas E, Makrakis E
Publication	*Int J Gynaecol Obstet*. 2009 Mar;104(3):223–225
Follow-up	1 pregnancy

Note	*During follow-up*:	LMW	IVIG
	Pregnancy	n = 40	n = 38
	Live birth	n = 29	n = 15
	Preterm delivery	n = 2	n = 1
	First trimester abortion	n = 11	n = 21
	Intrauterine death	n = 0	n = 2
	Birth weight, kg	3.134	3.232
	Vaginal delivery	n = 24	n = 11
	Cesarean delivery	n = 8	n = 2
Adverse events		LMW	IVIG
	Nausea, hypotension, and tachycardia	n = 0	n = 3
	Decrease in lumbar spine bone density	n = 0	Not analyzed
	Preterm vaginal delivery	n = 2	n = 1

Trial	Recurrent first trimester spontaneous abortion associated with antiphospholipid antibodies: a pilot study of treatment with intravenous immunoglobulin
Substance	**I. v. immunoglobulin 300 mg/kg every 3 weeks** After confirmation of pregnancy Until 16th to 17th week of pregnancy *Concomitant medication*: No aspirin No other medication
Result	The authors interpreted the results of this open study with intravenous immunoglobulins as promising
Patients	38 women with antiphospholipid syndrome • ≥ 3 consecutive abortions within the first trimester • Positive antiphospholipid antibodies
Authors	Marzusch K, Dietl J, Klein R, Hornung D, Neuer A, Berg PA
Publication	*Acta Obstet Gynecol Scand.* 1996;75(10):922–926

Note		
	Spontaneous abortions	n = 7
	Live Birth	n = 31
	Birth at weeks of gestation	37–42
	Birth weight	2´135–4´400 g

WAPS-Trial	A randomized clinical trial of high intensity Warfarin vs. conventional antithrombotic therapy for the prevention of recurrent thrombosis in patients with the antiphospholipid syndrome (WAPS) WAPS: Warfarin in the antiphospholipid syndrome		
Substance	**Warfarin High intensity therapy (INR range 3.0–4.5,** target 3.5, n = 54) **Aspirin 100 mg/day** (ASS, n = 55)		
Result	High intensity warfarin was not superior to low dose aspirin in preventing recurrent thrombosis in patients with antiphospholipid syndrome. It was associated with an increased rate of minor hemorrhagic complications		
Patients	109 patients with antiphospholipid syndrome • Previous thrombosis • No thrombosis during anticoagulation • No active hemorrhagic disorders		
Authors	Finazzi G, Marchioli R, Brancaccio V, Schinco P, Wisloff F, Musial J, Baudo F, Berrettini M, Testa S, D'Angelo A, Tognoni G, Barbui T		
Publication	*J Thromb Haemost.* 2005;3(5):848–853		
Note	*Outcome parameters*:		
		Warfarin	ASS
	Vascular death, major thrombosis	9.3%	5.5%
	Vascular death, major thrombosis or major hemorrhage	11.1%	9.1%
	Death	5.6%	3.6%
	Total thrombosis	11.1%	5.5%
	Ischemic stroke	n = 2	n = 2
	Transient ischemic attacks	n = 2	n = 1
	Deep venous thrombosis	n = 2	n = 0
	Pulmonary embolism	n = 1	n = 0
	Superficial thrombophlebitis	n = 1	n = 0
	Total hemorrhage	27.8%	14.6%
	Major hemorrhage	3.7%	5.5%
	Minor hemorrhage	27.8%	10.9%

Trial	A comparison of two intensities of warfarin for the prevention of recurrent thrombosis in patients with the antiphospholipid antibody syndrome
Substance	**Warfarin to achieve an INR of 2.0–3.0** (moderate intensity, n = 56) **Warfarin to achieve an INR of 3.1–4.0** (high intensity, n = 58) *Concomitant medication*: Aspirin was allowed
Result	High intensity warfarin was not superior to moderate intensity warfarin for thromboprophylaxis in patients with antiphospholipid antibodies and previous thrombosis
Patients	114 patients with antiphospholipid antibodies • Previous thrombosis • Not only IgM anticardiolipin antibodies • No clinically significant bleeding or diathesis • No thrombocytopenia < 50´000 /mm³ • No intracranial hemorrhage, stroke, or gastrointestinal bleeding ≤ 3 months • No pregnancy or planned pregnancy
Authors	Crowther MA, Ginsberg JS, Julian J, Denburg J, Hirsh J, Douketis J, Laskin C, Fortin P, Anderson D, Kearon C, Clarke A, Geerts W, Forgie M, Green D, Costantini L, Yacura W, Wilson S, Gent M, Kovacs MJ
Publication	*N Engl J Med.* 2003;349(12):1133–1138
Follow-up	2.7 years (mean)

Note	*Outcome parameters*:		
		High intensity (%)	Moderate intensity (%)
	Recurrent thrombosis	10.7	3.4

Adverse events		High intensity	Moderate intensity
	Major bleeding	n = 3	n = 4
	Any bleeding	n = 14	n = 11
	Myocardial infarction	n = 1	n = 0
	Deep vein thrombosis	n = 1	n = 0

Progressive Systemic Sclerosis

Corticosteroids

Trial	Intravenous dexamethasone pulse therapy in diffuse systemic sclerosis A randomized placebo-controlled study
Substance	**Dexamethasone i. v. 100 mg "pulse" therapy** (n = 17) **Placebo** (dextrose, n = 18) 1×/every month for 6 months *Concomitant medication*: No information provided
Result	Intravenous pulse dexamethasone treatment of diffuse systemic sclerosis lead to improvements of skin and lung manifestations
Patients	25 patients with diffuse systemic sclerosis • No patients with limited disease • Not pretreated with any immunosuppressive drug or corticosteroids
Authors	Sharada B, Kumar A, Kakker R, Adya CM, Pande I, Uppal SS, Pande JN, Sunderam KR, Malaviya AN
Publication	*Rheumatol Int*. 1994;14(3):91–94

(continued) ➜

R. Müller, J. von Kempis, *Clinical Trials in Rheumatology*,
DOI 10.1007/978-1-4471-2870-0_6, © Springer-Verlag London 2013

Note	*Change of:*		
		Dexamethasone	Placebo
	Total skin score	-4.5	+4.1
	Flexion index	-0.8	+2.9
	Maximum oral opening	-0.7	-0.5
	Extension index	+1.6	-0.4
	Functional disability score	-1.9	-0.6
	Frequency of Raynaud's phenomenon (times/day)	-3.1	-1.6
	ESR (mm/h)	-6.9	-1.6
	DLCO %	-15.8	-8.6%
	Tidal Volume	-0.6	+9.0
	FEV1	-2.0	-1.5
	Maximum mid-expiratory flow rate	+1.7	-1.6
Adverse events		Dexamethasone	Placebo
	Infections	n = 12	n = 6

Trial	Case–control study of corticosteroids and other drugs that either precipitate or protect from the development of scleroderma renal crisis
Substance	Corticosteroid use was determined prior to the onset of scleroderma renal crisis (SRC) in cases or prior to the first visit in controls. **Low dose corticosteroid use (equivalent of prednisone < 15 mg/day)** or High dose (average 21.5 mg prednisone/day). *Three groups of corticosteroid use were defined, as follows:* 1. Started during the 6 months prior to the event (renal crisis in cases or initial visit in controls) 2. Used continuously for more than 6 months prior to event; or 3. Used at any time after the onset of scleroderma, but not during the 6 months immediately prior to the event *Concomitant medication:* The effects of other drugs, including D-penicillamine, nonsteroidal antiinflammatory drugs (NSAIDs), calcium channel blockers, and angiotensin-converting enzyme (ACE) inhibitors, were also evaluated
Result	Antecedent high-dose corticosteroid therapy resulted in higher numbers of patients with renal crisis in this retrospective case–control of early diffuse scleroderma
Patients	Cases n = 110 Controls n = 110 Patients with SRC and scleroderma controls were matched according to the likelihood to develop renal crisis, and thus on sex, race, age, disease duration (6 months if renal crisis occurred during the first 4 years of symptoms, otherwise: 2 years), skin score, creatine phosphokinase levels, and palpable tendon friction rubs
Authors	Steen VD, Medsger TA Jr
Publication	*Arthritis Rheum.* 1998 Sep;41(9):1613–1619
Follow-up	110 cases with SRC between 1981 and 1993
Note	*Frequency of corticosteroid use in the 6 months prior to new renal crisis in cases and prior to the initial visit in controls (Values are the no. of positive patients. High dose was defined as ≥ 15 mg/day of prednisone equivalent; low dose as < 15 mg/day of prednisone equivalent. (+) = steroids present; (-) = no steroids).*

	Cases (+)/ controls (+)	Cases (+)/ controls (-)	Cases (-)/ controls (+)	Cases (-)/ controls (-)
New, high dose	5	35	8	62
New, low dose	3	15	8	84
Continuous dose	1	9	8	92
Any steroids	21	45	14	3

Trial	Cyclophosphamide with low or high dose Prednisolone for systemic sclerosis lung disease
Substance	**Prednisolone low doses** of (< 10 mg/day, n = 12) **Prednisolone high doses of 1 mg/kg/day** (max. 60 mg/day, n = 16) Tapered by 5 mg/day on alternating days each 2 weeks *Concomitant medication*: Cyclophosphamide intravenous pulses of 500 mg/m^2 Mesna in three separate doses
Result	A combination of intreavenous pulse cyclophosphamide with high doses of prednisolone was effective in improving the clinical, physiological, and radiological evolution of systemic sclerosis related interstitial lung disease
Patients	28 patients with systemic sclerosis • Related interstitial lung disease (ILD) • With FVC < 70% of predicted • FEV_1/FVC > 70% of predicted • No other disease affecting the lung
Authors	Pakas I, Ioannidis JP, Malagari K, Skopouli FN, Moutsopoulos HM, Vlachoyiannopoulos PG
Publication	*J Rheumatol.* 2002;29(2):298–304
Follow-up	12 months

Note — *Change of CT-Scan findings*:

	High dose prednisolone (%)	Low dose prednisolone (%)
Ground glass	-5.7	-1.1
Reticular pattern	-0.3	+5.9
Interstitial disease score	-6.0	+4.8

Change of pulmonary function tests:

	High dose prednisolone (%)	Low dose prednisolone (%)
TLC (% predicted)	+5.1	-1.0
FVC (% predicted)	+12.4	-0.7
DLCO (% predicted)	+7.3	+0.9
Skin involvement score	-5.4	-0.7

Adverse events

	High dose prednisolone	Low dose prednisolone
Death from end stage ILD during	–	n = 1
Leucopenia or other cytopenia	n = 0	n = 0
Scleroderma related renal crisis	n = 0	n = 0
Nausea and vomiting, typically lasting for 1–3 days respiratory tract infections	–	n = 3

ARIES Trial	Ambrisentan for the treatment of pulmonary arterial hypertension: results of the Ambrisentan in pulmonary arterial hypertension, randomized, double-blind, placebo-controlled, multicenter, efficacy (ARIES), study 1 and 2 ARIES: Ambrisentan in Pulmonary Arterial Hypertension, Randomized, Double-Blind, Placebo-Controlled, Multicenter, Efficacy Study
Substance	**Placebo** (n = 132) **Ambrisentan:** **ARIES 1: 5 mg/day** (n = 67) or 10 mg/day (n = 68) **ARIES 2: 2.5 mg/day** (n = 64) or 5 mg/day (n = 63) *Concomitant medication*: No bosentan No sitaxsentan No sildenafil No epoprostenol No iloprost No treprostinil
Result	Ambrisentan treatment of patients with pulmonary arterial hypertension improved exercise capacity. Ambrisentan was well-tolerated. It was associated with a low risk of aminotransferase abnormalities
Patients	269 (Aries 1) and 215 (Aries 2) patients • With pulmonary arterial hypertension (PAH), including (number not disclosed) secondary to connective tissue/autoimmune disease • No patients with 6-min walk distance < 150 m • No patients with 6-min walk distance > 450 m
Authors	Galiè N, Olschewski H, Oudiz RJ, Torres F, Frost A, Ghofrani HA, Badesch DB, McGoon MD, McLaughlin VV, Roecker EB, Gerber MJ, Dufton C, Wiens BL, Rubin LJ; Ambrisentan in Pulmonary Arterial Hypertension, Randomized, Double-Blind, Placebo-Controlled, Multicenter, Efficacy Studies (ARIES) Group
Publication	*Circulation*. 2008;117(23):3010–3019
Follow-up	12 weeks
Note	*Change of (ARIES 1)*:

Change of (ARIES 1):

	Placebo	5 mg ambrisentan	10 mg ambrisentan
6-min walk distance (m)	decreased	+31	+51

Improvements in World Health Organization functional class, Borg dyspnea score, and B-type natriuretic peptide

Change of:

	Placebo	2.5 mg ambrisentan	5 mg ambrisentan
6-min walk distance (m)	decreased	+32	+59

Improvements in time to clinical worsening, Short Form-36 score, Borg dyspnea score, and B-type natriuretic peptide

(continued) ➜

Adverse events *ARIES 1*

	Placebo (%)	5 mg ambrisentan (%)	10 mg ambrisentan (%)
Death	3	1	1
Hospitalization for PAH	3	3	3
Withdrawal because of other PAH treatment	1	0	1
Peripheral edema	10.4	26.9	28.4
Nasal congestion	3.0	6.0	10.4
Sinusitis	0	4.5	4.5
Flushing	0	3.0	1.5
Abdominal pain	1.5	3.0	3.0
Constipation	1.5	4.5	6.0
Palpitations	3.0	0.0	4.5
Dyspnea	3.0	6.0	4.5
Headache	20.9	17.9	19.4
Nasopharyngitis	1.5	7.5	3.2

ARIES 2

	Placebo (%)	2.5 mg ambrisentan (%)	5 mg ambrisentan (%)
Death	5	3	0
Hospitalization for PAH	14	5	3
Withdrawal because of other PAH treatment	0	0	0
Peripheral edema	10.8	3.1	9.5
Nasal congestion	0	1.6	4.8
Sinusitis	0	1.6	1.6
Flushing	1.5	6.3	4.8
Abdominal pain	0	3.1	3.2
Constipation	1.5	3.1	1.6
Palpitations	1.5	6.3	7.9
Dyspnea	3.1	1.6	4.8
Headache	6.2	7.8	12.7
Nasopharyngitis	0	0	3.2

ARIES Trial	Long-term ambrisentan therapy for the treatment of pulmonary arterial hypertension ARIES: Ambrisentan in Pulmonary Arterial Hypertension, Randomized, Double-Blind, Placebo-Controlled, Multicenter, Efficacy Study
Substance	*Clinical trial*: **Placebo** (n = 132) **Ambrisentan:** **ARIES 1:** 5 mg/day (n = 67) or 10 mg/day (n = 68) **ARIES 2:** 2.5 mg/day (n = 64) or 5 mg/day (n = 63) *Concomitant medication*: No bosentan No sitaxsentan No sildenafil No epoprostenol No iloprost No treprostinil *Long-term extension (first 24 weeks)*: Fixed dose *After week 24*: Randomized treatment assignment remained blinded Dose adjustments were permitted per investigator discretion Available doses: 1, 2.5, 5, and 10 mg 2.5 mg ambrisentan, finishing year 2 (n = 69) 5 mg ambrisentan, finishing year 2 (n = 126) 10 mg ambrisentan, finishing year 2 (n = 66)
Result	Ambrisentan treatment over 2 years was associated with sustained improvements in exercise capacity and a low risk of clinical worsening and death in patients with pulmonary arterial hypertension. Ambrisentan was well-tolerated
Patients	269 (Aries 1) and 215 (Aries 2) patients • With pulmonary arterial hypertension • No patients with-min walk distance < 150 m • No patients with-min walk distance > 450 m
Authors	Oudiz RJ, Galiè N, Olschewski H, Torres F, Frost A, Ghofrani HA, Badesch DB, McGoon MD, McLaughlin VV, Roecker EB, Harrison BC, Despain D, Dufton C, Rubin LJ; ARIES Study Group
Publication	*J Am Coll Cardiol.* 2009;54(21):1971–1981
Follow-up	2 years

(continued)

Note	Year 1:			
		Ambrisentan 2.5 mg	Ambrisentan 5 mg	Ambrisentan 10 mg
	Improvement of WHO class	17%	30%	38%
	No change of WHO class	72%	65%	48%
	Worsening of WHO class	11%	5%	15%
	Survival	n = 81	n = 153	n = 81
	Year 2:			
		Ambrisentan 2.5 mg	Ambrisentan 5 mg	Ambrisentan 10 mg
	Improvement of WHO class	17%	31%	41%
	No change of WHO class	62%	58%	45%
	Worsening of WHO class	21%	11%	15%
	Survival	n = 68	n = 121	n = 66
	Change of (end of first year):			
		Ambrisentan 2.5 mg	Ambrisentan 5 mg	Ambrisentan 10 mg
	6-min walking distance	+25 m	+28 m	+37 m
	Borg Dyspnea index	-0.08	-0.59	-0.51
	Change of (end of second year):			
		Ambrisentan 2.5 mg	Ambrisentan 5 mg	Ambrisentan 10 mg
	6-min walking distance	+7 m	+23 m	+28 m
	Borg Dyspnea index	+0.23	-0.33	-0.60

(continued)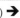

Adverse events		Ambrisentan 2.5 mg (%)	Ambrisentan 5 mg (%)	Ambrisentan 10 mg (%)
	Right ventricular failure	3.1	3.7	5.2
	Pulmonary hypertension	7.3	2.1	3.1
	Acute respiratory failure	0.0	1.1	2.1
	Cardiac arrest	1.0	1.1	0.0
	Cardiorespiratory arrest	1.0	1.1	0.0
	Pneumonia	1.0	0.5	1.0
	Diarrhea	0.0	1.1	0.0
	Dyspnea exacerbated	1.0	0.5	0.0
	Hemorrhage intracranial	0.0	0.0	2.1
	Hepatic enzyme increased	1.0	0.0	1.0
	Hypoxia	0.0	0.0	2.1
	Multiorgan failure	1.0	0.5	0.0
	Pyrexia	0.0	1.1	0.0
	Respiratory arrest	1.0	0.0	1.0
	Sudden death	0.0	0.5	1.0
	Syncope	2.1	0.0	0.0
	Vomiting	0.0	1.1	0.0
	Death	14	11	8

Trial	Experience with azathioprine in systemic sclerosis associated with interstitial lung disease		
Substance	**Azathioprine** **Plus low-dose prednisone** No information on the dosages used No information on concomitant medication		
Result	Azathioprine had an effect on dyspnea and on lung function parameters in this open study of patients with interstitial lung disease in systemic sclerosis		
Patients	11 patients with systemic sclerosis • Interstitial lung disease • FVC > 70% of the predicted and declining Nonsmokers		
Authors	Dheda K, Lalloo UG, Cassim B, Mody GM		
Publication	*Clin Rheumatol.* 2004;23(4):306–309		
Follow-up	18 months		
Note	*Respiratory function*:		

	Baseline	12 months	18 months
FVC predicted	54.25	63.38	60.0
Dyspnea score	1.55	0.50	0.43

Outcome parameters:

Patients improved during follow-up	n = 5
Patients remained stable during follow-up	n = 3
Mean dyspnea score improved	n = 8

Adverse events	Nausea	n = 1
	Leukopenia	n = 1
	Death	n = 1 (unknown cause)
	Carcinoma tongue	n = 1
	Pulmonary tuberculosis	n = 1

FAST-Trial	A multicenter, prospective, randomized, double-blind, placebo-controlled trial of corticosteroids and intravenous cyclophosphamide followed by oral Azathioprine for the treatment of pulmonary fibrosis in scleroderma FAST: Fibrosing Alveolitis in Skleroderma Trial
Substance	Induction therapy: **Prednisolone 20 mg on alternate days** **Plus 6 × 600 mg/sqm cyclophosphamide (CYC)/4 weeks** *Maintenance therapy*: **Azathioprine 2.5 mg/kg(AZA)/day** Started with 50 mg/day Increate to full dosage within 4 weeks (n = 22) **Placebo** (n = 23) *Pretreatment*: No prior AZA or CYC therapy for > 3 months No oral prednisolone ≥ 10 mg/day ≥ 3 months
Result	Patients treated with azathioprine did not improve significantly as compared to placebo treated patients. There was a trend toward better FVC values among patients treated with azathioprine
Patients	45 patients with systemic sclerosis (SSc) • SSc-associated pulmonary fibrosis • High resolution computer tomography: • ≥ 5% extend of the disease or ground glass attenuation or thoracoscopic lung biopsy • No treatment with AZA or CYC or high-dose oral corticosteroid therapy (30 mg of prednisolone), for > 3 months
Authors	Hoyles RK, Ellis RW, Wellsbury J, Lees B, Newlands P, Goh NS, Roberts C, Desai S, Herrick AL, McHugh NJ, Foley NM, Pearson SB, Emery P, Veale DJ, Denton CP, Wells AU, Black CM, du Bois RM
Publication	*Arthritis Rheum.* 2006;54(12):3962–3970
Follow-up	1 year

(continued) ➔

Note	Outcome parameters:		
		Azathioprine	Placebo
	Improvement on serial HRCT	40%	20%
	Change of:		
		Azathioprine	Placebo
	FVC (% predicted)	+2.4	-3.0
	DLCO (% predicted)	-3.3	-3.2
	TLC (% predicted)	-1.6	-2.4
	FEV1 (% predicted)	+1.7	-2.7
	Coefficient of gas transfer (% predicted)	+0.2	-4.8
	Dyspnea score (mean)	+1.05	+0.6
Adverse events		Azathioprine (%)	Placebo (%)
	Nausea	36.4	0
	Mood disturbance	18.2	0
	Oral ulcers	13.6	0
	Rash	13.6	0
	Abdominal findings	9.1	0
	Diarrhea	9.1	0
	Dyspepsia	4.5	0
	Respiratory tract infection	13.6	17.4
	Hematuria (baseline)	13.6	17.4
	Hematuria (end of follow-up)	45.5	26.1

Trial	Effects of the dual endothelin-receptor antagonist Bosentan in patients with pulmonary hypertension: a randomized placebo-controlled study
Substance	**Bosentan 2 × 62.5 mg/day (after 4 weeks then 2 × 125 mg/day, n = 21)**
	Placebo (n = 11)
	Prior medication:
	Stop any of treatments within 1 month of screening
	No epoprostenol within 1 month
	No glibenclamide or ciclosporin within 1 month
	Concomitant medication:
	Warfarin: 71% (bosentan), 73% (placebo)
	Diltiazem: 29% (bosentan), 18% (placebo)
	Amlodipine: 14% (bosentan), 36% (placebo)
	Previous medication:
	Active disease despite previous treatment with vasodilators, anticoagulants, diuretics, cardiac glycosides, or supplemental oxygen
Result	Bosentan increased exercise capacity and improved hemodynamics in patients with pulmonary hypertension
Patients	32 patients with pulmonary hypertension
	• Primary or associated with scleroderma
	• Functional classes III–IV (WHO classification)
	• Baseline 6-min walking distance 150–500 m
	• Mean pulmonary artery pressure > 25 mmHg
	• Pulmonary capillary wedge pressure < 15 mmHg
	• Pulmonary vascular resistance > 240 dyn s/cm^5
Authors	Channick RN, Simonneau G, Sitbon O, Robbins IM, Frost A, Tapson VF, Badesch DB, Roux S, Rainisio M, Bodin F, Rubin LJ
Publication	*Lancet*. 2001;358(9288):1119–1123
Follow-up	20 weeks
Note	*Change of*:

	Bosentan	Placebo
6-min walk test (m, week 12)	+70	-6
6-min walk test (m, week 20)	+77	-15
Cardiac index (L/min/m^2)	+0.5	-0.5
Pulmonary vascular resist. (dyn s/cm^5)	-223	+191
Pulmonary artery pressure (mmHg)	-1.6	+5.1
Mean right arterial pressure (mmHg)	-1.3	+4.9
Improvement to WHO class II	43%	9%

Trial	Bosentan therapy for pulmonary arterial hypertension
Substance	**Placebo** (n = 69) **Bosentan 2 × 62.5 mg/day** for 4 weeks *Followed by (bosentan treated patients only)*: Bosentan 2 × 125/day (n = 74) or Bosentan 2 × 250 mg/day (n = 70) for a minimum of 12 weeks *Concomitant medication*: Antithrombotic agents: 72% (placebo), 69% (125 mg bosentan), 71% (250 mg bosentan) Diuretics: 46% (placebo), 54% (125 mg bosentan), 56% (250 mg bosentan) Calcium-channel blockers: 52% (placebo), 45% (125 mg bosentan), 44% (250 mg bosentan) Supplemental oxygen at screening visit: 33% (placebo), 26% (125 mg bosentan), 31% (250 mg bosentan)
Result	Bosentan was beneficial and well-tolerated in patients with pulmonary arterial hypertension
Patients	213 patients with pulmonary arterial hypertension • WHO class III or IV • Despite anticoagulant treatment • Primary or associated with connective-tissue disease • 6-min walk test 150–450 m • Pulmonary artery pressure ≥ 25 mmHg • Capillary wedge pressure ≥ 15 mmHg • Pulmonary vascular resistance 240 dynx s/cm^5
Authors	Rubin LJ, Badesch DB, Barst RJ, Galie N, Black CM, Keogh A, Pulido T, Frost A, Roux S, Leconte I, Landzberg M, Simonneau G
Publication	*N Engl J Med*. 2002;346(12):896–903
Follow-up	16 weeks

 (continued) ➜

Note	Outcome parameters:			
		Placebo	Bosentan 125 mg	Bosentan 250 mg
	Improvement WHO III → II	28%	38%	34%
	Improvement WHO III → I	0%	3%	1%
	Clinical worsening	20%	7%	6%
	Death	3%	1%	0%
	Hospitalization or discontinuation for pulmonary arterial hypertension	13%	4%	4%
	Lack of clinical improvement leading to discontinuation	1%	0%	0%
	Worsening of pulmonary arterial hypertension leading to discontinuation	7%	4%	3%
	Receipt of Epoprostenol	4%	3%	3%
	Borg dyspnea index	+0.4	-0.1	-0.6
Adverse events		Placebo (%)	Bosentan 125 mg (%)	Bosentan 250 mg (%)
	Headache	19	19	23
	Dizziness	19	12	10
	Worsening of symptoms of pulmonary arterial hypertension	19	9	6
	Cough	12	5	6
	Dyspnea	10	3	7
	Syncope	6	8	10
	Flushing	4	9	9
	Abnormal hepatic function	3	4	14

RAPIDS-1-Trial	Digital ulcers in systemic sclerosis: prevention by treatment with Bosentan, an oral endothelin receptor antagonist RAPIDS: Randomized Placebo-controlled study on prevention of Ischemic Digital ulcers in Scleroderma
Substance	**Bosentan 2 × 62.5 mg/day** (n = 79) for 4 weeks • Increase of bosentan to 2 × 125 mg/day **Placebo** (n = 43) *Concomitant medication*: Continued treatment with oral vasodilating and immunosuppressive drugs: • Calcium channel blockers 58.1% (placebo), 41.8% (bosentan) • ACE inhibitors/Angiotensin II rec. antag. 25.6% (placebo), • 25.3% (bosentan) No treatment with parenteral prostanoids within the previous 3 months
Result	Bosentan was effective in preventing new digital ulcers and improving hand function in patients with systemic sclerosis
Patients	122 patients with systemic sclerosis and digital ulcers • 38% diffuse scleroderma • 62% limited scleroderma • Body weight > 40 kg
Authors	Korn JH, Mayes M, Matucci Cerinic M, Rainisio M, Pope J, Hachulla E, Rich E, Carpentier P, Molitor J, Seibold JR, Hsu V, Guillevin L, Chatterjee S, Peter HH, Coppock J, Herrick A, Merkel PA, Simms R, Denton CP, Furst D, Nguyen N, Gaitonde M, Black C
Publication	*Arthritis Rheum.* 2004;50(12):3985–3993
Follow-up	16 weeks

(continued)

Note	*Outcome parameters*:		
		Bosentan	Placebo
	New ulcers/patient	1.4	2.7
	New digital ulcers (% of the patients)	58%	61%
	≥ 4 new ulcers/patient with ulcers at baseline	13%	42%
	Study completed	n = 66	n = 37
	No difference in the healing of existing ulcers		

Adverse events	*All adverse events*:		
		Bosentan (%)	Placebo (%)
	Headache	16.5	16.3
	Liver function tests abnormal	11.4	0
	Upper respiratory tract infection	8.9	14.0
	Vomiting	8.9	9.3
	Diarrhea	8.9	2.3
	Infected skin ulcer	7.6	4.7
	Arthralgia	6.3	16.3
	Pain in limb	6.3	9.3
	Fatigue	5.1	7.0
	Nasopharyngitis	5.1	7.0
	Edema lower limb	5.1	7.0
	Flushing	5.1	2.3
	Constipation	5.1	0
	Esophageal reflux aggravated	5.1	0
	Other	83.5	72.1

	Serious adverse events:		
		Bosentan	Placebo
	Ventricular tachycardia	n = 2	n = 0
	Palpitations	n = 1	n = 0
	Dyspnea	n = 0	n = 1
	Acute high-altitude sickness	n = 0	n = 1
	Esophagitis	n = 0	n = 1
	Digital ischemia	n = 0	n = 1

BREATHE-1-Trial	Bosentan treatment for pulmonary arterial hypertension related to connective tissue disease: a subgroup analysis of the pivotal clinical trials and their open-label extensions BREATHE: Bosentan: Randomized Trial of Endothelin Receptor antagonist therapy for pulmonary arterial hypertension
Substance	**Bosentan 2 × 62.5 mg/day** for 4 weeks Increased to 2 × 125 or 2 × 250 mg for 8 or 12 weeks (n = 44) **Placebo** (n = 22) Followed by open label extension (n = 64) Bosentan monotherapy n = 40 Addition of prostanoids n = 1 Discontinued n = 19
Result	Short-term bosentan treatment patients with pulmonary arterial hypertension secondary to connective tissue disease with the subsequent addition of other PAH treatments, if required, was safe for long-term treatment and had a positive effect on outcome
Patients	66 patients with pulmonary arterial hypertension • Secondary to connective tissue disease (CTD) • World Health Organization (WHO) functional class III–IV 6-min walk test distance 150–500 m • Pulmonary arterial pressure > 25 mmHg • Pulmonary vascular resistance 0.240 dyn s/cm^5 • Pulmonary capillary wedge pressure < 15 mmHg (right heart catheterization) • No patients with vital capacity < 70% predicted • PAH/SSc n = 52 • SLE n = 8 • Overlap syndrome n = 4 • CTD (unclassified) n = 2
Authors	Denton CP, Humbert M, Rubin L, Black CM
Publication	*Ann Rheum Dis.* 2006;65(10):1336–1340
Follow-up	12–16 weeks, 1.6 years (mean) open label extension

Note		Bosentan	Placebo
	6-min walk distance at the end of the study (m)	+19.5	-2.6
	Change to epoprostenol	14%	16%
	Survival:		
	Bosentan 1 year	85.9%	
	Bosentan 2 year	73.4%	

Adverse events		Bosentan (%)	Placebo (%)
	Dizziness	18.2	4.5
	Lower limb edema	18.2	4.5
	Headache	15.9	22.7
	Fatigue	13.6	0
	Abnormal hepatic function	11.4	9.1

Trial	Improvement of vascular endothelial function using the oral endothelin receptor antagonist Bosentan in patients with systemic sclerosis
Substance	**Bosentan (2 × 62.5 mg/day, n = 12)** **Untreated control patients** (n = 12) *Concomitant medication*: Vasoactive and immunosuppressive therapy was continued
Result	Bosentan improved endothelial function without affecting hemodynamic parameters or endothelial activation-related processes
Patients	Systemic sclerosis (SSc) Patients • Pulmonary hypertension and/or • Digital ulcers • Decreased brachial artery ultrasound derived flow-mediated dilation (FMD%)
Authors	Sfikakis PP, Papamichael C, Stamatelopoulos KS, Tousoulis D, Fragiadaki KG, Katsichti P, Stefanadis C, Mavrikakis M
Publication	*Arthritis Rheum*. 2007;56(6):1985–1993
Follow-up	4 weeks
Note	*Change of*:

	Bosentan	Control
Flow-mediated dilation	+5.3%	0%
Systolic blood pressure (mmHg)	-3	-4
Diastolic blood pressure (mmHg)	-6	-6
Reactive hyperemia	+15%	-12%
Nitroglycerine-induced dilation	+5.7%	+5.3%
Augmentation index	-2.5%	+0.3%
Forearm blood flow (mL/min/100 mL)	+0.2	-0.1
Peripheral flow reserve	-0.3	-0.1
ICAM-1 (ng/mL)	+76	-67
E-selectin (ng/mL)	+6	+2
VEGF (pg/mL)	-19	-20
Endothelin 1 (pg/mL)	0	-0.4

BUILD-1-Trial	BUILD-1: a randomized placebo-controlled trial of Bosentan in idiopathic pulmonary fibrosis BUILD: Bosentan Use in Interstitial Lung Disease
Substance	**Bosentan oral 62.5 mg twice daily** for 4 weeks Increased to 125 mg twice daily thereafter (n = 74) **Placebo** (n = 84) *Concomitant medication*: No immunosuppressive drugs No cytotoxic drugs Prednisone ≤ 15 mg or equivalent No calcineurin inhibitors, fluconazole, and glyburide
Result	Bosentan treated patients with idiopathic pulmonary fibrosis did not show superiority over placebo. There was a trend in delayed time to death or disease progression, and improvement in quality of life, was observed with bosentan
Patients	Please note: trial shown here because of lack of trials in patients with pulmonary fibrosis secondary to connective tissue disease 158 patients with idiopathic pulmonary fibrosis Demonstrated by HRCT • Diagnosis ≤ 3 years before enrolment • Baseline 6-min walking distance between 150 and 499 m FVC ≥ 50% predicted • DLCO ≥ 30% predicted • RV > 120% • FEV1/FVC ≥ 65% • Echocardiographic assessment of pulmonary hypertension (systolic pulmonary pressure > 50 mmHg or tricuspid) • Regurgitation velocity > 3.2 m/s • No severe congestive heart failure • PaO_2 ≥ 55 mmHg
Authors	King TE Jr, Behr J, Brown KK, du Bois RM, Lancaster L, de Andrade JA, Stähler G, Leconte I, Roux S, Raghu G
Publication	*Am J Respir Crit Care Med* . 2008;177(1):75–81
Follow-up	12 months

(continued)

Note	Outcome parameters:		
		Bosentan	Placebo
	Disease progression or death	22.5%	36.1%
	Death	n = 3	n = 3
	Study not completed	33.8%	28.6%
	Change of:		
		Bosentan	Placebo
	6-min walk test (m)	-52	-34
	FVC	-6.4%	-7.7%
	DLCO	-4.3%	-5.8%
Adverse events		Bosentan (%)	Placebo (%)
	Cough	17.6	27.4
	Worsening of idiopathic pulmonary fibrosis	16.2	23.8
	Exacerbation of dyspnea	13.5	19.0
	Elevations in alanine aminotransferase	20.5	0

Trial	Long-term experience of Bosentan for treating ulcers and healed ulcers in systemic sclerosis patients	
Substance	**2 × 62.5 mg bosentan/day** for 28 days and a maintenance dose of 2 × 125 mg	
Result	Bosentan treatment of systemic sclerosis patients was a safe long-term alternative for treating the recurrence of skin ulcers	
Patients	15 patients with systemic sclerosis (SSc) suffering from digital ulcers • Diffuse cutaneous SSc 33.3% • Limited cutaneous SSc 66.6%	
Authors	García de la Peña-Lefebvre P, Rodríguez Rubio S, Valero Expósito M, Carmona L, Gámir Gámir ML, Beltrán Gutiérrez J, Díaz-Miguel C, Orte Martínez J, Zea Mendoza AC	
Publication	*Rheumatology (Oxford)*. 2008;47(4):464–466	
Follow-up	Median 24.7 months	
Note	*Change of:*	
	Modified Rodnan skin score	-1.8
	Oral opening (mm)	-3.4
	Mean hand flexion (mm)	+1.5
	Mean hand extension (mm)	-0.3
	Mean grip strength (mmHg)	-5.4
	No. of ulcers	-1.4
	No. of healed ulcers	-0.4
	Number of Raynaud's phenomenon episodes	-1.7
	Duration of Raynaud's phenomenon episodes (min)	-34.8
	Raynaud's phenomenon VAS (mm)	-50.0
	Overall disease VAS (mm)	+14.0
	Arthritis impact measurement scales	-0.6
	Scleroderma health assessment questionnaire	-0.1
Adverse events	Increase of transaminases (< 3 × normal values)	n = 3
	Myocardial infarction	n = 1
	Headache	n = 1
	Nasal congestion	n = 2
	Discomfort	n = 1
	Anemia	n = 2
	Infection of ulcers	n = 5
	Decrease of 1–2 points of hemoglobin	n = 6

Trial	No effects of Bosentan on microvasculature in patients with limited cutaneous systemic sclerosis
Substance	**Bosentan, 2 × 62.5 mg** 4 weeks Followed by 2 × 125 mg 12 weeks *Concomitant medication*: No prior use of bosentan Reliable method of contraception No prostanoids therapy during the last month No sympathectomy ≤ 12 months Calcium channel antagonists, ketanserin, angiotensin converting enzyme inhibitors were continued at a stable dosage
Result	Bosentan treatment of patients with limited cutaneous systemic sclerosis did not lead to structural improvement of microvascular system and function in this short-time mechanistic pilot study
Patients	15 patients with limited cutaneous systemic sclerosis • Digital pitting scars and/or ulceration • No current smoking or smoking ≤ 4 weeks
Authors	Hettema ME, Zhang D, Stienstra Y, Smit AJ, Bootsma H, Kallenberg CG
Publication	*Clin Rheumatol.* 2009;28(7):825–833
Follow-up	16 weeks with a follow-up period of 4 weeks
Note	*Change of*:

Baseline flux (arbitrary units)	-2.4
Plateau flux (arbitrary units)	+7.3
Absolute increase (arbitrary units)	+9.8
ACh-mediated vasodilatation	-31.3%
SNP-mediated vasodilatation	22.8
Plateau flux (arbitrary units)	29.1
Absolute increase (arbitrary units)	-2.6
Sodium nitroprusside-mediated vasodilatation	-151.3%
Number of capillaries	-0.5/3 mm

Trial	Long-term outcome of systemic sclerosis-associated pulmonary arterial hypertension treated with bosentan as first-line monotherapy followed or not by the addition of prostanoids or sildenafil
Substance	**2 × 62.5 mg bosentan/day** for 4 weeks Followed by 2 × 125 mg/day *Concomitant therapy*: Oral anticoagulants, to maintain an international normalized ratio of 1.5–2.5 Diuretics was permitted Oxygen therapy was permitted
Result	Bosenthan improved NYHA functional class and hemodynamic after 4 months of treatment and stabilized afterwards, with a poor overall long-term prognosis
Patients	49 consecutive patients with systemic sclerosis and pulmonary arterial hypertension • Diagnosis by the ACR preliminary classification criteria for SSc
Authors	Launay D, Sitbon O, Le Pavec J, Savale L, Tchérakian C, Yaïci A, Achouh L, Parent F, Jais X, Simonneau G, Humbert M
Publication	*Rheumatology (Oxford)*. 2010 Mar;49(3):490–500
Follow-up	12 months (NYHA, hemodynamics), 72 months (survival)
Note	*Patients with 4 month evaluation*:

	Baseline	4 months
NYHA functional class II vs. III/IV	6/38	16/28
6-min walking distance	272	285
mmRAP, mmHg	7	7
mPAP, mmHg	47	46
Cardiac index, L/min/m^2	2.49	2.87
Systolic index, mL/m^2	28.7	34.3
PVR, mmHg/Lmin	10.3	8.6
mSAP, mmHg	89	81
Heart rate	86	82

Patients with 12 month evaluation:

	Baseline	4 months	12 months
NYHA functional class II vs. III/IV	2/17	10/9	8/11
6-min walking distance	253	290	276
mmRAP, mmHg	9	8	8
mPAP, mmHg	51	48	48
Cardiac index, L/min/m^2	2.41	2.97	2.79
Systolic index, mL/m^2	29.4	38.8	37.7
PVR, mmHg/L min	11.6	7.9	9.1
mSAP, mmHg	92	85	86
Heart rate	86	79	77
Survival rate			
1 year	80%		
2 years	56%		
3 years	51%		

Trial	Randomized, prospective, placebo-controlled trial of bosentan in interstitial lung disease secondary to systemic sclerosis
Substance	**Bosentan 2 × 62.5 mg/d** Increased to 2 × 125 mg/d after 4 weeks (n = 77) **Placebo** (n = 86)
Result	No effect of bosentan on paramters of lung function was demonstrated
Patients	163 patients with limited systemic sclerosis and significant interstitial lung disease • HRCT: Reticular or ground glass changes extending at least to the venous confluence • DLCO of ≤ 80% of that predicted • 6-min walk distance of 150–500 m or • A distance of ≥ 500 m with a decrease in oxygen saturation (SpO2) of ≥ 4%. + 2 of the following 4 criteria: · • Worsening dyspnea • Worsening results of pulmonary function tests (FVC ≥ 7% and/ or worsening of DLCO ≥ 10%) • New areas of ILD on HRCT scan ≥ 5% of overall lung parenchyma (or 15% of a lobe) • Neutrophilia and/or eosinophilia in bronchoalveolar lavage fluid
Authors	Seibold JR, Denton CP, Furst DE, Guillevin L, Rubin LJ, Wells A, Matucci Cerinic M, Riemekasten G, Emery P, Chadha-Boreham H, Charef P, Roux S, Black CM
Publication	*Arthritis Rheum.* 2010 Jul;62(7):2101–2108
Follow-up	*12 months*
Note	*Change of:*

	Bosentan	Placebo
6-min walk distance	+16	+13
Worsening of pulmonary function test scores	n = 16	n = 20
Improved of pulmonary function test scores	n = 6	n = 11
FVC	-1.6%	-1.2%
DLCO	-1.3	-0.9

Adverse events	Bosentan (%)	Placebo (%)
Adverse events	97.4	94.2
Elevated liver aminotransferase levels	11.3	1.2

Trial	Immunosuppression with Chlorambucil, versus placebo, for scleroderma
	Results of a 3-year, parallel, randomized, double-blind study
Substance	**Placebo** (n = 32)
	Chlorambucil 0.05 mg/kg/day (n = 33)
	Chlorambucil 0.075 mg/kg/day after 6 months
	Chlorambucil 0.10 mg/kg/day after 1 year
	Concomitant medication:
	No immunosuppressive drugs > 3 months
	Prednisolone ≤ 15 mg
Result	Three years of treatment with chlorambucil did not improve signs and symptoms of this scleroderma population
Patients	65 patients with systemic sclerosis
	• Creatinine < 2 mg/dL
	• pO_2 > 55 torr
Authors	Furst DE, Clements PJ, Hillis S, Lachenbruch PA, Miller BL, Sterz MG, Paulus HE
Publication	*Arthritis Rheum.* 1989;32(5):584–593
Follow-up	*3 years*
Note	*Change of:*

	Chlorambucil	Placebo
Skin Score (max. 30)	-1.12	-0.27
Weight (kg)	-0.39	-0.31
DLCO (% of normal)	-1.73	-2.51
TLC (% of normal)	+0.72	-0.64
FVC (% of normal)	-0.14	-0.35
FEV (% of normal)	-0.25	+0.17
Creatinine clearance (mL/min)	-2.92	-4.55
Serum creatinine (mg%)	+0.01	-0.01
Proteinuria (mg/24 h)	+5.66	-2.70
Tender joint count	-0.06	-0.60

Adverse events		Chlorambucil	Placebo
	Lack of benefit	n = 4	n = 5
	Leucopenia	n = 21	n = 5
	Thrombocytopenia	n = 3	n = 1
	Gastrointestinal effects	n = 4	n = 4
	Infections	n = 6	n = 1
	Aplastic anemia	n = 0	n = 1
	Death	n = 9	n = 13
	Cancer	n = 0	n = 3

Trial	Ciclosporin in systemic sclerosis. Results of a 48-week open safety study in ten patients	
Substance	**Ciclosporin 1 mg/kg/day** (n = 10) **Placebo** (n = 13) *Concomitant medication*: Hypertension $\geq$ ACE inhibitor and/or decrease dosage CsA *Prior treatment*: No antimetabolite treatment $\leq$ 3 months No immunosuppressive treatment $\leq$ 3 months No colchicine $\leq$ 3 months No ACE inhibitors $\leq$ 3 months	
Result	Skin thickening decreased significantly in ciclosporin treated patients, while cardiac and pulmonary involvement remained unchanged. Adverse events were frequent and dose associated	
Patients	23 patients with systemic sclerosis • Duration of cutaneous involvement < 60 months • $\geq$ 21 years of age • No arterial hypertension (CsA group) • No $pO_2 \leq 55$ torr	
Authors	Clements PJ, Lachenbruch PA, Sterz M, Danovitch G, Hawkins R, Ippoliti A, Paulus HE	
Publication	*Arthritis Rheum.* 1993;36(1):75–83	
Follow-up	*48 weeks*	
Note	*Change of:*	

	Ciclosporin	Placebo
Skin Score	-2.9	-0.3
Joint count	-5.7	-5.1
Creatinine clearance (mL/min)	-27	-11
Serum creatinine (mg/dL)	+0.2	+0.07
Total lung capacity (%)	+0.5	-3.1
Vital capacity (%)	-1.2	-1.4
DLCO (%)	+1.7	-2.9

Adverse events		
Hypertrichosis	n = 6	
Tinnitus	n = 1	
Gastrointestinal upset	n = 1	
Rise in serum creatinine > 30%	n = 8	
Arterial hypertension	n = 2	
Coccidioidomycosis	n = 1	

Trial	Long-term evaluation of Colchicine in the treatment of scleroderma
Substance	**Colchicine** At the maximum tolerated individual doses Mean dose 10.1 mg/week Range 6–21 mg/week
Result	Colchicine treatment improved symptoms of scleroderma within three months
Patients	19 patients with scleroderma • Raynaud phenomenon n = 19 • Esophageal involvement n = 18 • Syndrome n = 4 • Progress. System Sclerosis n = 15
Authors	Alarcon-Segovia D, Ramos-Niembro F, Ibanez de Kasep G, Alcocer J, Tamayo RP
Publication	*J Rheumatol*. 1979;6(6):705–712
Follow-up	19–57 months (mean 39 months)
Note	*Percentage of patients with improvement of (%)*:
	Grip strength	17
	Finger palm distance	11
	Mouth opening	13
	Reappearance of hair	19
	Skins elasticity	19
	Raynaud's phenomenon	19
	Digital pitting microinfarcts	9
	Dysphagia	14
	Pulmonary function tests	9
	Skin biopsy	17
	Time on treatment before improvement (month):
	Grip strength	8.1
	Finger palm distance	10.0
	Mouth opening	13.0
	Reappearance of hair	19.6
	Skins elasticity	7.5 (observer's evaluation) 6.0 (patient's evaluation)
Adverse events	No significant adverse events
	Increased alkaline phosphatase (frequently)
	No leukopenia
	No gastrointestinal adverse events

Trial	Cyclophosphamide and low-dose Prednisone therapy in patients with systemic sclerosis (scleroderma) with interstitial lung disease
Substance	**Cyclophosphamide oral (1–2 mg/kg/day)** Plus low dose prednisone (< 10 mg/day) *Concomitant medication*: No information provided *Pretreatment*: No information provided
Result	Cyclophosphamide and low-dose prednisone therapy improved lung function in patients with systemic sclerosis with interstitial lung disease
Patients	14 patients with scleroderma and interstitial lung disease • Disease duration 23.1 months • Diffuse cutaneous scleroderma n = 9 • Limited cutaneous scleroderma n = 4 • SSc without scleroderma n = 1 • Active alveolitis proven by BAL • Minimum 2 standard deviation increase in the absolute number of macrophages, neutrophils, and/or eosinophils
Authors	Silver RM, Warrick JH, Kinsella MB, Staudt LS, Baumann MH, Strange C
Publication	*J Rheumatol*. 1993;20(5):838–844
Follow-up	24 months

Note		FVC (% predicted)	DLCO (% predicted)
	Baseline	51.4	54.5
	6 months	56.1	55.0
	12 months	58.3	51.9
	24 months	63.6	47.9

Adverse events	Leucopenia	n = 2	
	Thrombopenia	n = 1	
	Pneumonia	n = 1	
	Hemorrhagic cystitis	n = 2	
	Related malignancy	n = 1	

Trial	Intravenous Cyclophosphamide pulse therapy for the treatment of lung disease associated with scleroderma
Substance	**Cyclophosphamide 750 mg/m² monthly** i. v. pulse therapy for 12 months (n = 8) **Cyclophosphamide p. o. 2–2.5 mg/kg/day** (n = 8) *Concomitant medication*: Prednisone 10 mg/day Calcium channel blockers as needed H2 blockers as needed Omeprazole as needed
Result	Cyclophosphamide pulse therapy was effective in suppressing active alveolitis as demonstrated by ground glass appearance on HRCT
Patients	16 patients with systemic sclerosis and • Alveolitis detected by computed tomography • No pulmonary hypertension • Nonsmokers
Authors	Davas EM, Peppas C, Maragou M, Alvanou E, Hondros D, Dantis PC
Publication	*Clin Rheumatol.* 1999;18(6):455–461
Follow-up	12 months

Note: *HRCT score (following Wells et al.):*

	Oral cyclophosphamide	I. v. cyclophosphamide
Baseline	35%	+34.2%
6 months	31.5%	+30%
12 months	31.5%	+11.7%
Grade I (ground glass appearance)	n = 3	n = 8
Grade II (ground glass and reticular appearance)	n = 1	n = 0
Grade III (reticular appearance)	n = 4	n = 1

Change of (12 months):

	Oral cyclophosphamide (%)	I. v. cyclophosphamide (%)
FEV1	-1.1	+2.5
FVC	+1.0	+7.5
TLC	0	+8.9
DLCO	11.8	+16.5

Adverse events

	Oral cyclophosphamide	I. v. cyclophosphamide
Leucopenia	n = 3	–
Alopecia	n = 1	–
Nausea and vomiting	–	few, self limiting episodes

Trial	Cyclophosphamide pulse regimen in the treatment of alveolitis in systemic sclerosis	
Substance	**Cyclophosphamide 1'000 mg/m2 i. v./month** for 6 months plus **Prednisone 25 mg/day** for 1 month Followed by 5 mg prednisone/day for the remaining 5 months *Pretreatment*: No cytotoxic drugs No biologic ≤12 months	
Result	Cyclophosphamide pulse regimen seemed to stabilize alveolitis in the majority of cases	
Patients	23 patients with systemic sclerosis (SSc) • Diffuse SSc n = 17 • Limited SSc n = 6 • Alveolitis detected by BAL cell analysis • Recent deterioration in FVC	
Authors	Giacomelli R, Valentini G, Salsano F, Cipriani P, Sambo P, Conforti ML, Fulminis A, De Luca A, Farina G, Candela M, Generini S, De Francisci A, Tirri E, Proietti M, Bombardieri S, Gabrielli A, Tonietti G, Cerinic MM	
Publication	*J Rheumatol.* 2002;29(4):731–736	
Follow-up	6 months	
Note	*Outcome parameters*:	
	FVC no change	n = 13
	FVC Improvement (> 15% increase)	n = 8
	FVC decline	n = 2
	DLCO Improvement	n = 15
	DLCO no change	n = 4
	DLCO decline	n = 4
	Ground-glass aspect in HRCT stable	n = 8
	Ground-glass aspect in HRCT improvement	n = 10
	Ground-glass aspect in HRCT diffusion to other segments	n = 5
	Change of (bronchoalveolar lavage):	
		Baseline	6 months
	Recovery	53%	49%
	Cells/mL	460´000	285´000
	Macrophages	62%	78%
	Lymphocytes	16%	12%
	Neutrophils	4%	3%
	Basophils	0%	0.5%
	Eosinophils	0.4%	1%
Adverse events	Mild nausea	n = 4

Trial	Systemic sclerosis and interstitial lung disease: a pilot study using pulse intravenous methylprednisolone and Cyclophosphamide to assess the effect on high resolution computed tomography scan and lung function
Substance	**Cyclophosphamide 6 pulses of i. v. 15 mg/kg** **Plus i. v. methylprednisolone 10 mg/kg** The first 3 pulses were given at 3 weekly intervals The remaining 3 pulses were administered at 4 weekly intervals *Concomitant medication*: Proton pump inhibitor or H2 antagonist Patients were advised to drink 3 L of fluid on the day of the pulse 3 × 400 mg mesna tablets, 1 h pre-CYC and 4 and 12 h post-CYC metoclopramide or granisetron Amphoteracin Lisinopril (typically 2.5 mg daily)
Result	Intravenous cyclophosphamide of patients with systemic sclerosis stabilized lung disease. Stop or reduction of treatment resulted in deterioration of lung function in the majority of patients
Patients	14 consecutive patients with systemic sclerosis and lung involvement • A HRCT scan was performed • If the TLC was < 80% of the predicted • Or DLCO was < 75% of the predicted • Deterioration of DLCO and FVC • Abnormal HRCT: ground glass
Authors	Griffiths B, Miles S, Moss H, Robertson R, Veale D, Emery P
Publication	*J Rheumatol.* 2002;29(11):2371–2378
Follow-up	12–54 months
Note	*Outcome parameters*:

HRCT scan scores improved or stabilized	n = 13	
DLCO first 12 months	Remained stable	
Deterioration in DLCO 26 months	67% of patients	
Change of:		
Modified Rodnan skin score	17 → 13	

Adverse events	Death of cerebral hemorrhage	n = 1
	Death of generalized	n = 1
	Death of chest infection	n = 1

Trial	Effects of oral Cyclophosphamide and Prednisolone therapy on the endothelial functions and clinical findings in patients with early diffuse systemic sclerosis
Substance	**Cyclophosphamide oral 2–2.5 mg/kg/day** **Plus methylprednisolone 30 mg/every other day** Tapered by 2.5 mg every 6 weeks until 2.5 mg/every other day *Previous treatment*: No DMARDs No NSAIDs
Result	Combination therapy with cyclophosphamide plus prednisolone of patients suffering from early diffuse systemic sclerosis was effective
Patients	13 patients with early diffuse sytemic sclerosis • Disease duration was < 2 years • None of the patients was previously treated with DMARDs • All of them had diffuse cutaneous involvement • FVC ≥ 50% of predicted • DLCO ≥ 40% of • No congestive heart failure • No chronic obstructive lung disease
Authors	Apras S, Ertenli I, Ozbalkan Z, Kiraz S, Ozturk MA, Haznedaroglu IC, Cobankara V, Pay S, Calguneri M
Publication	*Arthritis Rheum.* 2003;48(8):2256–2261
Follow-up	12 months
Note	*Change of*:

	Baseline	Post treatment
Skin Score, median	48	32
ESR (mm/h)	52.3	17.2
White blood cell count (no/mm³)	8´300	6´290
Creatinine clearance (mL/min)	77.4	103.1
FVC (% of predicted)	76.4	86.2
DLCO (% of predicted)	64.3	76.3

Adverse events	No toxic effects

The Scleroderma Lung Study	Cyclophosphamide versus placebo in scleroderma lung disease
Substance	**Cyclophosphamide p. o.** ($\leq$ **2 mg/kg/day,** n = 79) **Placebo** (n = 79) Prednisone $\leq$ 10 mg/day *Previous medications*: No p. o. cyclophosphamide $\leq$ 2 i. v. cyclophosphamide courses No DMARDs
Result	Oral cyclophosphamide in patients with symptomatic scleroderma-related interstitial lung disease had a significant but modest beneficial effect on lung function, dyspnea, thickening of the skin, and the health-related quality of life

Patients	158 patients with scleroderma
	• Restrictive lung physiology
	• Dyspnea (Mahler dyspnea index Grade II)
	• FVC 45–85% of the predicted
	• DLCO $\geq$ 30% of the predicted
	• Non smokers $\geq$ 6 months
	• Evidence of inflammatory interstitial lung disease:
	  ° Bronchoalveolar lavage: neutrophilia $\geq$ 3% and/or
	  ° Eosinophilia of $\geq$ 2% or
	  ° HRCT: ground-glass opacity

Authors	Tashkin DP, Elashoff R, Clements PJ, Goldin J, Roth MD, Furst DE, Arriola E, Silver R, Strange C, Bolster M, Seibold JR, Riley DJ, Hsu VM, Varga J, Schraufnagel DE, Theodore A, Simms R, Wise R, Wigley F, White B, Steen V, Read C, Mayes M, Parsley E, Mubarak K, Connolly MK, Golden J, Olman M, Fessler B, Rothfield N, Metersky M; Scleroderma Lung Study Research Group
Publication	*N Engl J Med*. 2006;354(25):2655–2666

(continued)

Note	Change of:		
		Cyclophosphamide	Placebo
	FVC (% of predicted)	-1.0	-2.6
	Total lung capacity (% of predicted)	-0.3	-2.8
	DLCO (% of predicted)	-4.2	-3.5
	HAQ	-0.11	+0.16
	SF36 physical component	+0.7	-1.9
	SF36 mental component	+2.9	+0.1
	Skin-thickness score: Total score	-3.6	-0.9
	Diffuse	-5.3	-1.7
	Limited	-0.8	+0.2
Adverse events	Year 1:		
		Cyclophosphamide	Placebo
	Hematuria	n = 9	n = 3
	Leucopenia	n = 19	n = 0
	Neutropenia	n = 7	n = 0
	Anemia	n = 2	n = 0
	Pneumonia	n = 5	n = 1
	Death	n = 2	n = 3
	Year 2:		
		Cyclophosphamide	Placebo
	Hematuria	n = 1	n = 2
	Leucopenia	n = 0	n = 0
	Neutropenia	n = 0	n = 0
	Anemia	n = 2	n = 1
	Pneumonia	n = 1	n = 0
	Death	n = 4	n = 3

Trial	Oral Cyclophosphamide improves pulmonary function in scleroderma patients with fibrosing alveolitis: experience in one center
Substance	**Cyclophosphamide p. o. 2 mg/kg/day** for 1 year **Plus 25 mg prednisone/day** for 3 months Then tapered to 5 mg/day
Result	Oral cyclophosphamide treatment of scleroderma patients with active alveolitis was effective in ameliorating and/or stabilizing lung function, with beneficial effects lasting up to 1 year

Patients	33 scleroderma patients
	With active alveolitis:
	  • Presence of areas of ground-glass attenuation' on HRCT
	  • Recent deterioration in lung function
	  • Decline of TC $\geq$ 7%
	  • Decline of DLCO $\geq$ 7%
	  • No pulmonary hypertension (right ventricular systolic pressure > 40 mmHg)

Authors	Beretta L, Caronni M, Raimondi M, Ponti A, Viscuso T, Origgi L, Scorza R
Publication	*Clin Rheumatol.* 2007;26(2):168–172
Follow-up	24 months

(continued) ➔

Note	Outcome parameters (after 12 months):		
	Improvement of DLCO	63.6%	
	Stabilization of DLCO	24.2%	
	Deterioration of DLCO	12.1%	
	Improvement of VC	45.5%	
	Stabilization of VC	42.4%	
	Deterioration of VC	12.1%	
	Outcome parameters (after 24 months):		
		Improvement (%)	Deterioration (%)
	Response of DLCO dependent on initial radiological Grading (Wells): Grade I	76.2	0
	Grade II	50.0	40.0
	Grade III	0.0	0.0
	Response of VC dependent on initial radiological Grading (Wells): Grade I	52.4	9.5
	Grade II	40.0	10.0
	Grade III	0.0	50.0
	Change of (24 months):		
	Improvement of DLCO (mmol/min/kPa)	+0.26	
	DLCO (% predicted)	+6.9%	
	VC (l)	+0.06	
	VC (% predicted)	+4	
Adverse events	Reduction of white blood cell count < 3,000/mm³	n = 7	
	Alopecia	n = 1	
	Amenorrhea	n = 4	
	Hemorrhagic cystitis	n = 0	

Trial	A randomized unblinded trial of Cyclophosphamide vs. Azathioprine in the treatment of systemic sclerosis		
Substance	*Cyclophosphamide arm* n = 30: **Cyclophosphamide 2 mg/kg/day p. o.for 12 months** Then maintained on 1 mg/kg/day (Cyc) *Azathioprine arm* n = 30: **Azathioprine 2.5 mg/kg/day** for 12 months Then maintained on 2 mg/kg/day (Aza) *Concomitant medication*: 15 mg prednisone/day Tapered every month by 2.5 mg to 0 Reliable anticonception *Previous treatment*: No DMARDs Prednisolone in some patients NSAIDs in some patients		
Result	Cyclophosphamide treatment of patients with systemic sclerosis had more effect on skin, lung function, and joint pain than treatment with azathioprine		
Patients	60 patients with early, diffuse systemic sclerosis • Disease duration ≤ 12 months • No obstructive lung disease • No nephritis • No increased creatinine • No increased transaminases		
Authors	Nadashkevich O, Davis P, Fritzler M, Kovalenko W		
Publication	*Clin Rheumatol.* 2006;25(2):205–212		
Follow-up	18 months		
Note	*Change of (month 19)*:		
		Cyclophosphamide	Azathioprine
	Modified Rodnan skin score	-9.47	+0.2
	Attack frequency of Raynaud's phenomenon/day	-1.59	+0.41
	ESR (mm/h)	-14.6	+1.3
	FVC (% predicted)	+3.3	-11.1
	DLCO (% predicted)	0.0	-11.6
	Patients with arthralgias	-19	-5
Adverse events		Cyclophosphamide	Azathioprine
	Considerable hair loss	n = 3	n = 0
	Dyspepsia	n = 4	n = 2
	Leukopenia	n = 5	n = 2
	Nausea	n = 3	n = 3
	Otitis media	n = 0	n = 1

The Scleroderma lung study	Effects of 1-year treatment with Cyclophosphamide on outcomes at 2 years in scleroderma lung disease
Substance	**Cyclophosphamide p. o.** ($\leq$ 2 mg/kg/day, n = 79)
	Placebo (n =79)
	Prednisone $\leq$ 10 mg/day
	Treatment was discontinued after 12 months
	Previous medications:
	No oral cyclophosphamide
	No $\geq$ 2 i. v. cyclophosphamide
	No DMARDs
	Treatment during the second year:
	Finishing year 2: n = 57 (placebo) n = 56 (Cyc)
	Any off study drug: n = 14 (placebo) n = 10 (Cyc)
	Prednisone ($\geq$ 10 mg): n = 12 (average dose: 11.6 mg, Placebo), *n* = 10 (average dose: 14.0 mg, Cyc)
	Cyclophosphamide: n = 2 (average dose: 72.5 mg), n = 0 (Cyc)
	No patients received azathioprine or mycophenolate
Result	After stop of 1 of year treatment with cyclophosphamide lung function, skin scores, dyspnea, and health status/disability improved for several months. A sustained impact at 24 months was only seen for dyspnea.
Patients	158 patients with scleroderma
	• Restrictive lung physiology
	• Dyspnea (Mahler Dyspnea Index Grade II)
	• FVC 45–85% of the predicted
	• DLCO $\geq$ 30% of the predicted
	• Non smokers $\geq$ 6 months
	• Evidence of inflammatory interstitial lung disease:
	• Bronchoalveolar lavage: neutrophilia $\geq$ 3% and/or eosinophilia of $\geq$ 2% or
	• HRCT: ground-glass opacity
Authors	Tashkin DP, Elashoff R, Clements PJ, Roth MD, Furst DE, Silver RM, Goldin J, Arriola E, Strange C, Bolster MB, Seibold JR, Riley DJ, Hsu VM, Varga J, Schraufnagel D, Theodore A, Simms R, Wise R, Wigley F, White B, Steen V, Read C, Mayes M, Parsley E, Mubarak K, Connolly MK, Golden J, Olman M, Fessler B, Rothfield N, Metersky M, Khanna D, Li N, Li G; Scleroderma Lung Study Research Group
Publication	*Am J Respir Crit Care Med.* 2007;176(10):1026–1034
Follow-up	24 months

(continued) ➔

Note	Dissipation of beneficial effects on pulmonary function and health status after 18 months		
	Dissipation of beneficial effects on skin improvements after 12 months		
	Outcome parameters:		
		Cyclophosphamide	Placebo
	FVC < 70% predicted	n = 40	n = 37
	FVC ≥ 70% predicted	n = 29	n = 35
Adverse events		Cyclophosphamide	Placebo
	Leukopenia	n = 0	n = 0
	Neutropenia	n = 0	n = 0
	Hematuria	n = 1	n = 2
	Anemia	n = 2	n = 1
	Pneumonia	n = 1	n = 0
	Death	n = 4	n = 3

The scleroderma lung study	Treatment of scleroderma-interstitial lung disease with Cyclophosphamide is associated with less progressive fibrosis on serial thoracic high-resolution CT scan than placebo: findings from the scleroderma lung study		
Substance	**Cyclophosphamide p. o. ($\leq$ 2 mg/kg/day**, n = 79) **Placebo** (n =79) Prednisone $\leq$ 10 mg/day Treatment was discontinued after 12 months *Previous medications:* No oral cyclophosphamide No $\geq$ 2 i. v. cyclophosphamide pulses No DMARDs		
Result	Treatment of scleroderma-interstitial lung disease with cyclophosphamide was associated with treatment-related improvement in fibrosis scores on HRCT scans, which correlated with other pulmonary parameters		
Patients	158 patients with scleroderma • Restrictive lung physiology • Dyspnea (Mahler Dyspnea Index Grade II) • FVC 45–85% of the predicted • DLCO $\geq$ 30% of the predicted • Non smokers $\geq$ 6 months • Evidence of inflammatory interstitial lung disease • Bronchoalveolar lavage: ° Neutrophilia $\geq$ 3% and/or ° Eosinophilia of $\geq$ 2% or • HRCT: ground-glass opacity		
Authors	Goldin J, Elashoff R, Kim HJ, Yan X, Lynch D, Strollo D, Roth MD, Clements P, Furst DE, Khanna D, Vasunilashorn S, Li G, Tashkin DP		
Publication	*Chest.* 2009;136(5):1333–1340		
Follow-up	1 year		
Note	*Outcome parameters:*		

	Cyclophosphamide	Placebo
Fibrosis worse	n = 14	n = 26
Fibrosis not worse	n = 35	n = 23
Ground-glass opacities worse	n = 13	n = 16
Ground-glass opacities not worse	n = 36	n = 33
Honeycomb cysts worse	n = 3	n = 3
Honeycomb cysts not worse	n = 46	n = 46

Trial	High-dose prednisolone and bolus cyclophosphamide in interstitial lung disease associated with systemic sclerosis: a prospective open study		
Substance	**Prednisolone 1 mg/kg, with tapering to a dose of 7.5 mg/day** **Plus cyclophosphamide 6 monthly at 750 mg/m² intravenous** pulses were Followed by 3-monthly maintenance pulses		
Result	High-dose prednisolone with pulse cyclophosphamide led to improvement or stabilization of lung functions in patients with severe systemic sclerosis lung disease irrespective of presence of ground glass appearance on HRCT		
Patients	36 consecutive patients with systemic sclerosis and interstitial lung disease		
Authors	Wanchu A, Suryanaryana BS, Sharma S, Sharma A, Bambery P		
Publication	*Int J Rheum Dis.* 2009 Sep;12(3):239–242		
Follow-up	6 months		
Note		Baseline	6 months
	FVC (liter)	1.73	1.70
	FVC (% of the predicted)	63.26	65.89
	DLCO (% of the predicted)	39.08	41.29
Adverse events	Stopped, because of nausea	n = 1	
	Deterioration on treatment	n = 1	

Scleroderma Lung Study	Adverse events during the Scleroderma Lung Study
Substance	**Cyclophosphamide p. o.** (≤ **2 mg/kg/day,** n = 79)
	Placebo (n =79)
	Prednisone ≤ 10 mg/day
	Treatment was discontinued after 12 months
	Previous medications:
	No oral cyclophosphamide
	No ≥ 2 i. v. cyclophosphamide
	No DMARDs
	Treatment during the second year:
	Finishing year 2: n = 57 (placebo) n = 56 (Cyc)
	Any off study drug n = 14 (placebo) n = 10 (Cyc)
	Prednisone (≥ 10 mg) n = 12 (average dose: 11.6 mg, placebo), *n* = 10 (average dose: 14.0 mg, Cyc)
	Cyclophosphamide n = 2 (average dose: 72.5 mg), n = 0 (Cyc)
	No patients received azathioprine or mycophenolate
Result	Over two years, cyclophosphamide was associated with more adverse events than placebo
Patients	158 patients with scleroderma
	• Restrictive lung physiology
	• Dyspnea (Mahler Dyspnea Index Grade II)
	• FVC 45–85% of the predicted
	• DLCO ≥ 30% of the predicted
	• Non smokers ≥ 6 months
	• Evidence of inflammatory interstitial lung disease:
	• Bronchoalveolar lavage:
	° neutrophilia ≥ 3% and/or
	° eosinophilia of ≥ 2% or
	• HRCT: ground-glass opacity
Authors	Furst DE, Tseng CH, Clements PJ, Strange C, Tashkin DP, Roth MD, Khanna D, Li N, Elashoff R, Schraufnagel DE; Scleroderma Lung Study
Publication	*Am J Med*. 2011 May;124(5):459–467
Follow-up	2 years

(continued) ➜

Adverse events | *First year Adverse events/100 patient years*

	Cyclophosphamide	Placebo
Central nervous system	4.2	4.2
Constitutional	26.4	7.1
Ear, nose, and throat	13.9	4.2
Gastroenterological	29.1	22.7
Genitourinary	27.7	12.7
Hematologic	45.7	2.8
Infectious	18.0	4.2
Musculoskeletal	0	1.4
Neurologic	0	1.4
Psychological	1.4	0
Pulmonary	15.3	9.9
Skin	31.9	14.2
Total	215.9	84.1
Hematuria (year 1)	n = 8	n = 4

Second year Adverse events/100 patient years

	Cyclophosphamide	Placebo
Central nervous system	0	0
Constitutional	0	0
Ear, nose, and throat	0	0
Gastroenterological	4.9	1.6
Genitourinary	3.2	1.6
Hematologic	0	0
Infectious	0	0
Musculoskeletal	1.6	4.9
Neurologic	0	0
Psychological	0	0
Pulmonary	1.6	0
Skin	0	0
Total	14.6	8.1
Haematuria (year 2)	n = 2	n = 3

Serious adverse events (years 1 and 2):

	Cyclophosphamide	Placebo
Serious/possible/probable/ definitely treatment-related	n = 13	n = 8
Serious/unrelated to treatment	n = 34	n = 30
Total serious	n = 47	n = 38
Deaths related	n = 1	n = 1
Deaths unrelated	n = 5	n = 5
Cancer	n = 4	n = 3

Trial	Efficacy and safety of intravenous cyclophosphamide pulse therapy with oral prednisolone in the treatment of interstitial lung disease with systemic sclerosis: 4-year follow-up
Substance	**Cyclophosphamide 0.4 g/m²** i. v. per month for 2–6 months (IVCYC) **Plus prednisolone 0.8 mg/kg,** tapered to 2.5 mg/d daily for 2 weeks, and the dose was then increased to 10 mg/day as a maintenance dose. Patients whose interstitial lung disease improved after the second IVCYC treatment did not receive further IVCYC
Result	Intravenous cyclophosphamide with prednisolone was effective for active alveolitis in the first year
Patients	13 patients with systemic sclerosis and interstitial lung disease • High-resolution computed tomography: • Isolated ground-glass opacities • Honeycombing • Presence of ground-glass attenuation • Traction bronchiectasis and/or bronchiolectasis. *At least one of the following criteria*: 1. Elevation of serum KL-6 levels 2. FVC decrease of more than 10% 3. PaO$_2$ decrease of more than 5 mmHg 4. Increase in the percentage of lymphocytes, neutrophils, and eosinophils in bronchoalveolar lavage (BAL) fluid
Authors	Tochimoto A, Kawaguchi Y, Hara M, Tateishi M, Fukasawa C, Takagi K, Nishimagi E, Ota Y, Katsumata Y, Gono T, Tanaka E, Yamanaka H
Publication	*Mod Rheumatol.* 2011 Jun;21(3):296–301
Follow-up	4 years
Note	*Patient outcome*:

Improved	n = 7
Worsened	n = 5
Withdrawal	n = 1

Follow-up (severity score of ILD):

	Dyspnea	HRCT	%FVC	KL-6	Total
Baseline	1	3	1	1	7
3 months	0.5	2	1	1.5	4
6 months	0	2	1	1	4
12 months	0	2	1	1	4
24 months	0	2	1	1	3.5
36 months	0	2	1	1	3
48 months	0	2	1	1	3

Adverse events	Viral infectious myocarditis	n = 1
	Severe bone marrow suppression	n = 0
	Hemorrhagic cystitis	n = 0

Trial	D-Penicillamine therapy and interstitial lung disease in scleroderma. A long-term follow-up study		
Substance	**D-Penicillamine 750 mg/day** (range 250–1,250 mg/day, n = 17) **Prednisone 12.5 mg/day** (range 7.5–30 mg/day, n = 10) Background therapy: Colchicine n = 2 (D-penicillamine), n = 3 (placebo) NSAIDs if needed		
Result	D-Penicillamine treatment of patients with scleroderma associated interstitial lung disease had a beneficial effect		
Patients	27 scleroderma patients • With progressive disease • Pre-treated with D-Penicillamine for min. 6 months • Minimum 2 lung function measurements before		
Authors	de Clerck LS, Dequeker J, Francx L, Demedts M		
Publication	*Arthritis Rheum.* 1987;30(6):643–650		
Follow-up	Mean 4.7 years (range 0.75–11.0a, D-penicillamine) Mean 4.6 years (range 1.75–6.5a, prednisone)		
Note	*Outcome parameters*:		
		D-Penicillamine	Placebo
	DLCO > 10% lower than the initial value	n = 3	n = 5
	Change of:		
		D-Penicillamine (%)	Placebo (%)
	DLCO/lung volume	+1.2	-14.4
	DLCO	+0.5	-7.9
	TLC	-2.1	+0.2
	FEV1/FVC	-3.3	-0.5

Trial	High-dose vs. low-dose D-Penicillamine in early diffuse systemic sclerosis: analysis of a 2-year, double-blind, randomized, controlled clinical trial
Substance	**High-dose D-penicillamine (750–1,000 mg/day,** n = 66) **Low-dose D-penicillamine (125 mg every other day,** n = 68) *Concomitant medication*: Corticosteroids, ≤ 10 mg of prednisone/day (or equivalent) Safe contraceptive measures *Previous medication*: D-penicillamine, azathioprine, cyclophosphamide, methotrexate, chlorambucil, paraaminobenzoic acid, colchicine, or captopril had to be discontinued ≥ 1 month
Result	The effectivity of high and low-dose D-penicillamine was not different concerning the skin score and the frequencies of scleroderma renal crisis and mortality. High-dose D-penicillamine patients suffered from four times more adverse events leading to withdrawal
Patients	134 patients with systemic sclerosis • Early disease ≥ 18 months • Diffuse cutaneous scleroderma into a 2-year • No other rheumatic disease • No localized scleroderma, serious • No organ involvement: • DLCO < 45% predicted • Serum creatinine 2.0 mg/dL • Proteinuria > 500 mg/24 h • Intractable malabsorption
Authors	Clements PJ, Furst DE, Wong WK, Mayes M, White B, Wigley F, Weisman MH, Barr W, Moreland LW, Medsger TA Jr, Steen V, Martin RW, Collier D, Weinstein A, Lally E, Varga J, Weiner S, Andrews B, Abeles M, Seibold JR
Publication	*Arthritis Rheum.* 1999;42(6):1194–1203
Follow-up	24 months

(continued)

Note	*Outcome parameters*:		
		Low dose D-Penicillamine (%)	High dose D-Penicillamine (%)
	Physician's global assessment: Improved	86	59
	Change of:		
		Low dose D-Penicillamine	High dose D-Penicillamine
	Rodnan Skin Score	-6.7	-4.9
	DLCO (% predicted)	-2.9%	-0.5%
	FVC (% predicted)	+4%	+4.9%
	HAQ Disability Index (0–3.0 scale)	-0.19	-0.13
	Creatinine clearance (mL/min)	-1	-11
	Tender joint count (0–8 joints)	-0.73	-0.29
	CK (% of upper limit of normal)	+9%	+47%
	Left-hand spread (mm)	-4	-9
	Weight (kg)	-0.4	+0.4
	Right-hand spread (mm)	-1	-10
	Left-fist closure (mm)	-5	-4
	Right-fist closure (mm)	-8	-3
	Oral aperture (mm)	+3	+1
	New onset of organ involvement during follow-up (no. affecto/no at risk):		
		Low dose D-Penicillamine	High dose D-Penicillamine
	Lung	5/20	3/13
	Heart	5/33	5/24
	Kidney (chronic)	3/36	2/32
	Muscle	7/34	7/28
	Joint	7/23	8/17
Adverse events		Low dose D-Penicillamine	High dose D-Penicillamine
	Withdrawal because of adverse events	n = 4	n = 16
	Proteinuria (> 1 g)	n = 1	n = 7
	Rash	n = 0	n = 3
	Myasthennia gravis	n = 0	n = 1
	Low platelets	n = 1	n = 2
	Flu symptoms	n = 1	n = 1
	Stomatitis	n = 1	n = 2
	Death	n = 10	n = 5

Trial	Comparison of Methotrexate with placebo in the treatment of systemic sclerosis: a 24-week randomized double-blind trial, followed by a 24-week observational trial
Substance	**Methotrexate 15 mg/week** (increased to 25 mg/week if needed, n = 17) **Placebo** (n = 12) *Concomitant medication*: Corticosteroids ≤10 mg/day NSAIDs analgesics were permitted Nifedipene was permitted Ketanserine was permitted Cimetidine was permitted Omeprazole was permitted at stable doses All ≥ 8 weeks prior trial entry
Result	Low-dose methotrexate was more effective than placebo with regard to skin manifestations and serum creatinine
Patients	29 scleroderma patients • < 3 years from the first rememberable skin thickening • Patients with longer disease duration were also included if they had experienced a progression of skin thickening • Persistent digital ulcerations, or • Deterioration in pulmonary function during the last 6 months
Authors	van den Hoogen FH, Boerbooms AM, Swaak AJ, Rasker JJ, van Lier HJ, van de Putte LB
Publication	*Br J Rheumatol.* 1996;35(4):364–372
Follow-up	48 weeks

(continued)

Note	New organ involvement:		
		MTX	Placebo
	Cardiac involvement	n = 4	n = 3
	Creatinine clearance rate (mL/min)	+4.0	−3.0
	Esophageal	n = 13	n = 8
	Lung Fibrosis	n = 5	n = 4
	Change of:		
		MTX	Placebo
	Total skin score	-0.7	+1.2
	Extension index right (mm)	-2.1	-1.2
	Extension index left (mm)	-0.8	0.3
	Grip strength right (mmHg)	18.8	12.9
	Grip strength left (mmHg)	-0.5	-2.8
	Oral opening (mm)	-0.7	-0.2
	General health (0–100 mm VAS)	4.5	-1.0
	TLC (% predicted)	-1.1	-0.5
	VC (% predicted)	-2.7	-1.7
	DLCO	-0.03	-0.01
	ESR (Westergren, mm/h)	-0.71	+2.2
Adverse events		MTX	Placebo
	Progression of cardiopulmonary, gastrointestinal, and nephrological manifestations	n = 0	n = 1
	Renal failure due to scleroderma renal crisis	n = 2	n = 1
	Severe headache	n = 2	n = 0
	Death of cardiorespiratory	n = 1	n = 0
	Myocardial infarction	n = 1	n = 0
	Pancytopenia	n = 1	n = 0
	Liver enzyme abnormalities	n = 6	n = 0

Trial	A randomized, controlled trial of methotrexate versus placebo in early diffuse scleroderma
Substance	**Methotrexate 10 mg/week** (MTX, n = 35) Dosage was increased to a max. 15 mg/week in steps of 2.5 mg every 4 weeks **Placebo** (n = 36) *Concomitant medication*: Appropriate birth control Prednisone at 15 mg/day or equivalent stable within the last 2 months *Previous medication*: No current or past use of MTX No immunosuppressive therapy currently or within the last 3 months
Result	Treatment of early diffuse systemic sclerosis with methotrexate was only tendentially superior to placebo
Patients	71 patients with diffuse systemic sclerosis • Disease duration < 3 years • UCLA skin score ≥ 5 (maximum possible score = 30) • No overlap syndrome • No mixed connective tissue disease • No morphea, or linear scleroderma • No AST or bilirubin level > 2 times the upper limit of normal • No insulin-dependent diabetes mellitus • No uncontrolled hypertension or severe congestive heart failure • Forced expiratory volume in 1 s ≥ 40% • DLCO ≥ 40%
Authors	Pope JE, Bellamy N, Seibold JR, Baron M, Ellman M, Carette S, Smith CD, Chalmers IM, Hong P, O'Hanlon D, Kaminska E, Markland J, Sibley J, Catoggio L, Furst DE
Publication	*Arthritis Rheum.* 2001;44(6):1351–1358
Follow-up	12 months

(continued)

Note	*Outcome parameters*:		
		MTX	Placebo
	Oral opening (mm)	38.7	35.1
	HAQ pain (0–3)	1.1	1.0
	HAQ disability (0–3)	1.2	1.2
	Functional index (0–33)	8.3	7.5
	Grip strength right (mmHg)	160	146
	Grip strength left (mmHg)	156	142
	Flexion index right (mm)	68	84
	Flexion index (mm)	65	82
	DLCO (% predicted)	75.7	61.8
	Patient global assessment (VAS 10-cm)	4.2	4.3
	Change of (all patients):		
		MTX	Placebo
	UCLA Skin Score	-2.1	-0.3
	Rodnan skin score	-6.3	-1.1
	Physician's global assessment	-0.9	-0.3
	Change of (intent to treat analysis):		
		MTX	Placebo
	UCLA Skin Score	-1.3	-0.7
	Rodnan skin score	-4.1	-1.1
	Physician's global assessment	-0.2	-0.2
	Patient global assessment (VAS 10-cm)	0.0	-0.4
	DLCO (% predicted)	-3.7	-7.7

Trial	Methotrexate treatment in juvenile localized scleroderma: A randomized, double-blind, placebo-controlled trial
Substance	**Methotrexate 15 mg/m²/week** (n = 46), maximum 20 mg **Placebo** (n = 24) *Concomitant medication*: Prednisone (1 mg/kg/day, maximum 50 mg) tapered during the first 3 month
Result	Methotrexate was efficacious in the treatment of skin manifestations of juvenile localized scleroderma and was well-tolerated
Patients	70 patients with active juvenile localized scleroderma • Linear, generalized, or mixed subtype • No leukopenia < 3.0 × 10⁹/L • No thrombocytopenia • No < 100 × 10⁹/L, liver • No transaminase > 2 x the upper limit of normal • No creatinine clearance > 90 mL/min/1.73 m²
Authors	Zulian F, Martini G, Vallongo C, Vittadello F, Falcini F, Patrizi A, Alessio M, Torre FL, Podda RA, Gerloni V, Cutrone M, Belloni-Fortina A, Paradisi M, Martino S, Perilongo G
Publication	*Arthritis Rheum.* 2011 Jul;63(7):1998–2006
Follow-up	12 months

Note	Outcome parameters:	MTX	Placebo
	Completed study	67.4%	29.2%
	Relapse after initial	32.6%	70.8%
	New lesions	6.5%	16.7%
	Skin score rate (mean)	-0.21	+0.1
	Target lesion temperature	-44.4%	12.1%
	Skin Score Rate (mean)	+0.79	+1.1
	No. (%) of patients with new lesions	6.5%	16.7%

Adverse events		MTX	Placebo
	Mild side effects	56.5%	45.8%
	Patients with serious adverse events	n = 0	n = 0
	Patients with adverse events	56.5%	45.8%
	Alopecia	4.3%	0%
	Nausea	17.4%	0%
	Headache	10.9%	0%
	Fatigue	4.3%	0%
	Hepatotoxicity	6.5%	0%
	Weight gain (> 5% of body weight)	10.9%	41.7%
	Striae rubrae	8.7%	4.2%

Trial	A pilot study of Mycophenolate mofetil combined to intravenous methylprednisolone pulses and oral low-dose Glucocorticoids in severe early systemic sclerosis
Substance	**3 consecutive daily i. v. methylprednisolone pulses at 15 mg/kg Followed by five additional monthly i. v. methylprednisolone pulses 15 mg/kg** **Mycophenolate mofetil** (2 × 0.5 g/day for 1 week; then 2 × 1 g/day) Oral **prednisolone (5–10 mg/day)** *Concomitant medication*: ACE inhibitors in case of hypertension No other DMARDs *Previous medication*: Glucosteroids 25% Methotrexate 7% ACE inhibitors 14%
Result	The combination of mycophenolate mofetil, intravenous methylprednisolone and low-dose glucocorticoids achieved good clinical, functional, and radiological results in patients with severe early systemic sclerosis
Patients	16 patients with systemic sclerosis • Modified Rodnan total skin score ≥ 15 n = 9 • Active interstitial lung disease n = 7 • DLCO ≤ 75% of the predicted • Plus ground glass opacity on HRCT • Disease duration < 3a (first non-Raynaud manifestation) • Total skin score ≥ 15 • No scleroderma associated renal crisis Noserum creatinine ≥ 2 mg/dL • No vital capacity ≤ 50% • No left ventricular ejection fraction ≤ 40% • No DLCO ≤ 70% *Or bronchoalveolar lavage*: • ≥ 15% lymphocytes • ≥ 3% eosinophiles • ≥ 1% eosinophiles
Authors	Vanthuyne M, Blockmans D, Westhovens R, Roufosse F, Cogan E, Coche E, Nzeusseu Toukap A, Depresseux G, Houssiau FA
Publication	*Clin Exp Rheumatol.* 2007;25(2):287–292
Follow-up	12 months

(continued) ➔

Note	*Outcome parameters (all patients)*:	
	Total skin score responders	69%
	Responders of HAQ	50%
	Outcome parameters (interstitial lung's disease patients):	
	DLCO responders	71%
	FEV responders	86%
	VC responders	83%
	6-min walking distance responders	14%
	Ground glass appearance	-1.43
	Change of (all patients):	
	Total skin score	-7
	HAQ	-0.5
	SHAQ (VAS 1, Raynaud)	-10
	SHAQ (VAS 2, finger ulcers)	-6
	SHAQ (VAS 3, gastrointestinal)	-6
	SHAQ (VAS 4, lung)	-3
	SHAQ (VAS 5, overall)	-16
	SHAQ (VAS 6, pain)	-18
	CRP (mg/dL)	-1.5
	Change of (interstitial lung's disease patients):	
	VC (mL)	+345, +10% of the predicted
	FEV 1	+376 mL, +14% of the predicted
	DLCO	+13% of the predicted
	6-min walking distance (M)	+61
	Change of (skin patients):	
	Total skin score	−8
Adverse events	Enterocolitis	n = 1
	Varicella zoster virus	n = 1
	Bronchitis	n = 4
	Diarrhea	n = 4
	Nausea	n = 1
	Vertigo	n = 1
	Renal crisis	n = 0
	Hypertension	n = 4

Trial	5-fluorouracil in the treatment of scleroderma: a randomized, double-blind, placebo-controlled international collaborative study
Substance	**5-Fluorouracil 12 mg/kg/day** for 4 doses (max. 1'000 mg/day, n = 26) Followed by 4 × 6 mg/kg (≤ 800 mg/day) every 2 days **Placebo** (n = 20) *Concomitant medication:* Corticosteroids for inflammatory conditions (myositis, pericarditis) *Previous medication:* No D-penicillamine for 6 months No colchicine
Result	There was a modest benefit of 5 fluorouracil, but no improvement of visceral functions, in this open trial of patients with scleroderma
Patients	70 patients with limited systemic sclerosis • With evidence of visceral disease or digital ulcerations
Authors	Casas JA, Saway PA, Villarreal I, Nolte C, Menajovsky BL, Escudero EE, Blackburn WD, Alarcón GS, Subauste CP
Publication	*Ann Rheum Dis.* 1990;49(11):926–928
Follow-up	6 months

Note *Change of:*

	Placebo	5-FU
Total skin score	-1.7	-5.8
Skin weight (g)	-0.7	-3.7
Oral opening (mm)	-1.4	-0.2
Flexion index (mm)	-2.2	-0.7
Extension index (mm)	-0.65	-2.2
Functional score	-3.3	-2.1
Global assessment	0.9	1.52
Raynaud's score	0.0	-0.44
Ulcer (number)	0.25	-0.1
Esophageal involvement (score)	-0.1	0.0
Lung involvement (score)	0.2	-0.2
Heart involvement (score)	0.15	-0.23
Muscle involvement (score)	0.0	0.04

Adverse events

	Placebo (%)	5-FU (%)
Hemocytopenia	5	46
Leukopenia	5	42
Thrombocytopenia	0	4
Gastrointestinal symptoms	40	96
Angina pectoris	0	4
Pruritus	0	4
Total (patients)	50	96

Trial	Efficacy and safety of Etanercept in the treatment of scleroderma-associated joint disease
Substance	**Etanercept 50 mg/week** or Or **etanercept 2 × 25 mg/week** *Concomitant medication*: NSAIDs n = 18 MTX (dose range 2.5–25 mg/week) n = 15 Hydroxychloroquine n = 5 Prednisone (dose range 0.5–15 mg/day) n = 9 Minocycline n = 2
Result	Etanercept was effective in this retrospective analysis of patients with scleroderma associated synovitic disease
Patients	12 patients with limited systemic sclerosis • 6 patients with systemic sclerosis • All with inflammatory joint involvement
Authors	Lam GK, Hummers LK, Woods A, Wigley FM
Publication	*J Rheumatol.* 2007;34(7):1636–1637
Follow-up	Treatment duration 2–66 months
Note	*Outcome parameters*:	
	Positive result and decreasing synovitis	n = 15
	Sustained remission	n = 1
	Change of:	
	HAQ	-0.34
	Skin score	-2.69
	DLCO	-5.1%
	FVC	-1.4%
Adverse events	Opportunistic infections	n = 0
	Lupus like syndrome	n = 1

Trial	Rituximab in diffuse cutaneous systemic sclerosis: an open-label clinical and histopathological study
Substance	Rituximab 2 × 1´000 mg i. v. on day 0 and day 15 *Concomitant medication*: Low-dose prednisolone ≤ 10 mg/day at stable dose for ≥ 12 weeks Disease-modifying antirheumatic drugs (except methotrexate) stopped ≥ 12 weeks Methotrexate 15 mg/week was continued
Result	Rituximab was well-tolerated and seemed to have some efficacy for skin disease in diffuse cutaneous systemic sclerosis
Patients	8 patients with diffuse cutaneous systemic sclerosis • Disease duration ≤ 4 years • Modified Rodnan skin score ≥ 14 • Disease activity score ≥ 3 • FVC > 50% • DLCO > 40% • Left ventricular ejection fraction > 40%
Authors	Smith VP, Van Praet JT, Vandooren BR, Vander Cruyssen B, Naeyaert JM, Decuman S, Elewaut D, de Keyser F
Publication	*Ann Rheum Dis.* 2010;69(1):193–197
Follow-up	24 weeks

(continued)

Note	*Outcome parameters (histology):*			
		Baseline	After treatment, week 12	Normal reference
	Hyalinized collagen score	60	28	7.1
	Myofibroblast positivity	4/7	2/7	0/8
	Change of:			
	Total skin score	-10.5		
	DLCO (% of normal)	-0.3		
	Lung vital capacity (% of normal)	-4.5		
	Forced expiratory volume (% of normal)	-6.9		
	Systolic pulmonary artery pressure (mmHg)	-1.0		
	Left ventricular ejection fraction (% of normal)	-2.6		
	Creatinine clearance (mL/min per 1.73 m^2)	+8.8		
	Total SF-36	+9.9		
	HAQ-DI	-0.1		
	Disease activity score	-3.4		
Adverse events	Coronary artery bypass surgery	n = 1		
	Low grade fever occurring 2 weeks after the second infusion	n = 1		
	Infectious exacerbation of existing polyposis nasi	n = 1		
	Initiation of antihypertensive therapy	n = 1		
	Nausea and of depressive mood	n = 1		

Trial	B cell depletion with Rituximab in patients with diffuse cutaneous systemic sclerosis	
Substance	**Rituximab 2 × 1´000 mg** i. v., administered 2 weeks apart *Concomitant medication*: No immunosuppressive drugs (methotrexate n = 1 later in the study) Prednisone ≤ 10 mg/day No premedication *Infusion reactions*: Corticosteroids Acetaminophen Diphenhydramine	
Result	Rituximab treatment had little effect on the levels of systemic sclerosis-associated autoantibodies and no significant beneficial effect on skin disease. Treatment was safe and well-tolerated	
Patients	15 patients with diffuse cutaneous systemic sclerosis • First non-Raynaud's disease manifestation within 18 months of trial entry • DLCO > 50% of the predicted • FVC > 50% of the predicted • No significant cardiac arrhythmia • Ejection fraction > 40%	
Authors	Lafyatis R, Kissin E, York M, Farina G, Viger K, Fritzler MJ, Merkel PA, Simms RW	
Publication	*Arthritis Rheum.* 2009;60(2):578–583	
Follow-up	12 months	
Note	*Change of*:	
	Modified Rodnan skin thickness score	+0.5
	Forced vital capacity (% of predicted, 6 months)	+3.5
	DLCO (% of predicted, 6 months)	-1.9
	HAQ disability index	-0.12
	Visual analogue scale	-0.17
	Sedimentation rate (mm/h)	-10.9
	IgM (units/mL)	-21
	IgG (units/mL)	-0.85
	IgA (units/mL)	+4
Adverse events	Frequent infusion reactions	n = 7
	Mild hypotension	n = 2
	Urinary tract infection	n = 1
	Dental abscess	n = 1
	Flushing	n = 1
	Fatigue	n = 1
	Nausea/abdominal cramping	n = 1
	Rigors	n = 1
	Hand tingling	n = 1

Trial	Experience with rituximab in scleroderma: results from a 1-year, proof-of-principle study		
Substance	**Rituximab 1 cycle with 4 weekly 375 mg/m^2 infusions** at baseline and 1 additional cycle at 24 weeks (n = 8) **Placebo** (n = 6) *Previous medication*: No medications and/or dosage of treatment ≤ 12 months		
Result	Lung function improved with rituximab treatment		
Patients	14 patients with systemic sclerosis (SSc) • Positive for anti-Scl-70 • Presence of SSc-associated interstitial lung disease by HRCT of the chest or pulmonary function tests		
Authors	Daoussis D, Liossis SN, Tsamandas AC, Kalogeropoulou C, Kazantzi A, Sirinian C, Karampetsou M, Yiannopoulos G, Andonopoulos AP		
Publication	*Rheumatology (Oxford)*. 2010 Feb;49(2):271–280		
Follow-up	1 year		
Note	*Change after 1 year:*		
		RTX	Placebo
	Forced vital capacity (% median improvement)	10.25%	-5.04%
	Diffusing capacity of carbon monoxide (% median improvement)	19.46%	-7.5%
	Modified Rodnan Skin Score (% median improvement)	32.25%	20.28%
	HAQ (absolute change)	-0.375	-0.187
Adverse events	Respiratory tract infection n = 1 (RTX)		

Trial	Treatment of progressive systemic sclerosis by plasma exchange: long-term results in 40 patients
Substance	**Plasma exchange 30.7 sessions** (range 1–110)
	Centrifugation or filtration
	Replacement solution:
	Beginning 500 mL gelantine
	4% albumine 70% of the patients
	Fresh frozen plasma 5% of the patients
	Mixture albumine—fresh frozen plasma 25% of the patients
	Exchange volume 2.8 l (range 0.3–4.6 L)
	0.5–1 mg/kg prenisone with exchange n = 21
	2 mg/kg cyclophosphamide n = 9
	Chloraminophen n = 2
	Previous medication:
	Colchicine n = 12
	Antimalarial drugs n = 9
	D-Penicillamine n = 9
	Factor XIII n = 11
	Corticosteroids n = 19
	Cyclophosphamide n = 5
	Nitrated derivates n = 1
	Nifedipine n = 9
	Captopril n = 4
	Surgical sympathectomy n = 3
	Concomitant medication:
	Colchicine n = 4
	Antimalarial drugs n = 5
	D-Penicillamine n = 0
	Factor XIII n = 1
	Corticosteroids n = 21
	Cyclophosphamide n = 9
	Nitrated derivates n = 0
	Nifedipine n = 3
	Captopril n = 1
	Surgical sympathectomy n = 0
Result	Plasma exchange was effective in half of the patients with progressive systemic sclerosis but the effect was only short-lived

(continued) ➔

Patients	40 patients with scleroderma			
	Indication for plasma exchange:			
	• Necrosis of the limb	n = 9		
	• Lung involvement	n = 9		
	• Raynaud's syndrome	n = 5		
	• Joint involvement	n = 5		
	• Cardiac involvement	n = 4		
	• Sicca syndrome	n = 3		
	• Renal involvement	n = 1		
	• Retinal vasculitis	n = 1		
	• Malabsorption	n = 1		
Authors	Guillevin L, Amoura Z, Merviel P, Pourrat J, Bussel A, Sobel A, Khuy T, Houssin A, Alcalay D, Stroumza P et al.			
Publication	*Int J Artif Organs*. 1990;13(2):125–129			
Follow-up	14 years			
Note	*Positive effect on*:			
		3 months	12 months	> 12 months
	Scleroderma	8/13	2/13	1/11
	Necrosis of limbs	4/9	0/9	0/9
	Lung involvement	4/9	0/9	0/9
	Raynaud's phenomenon	3/5	0/5	0/9
	Joint involvement	4/5	0/5	1/5
	Cardiac involvement	2/4	0/4	0/4
	Sicca syndrome	0/3	0/3	0/3
	Retinal vasculitis	0/1	0/1	0/1
	Renal involvement	0/1	0/1	0/1
	Malabsorption	1/1	0/1	0/1
Adverse events	Venous thrombosis	n = 3		
	Vagal neuralgia/syncope	n = 12		
	Fever	n = 5		
	Allergic reactions	n = 4		
	Aggravated skin lesions	n = 3		

Trial	Phase I/II trial of autologous stem cell transplantation in systemic sclerosis: procedure related mortality and impact on skin disease
Substance	*Priming* (n = 40): Cyclophosphamide 4 g/m² + G-CSF (n = 29), cyclophosphamide alone (n = 1) G-CSF alone (n = 10) *Conditioning* (n = 37): Cyclophosphamide 150–200 mg/kg (n = 19) Cyclophosphamide 120 mg/kg + antithymocyte globulin +8 Gy total body iradiationl (n = 9) Cyclophosphamide 200 mg/kg + antithymocyte globulin (n = 4) Cyclophosphamide 200 mg/kg + CAMPATH-1 (n = 2) Cyclophosphamide 200 mg/kg + total lymphoid irradiation (n = 1) Other chemotherapy (n = 2) busulfan, cyclophosphamide with antithymocyte globulin; carmustine, fludarabine, and thiotepa
Result	Stem cell transplantation in systemic sclerosis had a marked impact on skin score and a trend toward stabilization of lung involvement. A higher procedure related mortality rate compared with patients with breast cancer and non-Hodgkin's lymphoma was observed
Patients	41 patients with systemic sclerosis • Predominantly diffuse skin disease • Limited disease n = 4 • Clinical overlap • Disease duration > 3 years • A high risk of further progression and mortality • Absence of severe irreversible internal organ damage • Patients with limited scleroderma with no life threatening pulmonary fibrosis or pulmonary hypertension *Organ involvement of patients*: • Lung 76% • Pulmonary hypertension 19% • Arterial hypertension 8% • Raynaud's phenomenon 93% • Renal 14% • Esophageal 58% • Gastrointestinal 11%
Authors	Binks M, Passweg JR, Furst D, McSweeney P, Sullivan K, Besenthal C, Finke J, Peter HH, van Laar J, Breedveld FC, Fibbe WE, Farge D, Gluckman E, Locatelli F, Martini A, van den Hoogen F, van de Putte L, Schattenberg AV, Arnold R, Bacon PA, Emery P, Espigado I, Hertenstein B, Hiepe F, Kashyap A, Kötter I, Marmont A, Martinez A, Pascual MJ, Gratwohl A, Prentice HG, Black C, Tyndall A
Publication	*Ann Rheum Dis.* 2001;60(6):577–584
Follow-up	4 years

(continued) ➔

Note	Skin score improvement > 25% (compared to baseline)	69%
	Skin score deterioration	7%
	VC improved (> 15%)	16%
	VC deteriorated (> 15%)	24%
	DLCO improved (> 15%)	9%
	DLCO deteriorated (> 15%)	39%
	Serum creatinine increase	57%
	Death	27% (total)
		17% (related to the procedure)
	Direct organ toxicity	$n = 4$
	Hemorrhage	n = 2
	Infection/neutropenic fever	n = 1
Reasons of death and survival time	Day 0	Sudden cardiac death
	Day 0	Neutropenic fever, pneumonia
	Day 0	Thrombopenia, pulmonary hemorrhagia
	Day 0	Disease progression
	Day 11	Diffuse alveolar hemorrhage
	Day 28	Interstitial Pneumonitis
	Day 40	Central nervous system bleeding
	Day 79	Interstitial pneumonitis
	Day 217	Pulmonary hypertension
	Day 242	Disease progression
	Day 527	Superior vena cava obstruction

Trial	High-dose immunosuppressive therapy and autologous hematopoietic cell transplantation for severe systemic sclerosis: long-term follow-up of the US multicenter pilot study
Substance	*Mobilization*:
	G-CSF 16 mcμ/kg/day s. c. to mobilized peripheral blood stem cells
	First apheresis day 4
	CD34-selection using a Isolex 300i device (Baxter, Irvine, CA)
	Autologous HC grafts were stored for treating engraftment failure or severe immunodeficiency after transplantation
	Induction therapy:
	Fractionated total body irradiation 800 cGy
	Cyclophosphamide 120 mg/kg
	Equine antithymocyte globulin 90 mg/kg
	Methylprednisolone 1 mg/kg i. v. together with ATG
	Prednisone 0.5 mg/kg/day on the start of conditioning to day 30 after hematopoietic cell transplantation
	Tapered over 1 month
	Graft transmission:
	CD34-selected autologous graft was infused
	5 mcg/kg/day G-CSF day 0 until neutrophil count $\geq 0.5 \times 10^9$/L for 3 days
	Infection prophylaxis:
	Trimethoprimsul
	Famethoxazole
	Acyclovir
	Fluconazole
Result	High-dose immunosuppressive therapy and autologous hematopoietic cell transplantation lead to a major reduction of the dermal fibrosis
Patients	34 patients with diffuse cutaneous systemic sclerosis
	• Disease duration ≤ 4 years
	• Modified Rodnan skin score ≥ 16
	• Significant visceral organ involvement
	• Decrease of DLCO $\geq 15\%$ 0 within 6 months
	• Decrease of FVC $\geq 15\%$ within 6 months
Authors	Nash RA, McSweeney PA, Crofford LJ, Abidi M, Chen CS, Godwin JD, Gooley TA, Holmberg L, Henstorf G, LeMaistre CF, Mayes MD, McDonagh KT, McLaughlin B, Molitor JA, Nelson JL, Shulman H, Storb R, Viganego F, Wener MH, Seibold JR, Sullivan KM, Furst DE
Publication	*Blood*. 2007;110(4):1388–1396
Follow-up	Max 5–8 years

(continued) ➔

Note	Outcome parameters:	
	Survival first year	n = 27
	(*final evaluation*):	
	mRSS	-22.08
	mHAQ	-1.03
	Dermal fibrosis rate	-3.1
	DLCO	-6.04%
	FVC	+2.11%
	Creatinine (mg/dL)	+0.25
	Ejection fraction	-2.37%
Adverse events	Fatal pulmonary toxicity	n = 2
	Renal crisis	n = 6
	Dialysis required	n = 2
	Supraventricular arrhythmia	n = 2
	Heart failure	n = 2
	Hypothyroidism	n = 1
	Myelodysplastic syndrome	n = 1
	Death	n = 12
	Treatment related	n = 8
	Disease related	n = 4
	EBV	3.7%
	HSV	11.1%
	CMV	25.9%
	VZV	22.2%
	BK Virus	3.7%
	Bacteremia	40.7%
	Urinary tract infections	11.1%
	Osteomyelitis	3.7%
	Cellulitis	3.7%
	Aspiration pneumonia	3.7%
	Aspergillus flavus	3.7%

ASSIST-Trial	Autologous nonmyeloablative hemopoietic stem cell transplantation compared with pulse cyclophosphamide once per month for systemic sclerosis (ASSIST): an open-label, randomized phase 2 trial ASSIST: American Scleroderma Stem cell versus Immune Suppression Trial
Substance	**Haemopoietic stem cell transplantation** group (HSCT, n = 10): *Mobilization*: I. v. cyclophosphamide (CYC, 2 g/m²) Plus 10 µg/kg subcutaneous filgrastim from day 5 after cyclophosphamide administration until apheresis *Conditioning regimen*: 200 mg/kg intravenous cyclophosphamide given in 4 equal fractions on day −5 to −2 Plus intravenous mesna 0.5 mg/kg i. v. rabbit antithymocyte globulin on day −5 1.5 mg/kg i. v. rabbit antithymocyte globulin on day −4 to −1 Plus methylprednisolone 1´000 mg on day −5 to −1 *Concomitant medication*: Oral lisinopril (2·5–10·0 mg per day) Subcutaneous filgrastim 10 µg/kg per Intravenous piperacillin-tazobactam or cefepime, and oral or intravenous aciclovir and fluconazole until d 12 after engraftment Trimethoprim-sulfamethoxazole 3x/week or Nebulized pentamidine inhaled 1x/month *Control group* (n = 9): Six cycles of intravenous cyclophosphamide (1.0 g/m² per month). *Previous medication*: ≤ 6 previous i. v. cyclophosphamide Total lung capacity ≤ 45% of predicted volume Left ventricular ejection fraction ≤ 40% Symptomatic cardiac disease
Result	Non-myeloablative autologous hemopoietic stem cell transplantation improved skin and pulmonary function for up to 2 years
Patients	Patients • ≤ 60 years with diffuse systemic sclerosis • mRSS ≥ 14 *Internal-organ involvement*: • DLCO ≤ 80% • Decline in FVC ≥ 10% in the previous 12 months • Pulmonary fibrosis or ground-glass appearance on high-resolution chest CT • Abnormal ECG • Gastrointestinal tract involvement
Authors	Burt RK, Shah SJ, Dill K, Grant T, Gheorghiade M, Schroeder J, Craig R, Hirano I, Marshall K, Ruderman E, Jovanovic B, Milanetti F, Jain S, Boyce K, Morgan A, Carr J, Barr W.
Publication	*Lancet.* 2011 Aug 6;378(9790):498–506
Follow-up	2 years

(continued)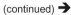

Note	*Change of:*				
		CYC 1 year	HCCT 1 year	6 months after switch to transplant	6 months after switch to transplant
	Predicted forced vital capacity (%)	-6%	+12%	+13%	+12%
	Predicted total lung capacity (%)	-9%	+4%	+6%	+5%
	Predicted DLCO corrected for hemoglobin (%)	-1%	+11%	0%	-4%
	Volume diseased lung (mL)	+98	-272	-243	-341
	Modified Rodnan skin score	+3	-13	-14	-17
	Quality of life				
		CYC 1 year	HCCT 1 year	6 months after switch to transplant	HRCT longest follow-up
	Quality of life, physical function	+7	+32	+36	+30
	Quality of life, physical role limitation	+7	+27	+50	+27
	Quality of life, body pain	-6	+21	+29	+27
	Quality of life, general heath perception	-23	+6	+59	+8
	Quality of life, vitality energy fatigue	+2	+13	+26	+15
	Quality of life, social function	-12	+22	+50	+24
	Quality of life, emotional role limitation	-41	+8	+34	+8
	Quality of life, mental health	+5	+9	+10	+2
	Quality of life, physical health	-6	+20	+40	+21
	Quality of life, mental health	-14	+12	+36	+12
	SF 36	-10	+17	+36	+17
Adverse events		CYC 1 year	HCCT 1 year		
	Cellulitis	n = 1	n = 0		
	Clostridium difficile	n = 0	n = 1		
	Micrococcus	n = 0	n = 1		
	Arrhythmias	n = 0	n = 2		
	Cytomegalovirus	n = 0	n = 1		

Raynaud's Phenomenon

Bosentan

Trial	Effect of the dual endothelin receptor antagonist bosentan on Raynaud's phenomenon secondary to systemic sclerosis: a double-blind prospective, randomized, placebo-controlled pilot study
Substance	**Bosentan 2 × 62.5 mg/day** for 4 weeks Followed by bosentan/day 2 × 125 mg/day for 12 weeks (n = 9) **Placebo** (n = 8) *Concomitant medication*: Vasodilator drugs for arterial hypertension were permitted Hand warmers or electric gloves were permitted No topical treatment with glyceryl nitrate *Previous medication*: No prostanoids ≤ 3 months No bosentan or other endothelin receptor blockers, phosphodiesterase-V-inhibitors No paraffin wax hand baths ≤ 4 weeks
Result	Bosentan was not effective for symptoms of secondary Raynaud's syndrome without pre-existing digital ulcers, but showed functional benefit in those patients
Patients	17 patients with Raynaud's phenomenon secondary to systemic sclerosis as defined by the ACR classification criteria, without preexisting active digital ulcers • Abnormal capillaries of the fingernail fold • ≥ 3 painful Raynaud's phenomenon attacks/week • No active digital ulcer or gangrene, abnormal hemostasis, platelet alterations and evidence of uncontrolled cardiovascular, pulmonary, hepatic or renal disease
Authors	Nguyen VA, Eisendle K, Gruber I, Hugl B, Reider D, Reider N
Publication	*Rheumatology (Oxford)*. 2010 Mar;49(3):583–587
Follow-up	16 weeks

(continued) ➜

R. Müller, J. von Kempis, *Clinical Trials in Rheumatology*,
DOI 10.1007/978-1-4471-2870-0_7, © Springer-Verlag London 2013

	Change at week 16:		
Note		Bosentan (%)	Placebo (%)
	Raynaud condition score	-31	-36
	Raynaud's phenomenon pain	+531	-27
	Raynaud's phenomenon attacks	-30	-57
	HAQ-DI	-39	+51
	United Kingdom functional score	-5	-35
Adverse events	Peripheral edema	n = 1	

Trial	Bosentan treatment of digital ulcers related to systemic sclerosis: results from the RAPIDS-2 randomized, double-blind, placebo-controlled trial
Substance	**Bosentan 2 × 62.5 mg/day** for 4 weeks Bosentan 2 × 125 mg/day (n = 98) **Placebo** (n = 90; total 24 weeks) *Concomitant medication*: Contraception was obligatory Systemic antibiotics Analgesics Topical treatments for wound care No required parenteral, oral or inhaled prostanoid *Previous medication*: No intravenous prostanoids ≤ 3 months No phosphodiesterase inhibitors
Result	Bosentan treatment was well-tolerated and reduced the occurrence of new digital ulcers but had no effect on their healing
Patients	188 patients with systemic sclerosis as defined by the preliminary ACR classification criteria • With at least 1 active digital ulcer ("cardinal ulcer" ≥ 2 mm with visible depth and loss of dermis)
Authors	Matucci-Cerinic M, Denton CP, Furst DE, Mayes MD, Hsu VM, Carpentier P, Wigley FM, Black CM, Fessler BJ, Merkel PA, Pope JE, Sweiss NJ, Doyle MK, Hellmich B, Medsger TA Jr, Morganti A, Kramer F, Korn JH, Seibold JR
Publication	*Ann Rheum Dis.* 2011 Jan;70(1):32–38
Follow-up	24 weeks
Note	No difference between bosentan and placebo treatments in the time to healing of the cardinal ulcer at 24 weeks

At week 12:

	Bosentan	Placebo
New digital ulcers	0.8	1.3

At week 24:

	Bosentan	Placebo
New digital ulcers	1.9	2.7
No new digital ulcer	33.7%	29.2%
One or more new digital ulcer	66.3%	70.8%
Max number of new digital ulcers	n = 10	n = 16
Healing of all digital ulcers	36.8%	39.3%
Patient-rated measures of overall hand pain	-1.7	-1.6

(continued)

Adverse events		Bosentan (%)	Placebo (%)
	All patients with ≥ 1 adverse event	86.5	84.4
	Peripheral edema	18.8	4.4
	Elevated aminotransferases	12.5	2.2
	Arthralgia	10.4	6.7
	Headache	9.4	12.2
	Infected skin ulcer	9.4	6.7
	Upper respiratory tract infection	8.3	7.8
	Diarrhea	6.3	8.9
	Pain in extremities	6.3	4.4
	Nausea	5.2	12.2
	Skin ulcer/disease progression	5.2	7.8
	Urinary tract infection	5.2	3.3
	Dermatitis	5.2	2.2
	Other	81.3	77.8
	All patients with ≥ 1 serious adverse event	9.4	16.7

Trial	A randomized double-blind trial of Diltiazem in the treatment of Raynaud's phenomenon	
Substance	*1 week placebo prior to randomization*: **Diltiazem 3 × 120 mg/day** **Placebo** *Crossover after 2 weeks* No information on concomitant medication and precise numbers in each group	
Result	Diltiazem in the treatment of Raynaud's phenomenon was effective, especially in patients with idiopathic vasospastic disease	
Patients	16 patients with Raynaud's phenomenon • Progressive systemic sclerosis n = 7 • Rheumatoid arthritis n = 2 • Systemic lupus erythematosus n = 1 • Idiopathic Raynaud's phenomenon n = 6	
Authors	Kahan A, Amor B, Menkes CJ	
Publication	*Ann Rheum Dis.* 1985;44(1):30–33	
Follow-up	4 weeks	
Note	*Outcome parameters*:	

	Diltiazem	Placebo
Marked or moderate improvement	n = 9	n = 3

Frequency of attacks/2 weeks:

	Diltiazem	Placebo
All patients	12.6	18.9
Idiopathic Raynaud's phenomenon patients	8.5	16.3
PSS+RA+SLE patients	15.1	20.4

Severity of attacks (VAS 0–10):

	Diltiazem	Placebo
All patients	4.2	6.2
Idiopathic Raynaud's phenomenon patients	2.6	5.4
PSS+RA+SLE patients	5.1	6.6

Adverse events	Diltiazem	Placebo
Headache	n = 2	n = 0
Flushing	n = 2	n = 0
Dizziness	n = 1	n = 0
Nausea	n = 2	n = 1
Ankle edema	n = 1	n = 0
Light-headedness	n = 0	n = 1

Trial	A double-blind placebo-controlled crossover randomized trial of Diltiazem in Raynaud's phenomenon				
Substance	**Diltiazem 3 × 60 mg/day** **Placebo** No information on the concomitant medication Initial basal line observation 4 weeks study first phase 4 weeks crossover				
Result	Diltiazem was effective the treatment of intermittent digital vasospasm				
Patients	30 patients with bilateral Raynaud's phenomenon • Secondary disease n = 9 • Systemic sclerosis n = 4 • Mixed connective tissue disease n = 4 • SLE n = 2				
Authors	Rhedda A, McCans J, Willan AR, Ford PM				
Publication	*J Rheumatol.* 1985;12(4):724–727				
Follow-up	10 weeks				
Note	Drop out	n = 8			

Change of:

	Placebo first	After change to diltiazem	Diltiazem first	After change to placebo
Frequency of attacks (attacks/month)	-4.6	-22.9	-12.0	0.0
Duration of attacks (min/month)	-159.7	-443.6	-230.8	+27.7

Adverse events		Diltiazem	Placebo
	Headache	n = 1	n = 0
	Rash	n = 1	n = 0

Trial	Inefficacy of Diltiazem in the treatment of Raynaud's phenomenon with associated connective tissue disease: a double-blind placebo-controlled study		
Substance	**Diltiazem 3 × 60 mg/day** (n = 14) **Placebo** (n = 14) for 2 weeks Patient groups were crossed over after 2 weeks No information on concomitant medication		
Result	Diltiazem treatment in Raynaud's phenomenon patients was inefficient		
Patients	15 patients suffering from Raynaud's syndrome with associated connective tissue disorder • SLE n = 8 • Systemic sclerosis n = 4 • Mixed connective tissue disease n = 1		
Authors	da Costa J, Gomes JA, Espirito Santo J, Queirós M		
Publication	*J Rheumatol* 1987;14(4):858–859		
Follow-up	4 weeks		
Note	*Outcome parameters*:	Diltiazem	Placebo
	Number of vasospastic attacks improved	n = 12	n = 11
	Patient assessed drug as effective	n = 4	n = 6
	Digital rheography improved	n = 8	n = 7

Trial	Topical Glyceryl trinitrate as adjunctive treatment in Raynaud's disease
Substance	**Glyceryl trinitrate 1% ointment** **Placebo** Applied to one hand only for 6 weeks, contralateral hand as internal control Crossover for another 6 weeks *Background medication*: Guanethidine 10 mg/day n = 3 Methyldopa 1–2 g/day n = 10
Result	The frequency and severity of attacks and of size of ulcers were lower with topical glyceryl trinitrate compared to placebo in Raynaud's disease associated with connective tissue disease
Patients	17 patients with bilateral Raynaud's disease • Secondary to "collagen" disease • Systemic sclerosis n = 13 • SLE n = 3 • RA n = 1 • Oral sympatholytic agents at the maximum levels patients could tolerate
Authors	Franks AG Jr
Publication	*Lancet.* 1982;1(8263):76–77
Follow-up	12 weeks

Note	*Outcome parameters*:		
		Glyceryl trinitrate	Placebo
	Reduction of number of Raynaud's attacks	n = 13	n = 6
	Reduction of severity of Raynaud's attacks	n = 11	n = 1
	Size of ulcerations improved	n = 7	n = 1
Adverse events	Headache	(no frequencies were listed)	
	Postural hypotension		
	Abnormal sensations in the untreated hand		

Trial	Objective relief of vasospasm by glyceryl trinitrate in secondary Raynaud's phenomenon			
Substance	**Topical glyceryl trinitrate**			
Result	An objective response to topical glyceryl trinitrate by digital plethysmography was shown in patients with secondary, but not with primary Raynaud's syndrome			
Patients	17 patients with Raynaud's phenomenon • Secondary Raynaud's phenomenon n = 10 • Scleroderma n = 5 • SLE n = 4 • Overlap syndrome n = 1			
Authors	Coppock JS, Hardman JM, Bacon PA, Woods KL, Kendall MJ			
Publication	*Postgrad Med J.* 1986 Jan;62(723):15–18			
Follow-up	30 min			
Note	*Change of finger systolic pressure*			

	Glyceryl trinitrate		Placebo	
	30°C	15°C	30°C	15°C
All patients	24	16	12	0
Primary Raynaud's phenomenon	24	0	16	0
Secondary Raynaud's phenomenon	22.5	31.5	4.5	-3.5

Adverse events	Headache n = 4 (glyceryl trinitrate)

Trial	Sustained-release transdermal glyceryl trinitrate patches as a treatment for primary and secondary Raynaud's phenomenon		
Substance	**Glyceryl trinitrate patches** (GTN, 0.2 mg/h) **Placebo patches** For 7 days followed by a crossover Patients were asked not to smoke		
Result	Glyceryl trinitrate patches were effective in reducing the number and severity in both primary and secondary Raynaud's syndrome patients. Headaches were frequent		
Patients	Patients with primary Raynaud's disease (n = 21) and Patients with Raynaud's phenomenon secondary to systemic sclerosis according to the ACR criteria (n = 21)		
Authors	Teh LS, Manning J, Moore T, Tully MP, O'Reilly D, Jayson MI		
Publication	*Br J Rheumatol.* 1995 Jul;34(7):636–641		
Follow-up	14 days		
Note	*Comparison of treatment*		
		Primary Raynaud	Secondary Raynaud
	Baseline vs. GTN	p = 0.002	p = 0.011
	Baseline vs. placebo	p = 0.245	p = 0.116
	GTN vs. placebo	p = 0.013	p = 0.046
	Statistical analysis of severity of attacks comparing placebo vs. active treatment:		
		Primary Raynaud	Secondary Raynaud
	Numbness	p = 0.002	p = 0.009
	Pain	p = 0.004	p = 0.034
	Color change	p = 0.0013	p = 0.012
	Overall severity	p = 0.002	p = 0.036
	Distal dorsal temperature difference	p = 0.72	p = 0.65
	Initial temperature of the digits at 0 min 0°C	p = 0.62	p = 0.083
	Percentage recovery of temperature at 10 min	p = 0.22	p = 0.11
	Tlog before max. Onset of temperature recovery (min)	p = 0.64	0.48
Adverse events		GTN	Placebo
	Headache	n = 26	n = 10
	Flushing	n = 6	n = 5
	Nausea	n = 5	n = 2
	Palpitations	n = 4	n = 2
	Dizziness	n = 4	n = 1
	Tingling in hands	n = 1	n = 0
	Skin irritation	n = 1	n = 0
	Headaches leading to withdrawal	n = 8	

Trial	Disease-modifying effects of long-term cyclic iloprost therapy in systemic sclerosis. A retrospective analysis and comparison with a control group		
Substance	**Iloprost, 6-h continuous i. v. infusion at the maximal tolerated dose (mean ± DS: 1.25 ± 0.45 ng/kg/min) on 5 consecutive days, followed by 1× every 3 weeks (maintainance)**		
	Concomitant medication:		
	Low dose corticosteroids		
	Calcium-channel blockers		
	Other vasodilators		
	Low dose aspirin		
	i. v. cyclophosphamide for interstitial lung disease if needed		
	D-penicillamine		
	Ciclosporin A		
Result	There were less ulcers in a majority of patients, but not in all, at the end of the observations period in this open trial not only addressing iloprost's effects on Raynaud's syndrome		
Patients	56 consecutive SSc patients		
	Compared with 56 control patients		
Authors	Airò P, Rossi M, Scarsi M, Danieli E, Grottolo A, Zambruni A		
Publication	*Clin Exp Rheumatol.* 2007 Sep-Oct;25(5):722–727		
Follow-up	4 years		
Note	Still receiving iloprost (end of follow-up)	n = 34	
	Iloprost discontinued	n = 22	
		Disease improvement	n = 6
		Death	n = 8
		Lack of compliance	n = 2
		Renal crisis	n = 2
		Ischemic cardiopathy	n = 2
		Pregnancy	n = 1
		Neoplasm	n = 1
	Patients with ischemic ulcers at the start	n = 47	
	No lesions at the last observation	n = 29	
	Decrease in the Raynaud's phenomenon	VAS 10/10 → 5/10	
	Change in HAQ score	0.9 → 1.1	
	Decrease in modified Rodnan skin thickness score	23 → 18	
	Change of:		
		Iloprost	Controls
	FVC loss/year	-2.4%	-3.2%
	DLCO loss/year	-2.1%	-2.6%
	Receiving cyclophosphamide during follow-up	n = 10	n = 16

(continued) ➜

Adverse events	Iloprost	Controls
Active ILD	n = 4	n = 6
Isolated PAH	n = 0	n = 2
Renal crisis	n = 2	n = 1
Deaths (total)	n = 8	n = 7
Deaths (disease-related)	n = 4	n = 6
Deaths (for other causes)	n = 4	n = 1

Trial	Prolonged increase in digital blood flow following iloprost infusion in patients with systemic sclerosis
Substance	**Iloprost, 8-h infusions of (2 ng/kg/min) on 3 consecutive days** *Concomitant medication:* Vasoactive drugs (channel calcium antagonists, antiplatelet activity, nonsteroidal antiinflammatory agents) discontinued ≥ 2 weeks before admission
Result	Digital blood flow increased and number of cutaneous lesions decreased following an infusion of iloprost given for 8 h on 3 consecutive days, with effects persisting for 10 weeks
Patients	13 patients with Raynaud's phenomenon secondary to systemic sclerosis
Authors	Rademaker M, Thomas RH, Provost G, Beacham JA, Cooke ED, Kirby JD
Publication	*Postgrad Med J.* 1987;63(742):617–620
Follow-up	10 weeks
Note	*Outcome parameters:*

Subjective improvement		n = 9
Decrease of digital peripheral vascular resistance		n = 9
Cutaneous lesions:		
Onset		n = 26
2 weeks		n = 14
10 weeks		n = 7

Trial	Infusion of iloprost, a prostacyclin analogue, for treatment of Raynaud's phenomenon in systemic sclerosis
Substance	**Iloprost 2.0 mg/kg/min for 6 h (n = 11) on 3 consecutive days** **Placebo** (n = 9) No information on concomitant medication and on crossover schedule
Result	Iloprost significantly reduced the number and the severity of attacks compared with placebo
Patients	29 patients with severe Raynaud's phenomenon • Systemic sclerosis n = 26 • Idiopathic Raynaud's phenomenon n = 3
Authors	McHugh NJ, Csuka M, Watson H, Belcher G, Amadi A, Ring EF, Black CM, Maddison PJ
Publication	*Ann Rheum Dis.* 1988;47(1):43–47
Follow-up	6 weeks

Note	*Change of:*		
		Iloprost (%)	Placebo (%)
	No. of attacks a week	-30	-2
	Duration	-9	+26
	Severity	-20	-1
	Painful attacks	-16	-11

Adverse events		Iloprost
	Headache	n = 18
	Facial flushing	n = 6
	Nausea	n = 14
	Vomiting	n = 7
	Diarrhea	n = 5

Trial	Comparison of intravenous infusions of Iloprost and oral Nifedipine in treatment of Raynaud's phenomenon in patients with systemic sclerosis: a double-blind randomized study
Substance	**Iloprost i. v. 0.5 ng/kg/min,** increased by 0.5 ng/kg/min every 15 min to max. 2.0 ng/kg/min for 8 h on 3 consecutive days Plus 1 single infusion at week 8 (n = 12) **Nifedipine 30 mg/day,** increased to 60 mg/day after 4 weeks (n = 11) *Concomitant therapy:* Adequate contraception
Result	Iloprost and nifedipine were both beneficial in the treatment of Raynaud's phenomenon. Nifedipine-associated adverse events were common. Short-term infusions of iloprost provided long-lasting relief of symptoms. Side effects occurred only during the infusions and were dose-dependent
Patients	23 patients with Raynaud's phenomenon • Associated with systemic sclerosis • Typical for systemic sclerosis on capillaroscopy of the fingernail fold
Authors	Rademaker M, Cooke ED, Almond NE, Beacham JA, Smith RE, Mant TG, Kirby JD
Publication	*BMJ.* 1989;298(6673):561–564
Follow-up	16 weeks

Note	*Change of:*	Iloprost	Nifedipine
	Number of skin lesions	-2.9	-2.9
	Number of attacks	-55.4%	-41.5%
	Severity of attacks	-34.6%	-31.5%
	Duration of attacks	-46.8%	-44.7%

Adverse events		Iloprost (%)
	Headache	> 50
	Nausea	> 50
	Vomiting	> 50

Trial	A double-blind, randomized, multicentre comparison of two doses of intravenous Iloprost in the treatment of Raynaud's phenomenon secondary to connective tissue diseases
Substance	**Iloprost 0.5 ng/kg/min** (n = 28, low dose) **Iloprost 2 ng/kg/min** (n = 27, standard dose), both on 3 consecutive days 10 mL/h with increments of 10 mL/h every 15 min until infusion rates reached 0.5 ng/kg/min and 2 ng/kg/min, respectively No information on concomitant medication
Result	Iloprost reduced the severity of Raynaud's phenomenon and encouraged ulcer healing. Low dose treatment was associated with fewer side effects and was better tolerated
Patients	55 patients with Raynaud's phenomenon • > 7 attacks/week • Systemic sclerosis n = 32 • Limited cutaneous scleroderma n = 11 • Mixed connective tissue disease n = 5 • Rheumatoid arthritis n = 1 • Sjoegren's syndrome n = 1 • Childhood dermatomyositis n = 1 • No definite diagnosis n = 3
Authors	Torley HI, Madhok R, Capell HA, Brouwer RM, Maddison PJ, Black CM, Englert H, Dormandy JA, Watson HR
Publication	*Ann Rheum Dis.* 1991;50(11):800–804
Follow-up	8 weeks

Note	*Outcome parameters:*	Low dose iloprost	Standard dose iloprost
	Ulcer healing	44%	39%
	New lesions	n = 3	n = 6
	Patients' subjective improvement	41%	68%
	Change of:	Low dose iloprost	Standard dose iloprost
	Frequency of Raynaud's attacks	-28%	-37%
	Duration of Raynaud's attacks (min)	-20	-46
	Severity of Raynaud's attacks (VAS)	-10	-23

Adverse events		Low dose iloprost	Standard dose iloprost
	Flushing	n = 3	n = 3
	Headache	n = 8	n = 20
	Nausea	n = 1	n = 13
	Vomiting	n = 0	n = 8
	Diarrhea	n = 0	n = 7
	Abdominal cramps	n = 0	n = 6
	Painful eyes	n = 0	n = 1
	Dizziness	n = 0	n = 2
	Drowsiness	n = 1	n = 0
	Tingling fingers	n = 1	n = 3
	Patients reporting any side effect	n = 9	n = 21

Trial	Placebo-controlled study showing therapeutic benefit of Iloprost in the treatment of Raynaud's phenomenon
Substance	**Iloprost 3×0.5 ng/kg/min over 6 h, on 3 consecutive days** (increased every 30 min to max. 2 ng/kg/min) **Placebo** Crossover after 6 weeks *Previous therapy*: Nifedipine n = 7 (benefit n = 2) Naftidrofuryl n = 1 (benefit n = 1) PGE1 n = 5 (benefit n = 2) Oxerutins n = 1 (benefit n = 0) Thymoxamine n = 2 (benefit n = 1) Sympathectomy n = 3 (benefit n = 1) Evening primrose oil n = 1 (benefit n = 1) Nicotinic acid n = 5 (benefit n = 2)
Result	Treatment with iloprost reduced the frequency and duration of Raynaud's phenomenon attacks
Patients	13 patients with Raynaud's phenomenon • Primary Raynaud phenomenon n = 8 • Systemic sclerosis n = 4 • Mixed connective tissue disease n = 1
Authors	Kyle MV, Belcher G, Hazleman BL
Publication	*J Rheumatol.* 1992;19(9):1403–1406
Follow-up	2×6 weeks

Note	*Change of (week 6)*:	Placebo	Iloprost
	Frequency of attacks	-24.5	-44.4
	Duration of attacks	-54.3	-12.2
	Severity of attacks	+0.1	-9.5

Adverse events	Headache	n = 5	
	Flushing	n = 2	
	Nausea	n = 4	
	Vomiting	n = 1	
	Diarrhea	n = 2	

Trial	Intravenous Iloprost treatment of Raynaud's phenomenon and ischemic ulcers secondary to systemic sclerosis		
Substance	**Iloprost i. v. (0.5–2.0 ng/kg/min,** n = 18) by continuous infusion for 6 h on 5 consecutive days **Placebo** (n = 17) No information on concomitant medication		
Result	Iloprost was effective in the treatment of digital ulcers in systemic sclerosis and was associated with evidence of prolonged physiologic improvement		
Patients	35 patients with Raynaud's phenomenon • Secondary to systemic sclerosis • With digital ischemic ulcerations n = 11 • ≥ 8 symptomatic episodes of Raynaud's phenomenon/week		
Authors	Wigley FM, Seibold JR, Wise RA, McCloskey DA, Dole WP		
Publication	*J Rheumatol.* 1992;19(9):1407–1414		
Follow-up	10 weeks		
Note	*Outcome parameters*:		
		Iloprost	Placebo
	Complete healing of all cutaneous lesions	86%	0%
	Critical ischemic temperature (°C)	21.6 → 17.8	21.4 → 20.1
	Change of:		
		Iloprost	Placebo
	Duration of attacks (min)	+2	-22.6
	Severity of attacks (VAS 0–4)	-0.17	-0.27
	Recovery (°C/min)	+0.29	+0.10
Adverse events		Iloprost (%)	Placebo (%)
	Headache	100	47
	Nausea	78	6
	Pain	50	0
	Vomiting	50	0
	Vasodilatation	33	0
	Injection-site reaction	28	1
	Diarrhea	17	0
	Dizziness	17	24
	Abdominal pain	17	0
	Myalgia	11	0
	Chest pain	11	0

Trial	Intravenous Iloprost infusion in patients with Raynaud's phenomenon secondary to systemic sclerosis. A multicenter, placebo-controlled, double-blind study
Substance	**Iloprost, sequential, 6-h i. v. infusions of (0.5–2.0 ng/kg per min, n = 64)** **Placebo** (n = 67), both for 5 days Prior use of nifedipine n = 26
Result	Iloprost was effective as short-term treatment of severe Raynaud's phenomenon in patients with systemic sclerosis
Patients	131 patients with systemic sclerosis (101 women, 30 men) • Min. 8 attacks/week • ≥ 1 finger cutaneous ischemic lesion
Authors	Wigley FM, Wise RA, Seibold JR, McCloskey DA, Kujala G, Medsger TA Jr, Steen VD, Varga J, Jimenez S, Mayes M, Clements PJ, Weiner SR, Porter J, Ellman M, Wise C, Kaufman LD, Williams J, Dole W
Publication	*Ann Intern Med.* 1994;120(3):199–206
Follow-up	9 weeks
Note	*Physician's overall assessment*:

	Iloprost (%)	Placebo (%)
Great improvement	12.5	4.5
Improved	48.4	22.4
Same	32.8	56.7
Worse	6.3	16.4

Change of:

	Iloprost (%)	Placebo (%)
Raynaud severity score	-34.8	-19.7
Frequency of Raynaud attacks	-39.1	-22.2
Number of Raynaud attacks	-44.86	-27.21
Global Raynaud severity score	34.8	19.7
Physician's overall rating	60.9	26.9
HAQ	-6.71	+9.17

(continued) ➜

Adverse events	Iloprost (%)	Placebo (%)
Headache	84	31
Flushing	50	9
Nausea	45	16
Jaw pain	23	3
Diarrhea	20	3
Vomiting	19	3
Injection-site reactions	14	0
Abdominal pain	11	9
Dizziness	8	10
Myalgia	8	0
Nausea and vomiting	8	1
Injection-site pain	8	0
Dyspepsia	6	6
Paresthesia	6	1
Dry mouth	5	1
Flatulence	5	1
Hypertonia	5	0
Injection-site inflammation	5	1
Back pain	5	1
Phlebitis	5	0
Arthralgia	3	1
Chills	3	3
Circumoral paresthesia	3	0
Taste perversion	3	1
Amblyopia	2	1
Asthenia	2	1
Eructation	2	0
Gastrointestinal disorder	2	0
Hyperkinesia	2	0
Hypotension	2	0
Postural hypotension	2	1
Abnormal liver function	2	0
Neck pain	2	0
Increased sweating	2	1
Arrhythmia	0	3
Dyspnea	0	3
Injection-site edema	0	1
Peripheral edema	0	3
Chest pain	0	1
Vertigo	0	1

Trial	Oral Iloprost as a treatment for Raynaud's syndrome: a double-blind multicenter placebo-controlled study		
Substance	**Iloprost 2 × 50 −150 µg/day** p. o. (n = 32) **Placebo** (n = 31) Both applied for 10 days 14 days washout of vasoactive substances		
Result	Oral administration of iloprost displayed a trend in favor of iloprost in this short-term follow-up study		
Patients	63 Patients with Raynaud's syndrome secondary to systemic sclerosis		
Authors	Belch JJ, Capell HA, Cooke ED, Kirby JD, Lau CS, Madhok R, Murphy E, Steinberg M		
Publication	*Ann Rheum Dis.* 1995;54(3):197–200		
Follow-up	10 days treatment plus 14 days follow-up		
Note	*Global opinion*:		
		Placebo (%)	Iloprost (%)
	Symptoms unchanged	60%	−
	Symptoms improved	−	60%
	Change of duration of Raynaud's attacks:		
		Placebo (%)	Iloprost (%)
	End of treatment	-24	-40
	After 2 weeks follow-up	-25	-25
	Change of painful attacks:		
		Placebo	Iloprost
	End of treatment	-23	+1
	After 2 weeks follow-up	-7	-27
Adverse events		Placebo	Iloprost
	Headache leading to withdrawal	n = 0	n = 3
	Headache, flushing, and nausea	61%	97%

Trial	Oral Iloprost treatment in patients with Raynaud's phenomenon secondary to systemic sclerosis: a multicenter, placebo-controlled, double-blind study
Substance	**Iloprost 2×50 µg/day** p. o. (n = 157) **Placebo** (n = 151) *Previous medication:* No prostanoid therapy (including misoprostol) ≤ 2 months No prior ciclosporin
Result	Oral iloprost treatment of Raynaud's phenomenon secondary to scleroderma was equally effective as placebo
Patients	308 patients with scleroderma (272 women, 36 men, mean age 49 years) • And Raynaud's phenomenon • ≥ 6 Raynaud attacks/week
Authors	Wigley FM, Korn JH, Csuka ME, Medsger TA Jr, Rothfield NF, Ellman M, Martin R, Collier DH, Weinstein A, Furst DE, Jimenez SA, Mayes MD, Merkel PA, Gruber B, Kaufman L, Varga J, Bell P, Kern J, Marrott P, White B, Simms RW, Phillips AC, Seibold JR
Publication	*Arthritis Rheum.* 1998;41(4):670–677
Follow-up	12 weeks
Note	*Outcome parameters:*

	Placebo (%)	Iloprost (%)
Improvement in duration of Raynaud's phenomenon attacks > 50%	41.7	45.9
Improvement in duration of Raynaud's phenomenon attacks > 50%	24.5	24.8
Improvement in Raynaud's condition score > 50%	24.5	35.0

Change of:

	Placebo (%)	Iloprost (%)
Duration of Raynaud attacks	-21.13	-24.06
Frequency of Raynaud attacks	-15.38	-24.12
Raynaud's condition score	-21.46	-29.18

(continued) ➔

Adverse events	Placebo (%)	Iloprost (%)
Headache	28.9	67.3
Flushing	6.0	31.4
Nausea	11.4	22.4
Dizziness	9.4	18.6
Diarrhea	10.7	13.5
Skin ulcers	13.4	11.5
Asthenia	5.4	10.9
Abdominal pain	3.4	9.6
Myalgia	6.0	9.0
Vascular disorder	9.4	8.3
Cough increase	8.7	8.3
Pain	12.8	7.7
Dyspepsia	8.7	7.7
Infection	6.7	7.1
Rhinitis	5.4	7.1
Flu syndrome	4.7	7.1
Upper respiratory infection	7.4	6.4
Vomiting	6.4	6.4
Arthralgias	4.7	5.8
Trismus	1.3	5.1
Sinusitis	6.0	3.2

Trial	Oral Iloprost in Raynaud's phenomenon secondary to systemic sclerosis: a multicenter, placebo-controlled, dose-comparison study
Substance	**Placebo** (n = 35) **Iloprost 50 mg/day** p. o. (n = 33) **Iloprost 100 mg/day** p. o. (n = 35) No information on concomitant medication
Result	Oral iloprost was effective with regard to duration and frequency of attacks in Raynaud's phenomenon secondary to systemic sclerosis
Patients	103 patients with Raynaud's phenomenon • Secondary to systemic sclerosis
Authors	Black CM, Halkier-Sørensen L, Belch JJ, Ullman S, Madhok R, Smit AJ, Banga JD, Watson HR
Publication	*Br J Rheumatol.* 1998;37(9):952–960
Follow-up	12 weeks

Note	*Outcome parameters*:			
		Placebo	Iloprost 50 μg	Iloprost 100 μg
	Improvement	44%	57%	64%
	Healing of digital cutaneous lesions	n = 1/7	n = 1/8	n = 3/7
	Change of:			
		Placebo (%)	Iloprost 50 μg (%)	Iloprost 100 μg (%)
	Duration of Raynaud's attacks	-9	-60	-60
	Frequency of Raynaud's attacks	-15	-46	-50
	Raynaud's condition score	-15	-38	-60

(continued)

Adverse events		Placebo (%)	Iloprost 50 µg (%)	Iloprost 100 µg (%)
	Headache	40	79	86
	Flushing	17	27	46
	Nausea	3	30	37
	Flu syndrome	31	9	14
	Dizziness	17	6	14
	Vomiting	6	9	20
	Diarrhea	3	9	20
	Pain in extremity	3	12	14
	Asthenia	3	9	14
	Dyspepsia	9	9	9
	Rash	3	6	14
	Trismus	0	6	17
	Infection	11	9	3
	Pharyngitis	0	12	6
	Any adverse events	80	86	97
	Treatment discontinuation due to adverse events	6	27	51

Trial	Effects of long-term cyclic Iloprost therapy in systemic sclerosis with Raynaud's phenomenon. A randomized, controlled study
Substance	**Iloprost i. v., infusions (2 ng/kg/min)** on 5 consecutive days over a period of 8 h/day and subsequently for 8 h on 1 day every 6 weeks (n = 29) **Nifedipine (40 mg/day,** n = 17)
Result	Cyclic intravenous iloprost infusions were able to control vasospastic disease. It also seemed to reduce the skin score
Patients	46 patients with systemic sclerosis and Raynaud's phenomenon
Authors	Scorza R, Caronni M, Mascagni B, Berruti V, Bazzi S, Micallef E, Arpaia G, Sardina M, Origgi L, Vanoli M
Publication	*Clin Exp Rheumatol.* 2001;19(5):503–508
Follow-up	12 months

Note	*Change of:*	Ilomedin	Nifedipine
	Reduced the skin score	-4.0	+1.34
	Raynaud's phenomenon severity score	-0.95	-0.75
	DLCO (% of the predicted normal value)	-2.8	-13.0
	Total skin score	-12.2	+6.3
Adverse events		Ilomedin (%)	Nifedipine (%)
	Headache	100	24
	Nausea, Vomiting	83	0
	Jaw pain	69	0
	Myalgia	34	0
	Diarrhea	28	0
	Chills	17	0
	Hypotension	14	29
	Arrhythmia	7	0
	Hyperkinesia	3	0
	Tachycardia	0	6

Trial	Comparison between Iloprost and Alprostadil in the treatment of Raynaud's phenomenon		
Substance	**Iloprost i. v., 8–30 µg/day** (n = 11) **Alprostadil i. v., 20 µg/h** (n = 10), cyclically 5 consecutive days, followed by 1 day every 30 days No information on concomitant medication		
Result	Iloprost and alprostadil were both effective in connective tissue disease-associated Raynaud's phenomenon, without significant differences in either clinical efficacy or circulating biomarkers		
Patients	21 women with connective tissue disease-associated Raynaud's phenomenon • Meeting the ACR-criteria of systemic sclerosis n = 18 • MCTD n = 3 • > 3 Raynaud's attacks/s and/or digital ischemic changes		
Authors	Marasini B, Massarotti M, Bottasso B, Coppola R, Papa ND, Maglione W, Comina DP, Maioli C		
Publication	*Scand J Rheumatol.* 2004;33(4):253–256		
Follow-up	60 days		
Note	*Outcome parameters*:		

		Iloprost (%)	Alprostadil (%)
	Raynaud's phenomenon improved	45	90
	Improvement of ulcers	60	40

Change of:

		Iloprost	Alprostadil
	Skin score	-2.2	+1.2
	Circulating von Willebrand factor (mU/dl)	-6.2%	-9.4%
	Tissue plasminogen activation (ng/mL)	-0.9	+1.6
	Thrombomodulin (ng/mL)	-0.6	+0.2
	Pro-collagen N terminal peptide (µg/mL)	-0.1	+0.2

Adverse events		Iloprost	Alprostadil
	Headache	n = 6	n = 0
	Nausea	n = 3	n = 0
	Vomiting	n = 1	n = 0
	Injection-site reaction	n = 0	n = 1

Trial	Low vs. high dose Iloprost therapy over 21 days in patients with secondary Raynaud's phenomenon and systemic sclerosis: a randomized, open, single-center study		
Substance	**Iloprost i. v., 2 ng/kg body weight per minute** (n = 25) **Iloprost i. v., low dose (0.5 ng/kg/min)** intravenous administration (n = 25), applied for 6 h daily over 21 days No information on concomitant medication		
Result	Low dose Iloprost was equally effective as high dose iloprost in long-term treatment and was very effective in the therapy of digital ulcers		
Patients	50 patients with systemic sclerosis • Stable immunosuppression or vasoactive therapies for 3 months • Current smokers, patients with a history of gastric ulcer ≤ 3 months Cardiac ejection fraction < 25% *No severe organ involvement or other uncontrolled disease*: • Angina pectoris • Severe anemia • Coagulopathies • Azotemia • Cerebral infarction during the last 6 months • Malignant diseases		
Authors	Kawald A, Burmester GR, Huscher D, Sunderkötter C, Riemekasten G		
Publication	*J Rheumatol.* 2008;35(9):1830–1837		
Follow-up	12 months		
Note	*Outcome parameters*:		
		High dose iloprost (%)	Low dose iloprost (%)
	Reduction of digital ulcers	76.2	61.0
	Reduction in frequency of Raynaud's phenomenon	46	42
	Modified Rodnan skin score	Unchanged both regimen	
	No response to treatment	12	12
Adverse events		High dose iloprost (%)	Low dose iloprost (%)
	Flushing	48	40
	Headache	24	12
	GI symptoms like nausea or vomiting	12	4

Trial	Controlled trial of Nifedipine in the treatment of Raynaud's phenomenon
Substance	**Nifedipine 4×10 mg/day** (n = 8) **Placebo** (n = 8) Crossover after 2 weeks No concomitant vasoactive substance
Result	Nifedipine was effective in 12 out of 17 patients
Patients	Patients with moderate to severe Raynaud's phenomenon n = 17 • Idiopathic Raynaud's phenomenon n = 5 • Systemic sclerosis n = 11 • Min. 1 attack/day
Authors	Smith CD, McKendry RJ
Publication	*Lancet.* 1982;2(8311):1299–1301
Follow-up	6 weeks

Note	*Outcome parameters*:	Nifedipine	Placebo
	Patient sore of effectiveness	5.3	1.3
	Change of:	Nifedipine	Placebo
	Frequency of attacks	-1.5	-0.3
	Severity of attacks	-2.4	+0.6

Adverse events		Nifedipine	Placebo
	Flushing	n = 5	n = 1
	Headache	n = 4	n = 0
	Sensation of light headed	n = 3	n = 0
	Ankle swelling	n = 3	n = 0

Trial	Controlled double-blind trial of Nifedipine in the treatment of Raynaud's phenomenon		
Substance	**Nifedipine 3 × 20 mg/day** **Placebo** Patient groups were crossed over after 2 weeks and crossed back after another 2 weeks No information on concomitant medication		
Result	Treatment of patients with nifedipine lead to a decrease in the frequency of attacks and moderate improvement in symptoms		
Patients	15 patients with symptomatic Raynaud's syndrome • Systemic sclerosis n = 9 • SLE n = 1 • No systemic disease n = 5 • Bilateral episodes		
Authors	Rodeheffer RJ, Rommer JA, Wigley F, Smith CR		
Publication	*N Engl J Med.* 1983;308(15):880–883		
Follow-up	4 weeks		
Note	*Outcome parameters*:		
		Nifedipine	Placebo
	Moderate or marked improvement	60%	13%
	Minimal improvement, change, or worse	40%	87%
	Attack rate/2 weeks	14.7	10.8
Adverse events		Nifedipine (%)	Placebo (%)
	Headache	80	20
	Lightheadedness	33	7

Trial	Comparison of intravenous infusions of iloprost and oral nifedipine in treatment of Raynaud's phenomenon in patients with systemic sclerosis: a double blind randomized study
Substance	**0.5 ng/kg/min iloprost** (n = 13) Increased by 0.5 ng/kg/min every 15 min to a maximum of 2.0 ng/kg/min for 8 h on 3 consecutive days Nifedipine 30 mg/day (n = 12) Increased to 60 mg/day after 4 weeks for another 12 weeks
Result	Both iloprost and nifedipine were beneficial in the treatment of Raynaud's phenomenon. Side effects with nifedipine were common
Patients	25 patients with primary Raynaud's phenomenon
Authors	Rademaker M, Cooke ED, Almond NE, Beacham JA, Smith RE, Mant TG, Kirby JD
Publication	*BMJ.* 1989 Mar 4;298(6673):561–564
Follow-up	16 weeks
Note	Both regimens produced a reduction in the number, duration, and severity of attacks of Raynaud's phenomenon

Change of (week 16):

	Iloprost	Nifedipine
Number of digital lesions	-2.9	-2.9
Number of attacks	-55.4	-41.5
Duration of attacks	-46.8	-44.7
Severity of attacks	-34.6	-31.5

Hand temperature and digital and microcirculatory blood flow were increased with iloprost but not with nifedipine.

Adverse events	Iloprost	Nifedipine
Peripheral edema	n = 0	n = 1
Headache	≥ half of the iloprost treated patients	n = 2
Nausea	≥ half of the iloprost treated patients	n = 0
Vomiting	≥ half of the iloprost treated patients	n = 0

Trial	Controlled double-blind trial of the clinical effect of nifedipine in the treatment of idiopathic Raynaud's phenomenon	
Substance	**Placebo** (n =13) **Nifedipine 20 mg/day** (n = 12)	
Result	Nifedipine was effective in the treatment of idiopathic Raynaud's phenomenon, but side effects were frequent	
Patients	27 patients with primary Raynaud's phenomenon	
Authors	Gjørup T, Kelbaek H, Hartling OJ, Nielsen SL	
Publication	*Am Heart J.* 1986 Apr;111(4):742–745	
Follow-up	2 × 14 days with crossover	
Note	Nifedipine significantly reduced frequency and severity of attacks 19 of 21 patients preferred nifedipine to placebo	
Adverse events	Total adverse events	n = 16
	Headache	n = 11
	Flushing	n = 6
	Palpitation	n = 2

Trial	A randomized double-blind crossover trial of Nifedipine in the treatment of primary Raynaud's phenomenon
Substance	**Nifedipine 2 × 5 mg/day** (dose increased to 2 × 15 mg/day within 3 weeks, n = 22) **Placebo** (n = 23) No concomitant medication for Raynaud's phenomenon was allowed
Result	Nifedipine was effective in primary Raynaud's phenomenon in most patients but side effects were common
Patients	23 women with primary Raynaud's phenomenon • Disease duration > 2 years
Authors	Corbin DO, Wood DA, Macintyre CC, Housley E
Publication	*Eur Heart J.* 1986;7(2):165–170
Follow-up	4 weeks

Note

Outcome parameters:

	Nifedipine	Placebo
Number of attacks of Raynaud's phenomenon	2.3	5.0
Systolic blood pressure	109.5/68.1	109.6/68.6

Drug compliance:

	Nifedipine 45 mg	Nifedipine 30 mg	Nifedipine 15 mg	Placebo
Good	n = 10	n = 0	n = 3	n = 15
Moderate	n = 5	n = 2	n = 0	n = 6
Poor	n = 0	n = 2	n = 0	n = 2

Adverse events

	Nifedipine (%)	Placebo (%)
Headache	26	9
Ankle swelling	22	0
Flushing	52	0
Palpitations	9	0
Nausea	17	4
Parasthesia	35	0
Dizziness	13	0
Chest pain	0	0

Trial	Nifedipine in the treatment of Raynaud's phenomenon in patients with systemic sclerosis
Substance	**Nifedipine 3 × 10 mg/day** (n = 5) **Placebo** (n = 5), both for 6 weeks After a 2 week wash out period Patient groups were crossed over and followed again for 6 weeks
Result	Patients with idiopathic Raynaud's phenomenon responded better to nifedipine than patients with disease secondary to systemic sclerosis
Patients	10 patients with Raynaud's phenomenon • Secondary to systemic sclerosis
Authors	Meyrick Thomas RH, Rademaker M, Grimes SM, MacKay A, Kovacs IB, Cook ED, Bowcock SM, Kirby JD
Publication	*Br J Dermatol.* 1987;117(2):237–241
Follow-up	14 weeks
Note	*Outcome parameters*:

	Placebo	Nifedipine
Duration of Raynaud's attacks (min)	29.7	18.7
Number of attacks/day	1.6	1.3
Percentage of mild attacks	32.4	50.3
Percentage of moderate attacks	48.9	37.2
Percentage of severe attacks	18.7	12.5
Percentage of pain free attacks	49.5	59.3

Trial	Sildenafil in the treatment of Raynaud's phenomenon resistant to vasodilatory therapy
Substance	**Sildenafil 2 × 50 mg/day** **Placebo** b.i.d., both for 4 weeks Fixed dose, crossover study, 1 week wash out period in between the two treatment periods of 4 weeks each All vasoactive substances were stopped before the trial Concomitant substances for rheumatological disease remained unchanged
Result	Sildenafil was an effective and well-tolerated treatment in patients with Raynaud's phenomenon
Patients	18 patients with symptomatic secondary Raynaud's phenomenon • Resistant to vasodilatory therapy with at least two agents • Regular occurrence of painful Raynaud attacks • Systemic sclerosis, n = 14 • Mixed connective tissue disease, n = 2 • No connective tissue disease, n = 2
Authors	Fries R, Shariat K, von Wilmowsky H, Böhm M
Publication	*Circulation*. 2005;112(19):2980–2985
Follow-up	9 weeks
Note	*Outcome parameters*:

	Sildenafil	Placebo
Frequency of Raynaud attacks	35	52
Cumulative attack duration (min)	581	1,046
Mean capillary flow velocity	+0.31	+0.07

Adverse events	Sildenafil
Headache	n = 3
Muscle pain	n = 1
Swelling of the nasal mucosa	n = 1
Transient facial sensation of heat	n = 3
Mild nausea	n = 2
Dizziness	n = 1
Blood pressure and heart rate	No significant effect

Trial	Modified-release sildenafil reduces Raynaud's phenomenon attack frequency in limited cutaneous systemic sclerosis		
Substance	**Sildenafil 100 mg day for 3 days** **Followed by modified-release sildenafil 200 mg/day** (n = 30) **Placebo** (n = 27)		
Result	Treatment with sildenafil reduced attack frequency in patients with Raynaud's phenomenon secondary to limited systemic sclerosis and was well-tolerated		
Patients	57 patients with Raynaud's phenomenon • Secondary to limited systemic sclerosis as confirmed by the investigator • ≥ 7 Raynaud's phenomenon attacks per week with attacks on ≥ 5 days • No hemodynamic instability or systolic arterial pressure < 95 mmHg		
Authors	Herrick AL, van den Hoogen F, Gabrielli A, Tamimi N, Reid C, O'Connell D, Vázquez-Abad MD, Denton CP		
Publication	*Arthritis Rheum.* 2011 Mar;63(3):775–782		
Follow-up	28 days		
Note	*Change of*		

		Sildenafil	Placebo
	Attacks	-44.0%	-18.1%
	Mean number of attacks per week	-5.7	-11.8
	Raynaud's condition score	-1.2	-0.7
	Raynaud's phenomenon pain score	-0.8	-0.9
	Duration of attacks (minutes)	-7.0	-2.8
	Peripheral arterial tonometric-reactive hyperemic responses	0.0	-0.3
	Soluble vascular cell adhesion molecule (ng/mL)	+39.0	-41.0
	Soluble intercellular adhesion molecule (ng/mL)	-2.1	-5.0
	N-terminal type I procollagen propeptide (ng/mL)	+1.1	-1.5

Adverse events	*Adverse events/number of treatment- related adverse events:*		

		Sildenafil	Placebo
	Headache	15/12	8/6
	Dyspepsia	7/5	3/2
	Flatulence	3/1	1/0
	Arthralgia	3/0	0/0
	Myalgia	2/2	3/1
	Respiratory tract infection	3/0	1/0

Adverse events leading to discontinuation:

		Sildenafil	Placebo
	Allergic reaction	n = 1	n = 0
	Headache and myalgia	n = 1	n = 0
	Headache, chest pain, and facial edema	n = 1	n = 0
	Headache, palpitations, and nontreatment-related arthralgia	n = 1	n = 0

Trial	Randomized placebo-controlled crossover trial of tadalafil in Raynaud's phenomenon secondary to systemic sclerosis.		
Substance	*Crossover design*: **Tadalafil 20 mg/day** **Placebo** *Concomitant medication*: No nitrates or nitrites No calcium channel blockers No PDE-5 inhibitors No sympatholytic drugs No arginine No papaverine No other vasodilators		
Result	Tadalafil was safe and well-tolerated but showed no efficacy in comparison to placebo		
Patients	39 patients suffering from systemic sclerosis according to the ACR criteria • ≥ 6 Raynaud attacks/week with a run in period of 2 weeks • During October and November • No active smoking status, hepatobiliary disease, serum creatinine > 1.8 mg/dL, myocardial infarction or unstable angina, congestive heart failure		
Authors	Schiopu E, Hsu VM, Impens AJ, Rothman JA, McCloskey DA, Wilson JE, Phillips K, Seibold JR		
Publication	*J Rheumatol.* 2009 Oct;36(10):2264–2268		
Follow-up	2 weeks run in phase 4 weeks randomized trial 2 weeks wash out 4 weeks randomized trial with crossover therapy		
Note	*Change of*:		
		Tadalafil	Placebo
	Raynaud condition score (cm)	-1.33	-1.23
	Raynaud phenomenon (frequency/day)	-0.85	-0.83
	Raynaud phenomenon duration (min)	-12.81	-6.42
Adverse events		Tadalafil	Placebo
	Headache	n = 6	n = 7
	Back pain	n = 7	n = 2
	Fluid retention	n = 2	n = 1
	Vasomotor changes	n = 2	n = 2
	Fatigue	n = 1	n = 1
	Sleep disturbances	n = 2	n = 0
	Palpitations	n = 2	n = 0

Trial	Efficacy of tadalafil in secondary Raynaud's phenomenon resistant to vasodilator therapy: a double-blind randomized crossover trial
Substance	**Tadalafil 20 mg on alternate days for 6 weeks** **Placebo** *Concomitant medication*: Vasodilators for ≥ 6 weeks *Crossover*: After 7 days of wash out followed again for 6 weeks with crossed over therapy *Previous medication*: After 2 week run-in period Vasodilators for at least 3 months No nitrates No alpha blockers No phosphodiesterase inhibitors No prostacyclins or endothelin antagonists
Result	Symptoms of Raynaud's phenomenon improved after tadalafil as add-on therapy, digital ulcers healed and were prevented
Patients	25 patients with Raynaud's phenomenon (RP) • ≥ 4 Raynaud's phenomenon attacks (episode of pallor or cyanosis with or without associated pain and tingling or numbness) per week in the 2 weeks before inclusion • No current smokers
Authors	Shenoy PD, Kumar S, Jha LK, Choudhary SK, Singh U, Misra R, Agarwal V
Publication	*Rheumatology (Oxford)*. 2010 Dec;49(12):2420–2428
Follow-up	13 weeks

(continued)

		Mean frequency of daily episodes	Average daily duration (min)	
Note	*Effect of tadalafil on RP symptoms:*			
	Baseline	3.47	46.34	
	Placebo	3.37	54.89	
	Tadalafil	2.29	33.81	
	Change of:			
		Baseline	Placebo	Tadalafil
	HAQ	0.94	0.99	0.76
	Physician global assessment	Not available	8.98	6.13
	Patient global assessment	Not available	9.19	5.60
	Flow-mediated dilatation	7.27	7.28	14.41
	Scleroderma-specific HAQ (SHAQ) Pain	1.73	1.68	1.27
	SHAQ limitation of activity due to RP	1.95	1.91	0.94
	SHAQ limitation of activity due to finger ulcer	1.31	1.3	0.69
	SHAQ limitation of activity due to GI problems	1.14	1.30	1.06
	SHAQ limitation of activity due to breathing problems	1.15	1.14	0.87
	SHAQ limitation of activity due to the disease as a whole	2.12	1.92	1.26
	QoL physical function	34.4	35.20	38.28
	QoL role physical	32.37	32.89	32.98
	QoL body pain	36.09	38.04	40.81
	QoL general health	31.70	34.27	34.11
	QoL vitality	38.3	41.41	42.33
	QoL social functioning	38.65	37.29	36.83
	QoL role emotional	30.45	31.27	30.95
	QoL mental health	36.15	37.22	40.38
	QoL physical component summary	34.77	36.26	37.82
	QoL mental component summary	36.38	37.15	37.65
	Healing of digital ulcers	–	n = 3	n = 24
	New digital ulcers	–	n = 13	n = 1
	Five digital ulcers in 2 patients: all healed during tadalfil treatment			

		Tadalafil (%)	Placebo (%)
Adverse events	Headache	37.5	41.7
	Dizziness	20.8	16.7
	Nasal stuffiness	29.2	16.7
	Flushing	8.3	4.2
	Muscle pain	12.5	83
	Rhinorrhea	16.7	8.3
	Heaviness of lids	16.7	0
	Vertigo	4.2	0
	Insomnia	0	8.3
	Central serous retinopathy	0	4.2
	Persistent erection	4.0	0
	Itching	8.3	4.2

Dermato/Polymyositis

Corticosteroids

Trial	Childhood dermatomyositis: Clinical course of 36 patients treated with low doses of corticosteroids	
Substance	Low doses of corticosteroids (**prednisolone 1 mg/kg/day**, n = 36)	
	Additional treatment with DMARDs (n = 13):	
	Ciclosporin (n = 4)	
	Methotrexate (n = 2)	
	I. v. immunoglobulins (n = 2)	
	Methotrexate plus ciclosporin (n = 1)	
Patients	36 patients with juvenile dermatomyositis	
	• Diagnosed according to the criteria of Bohan and Peter	
Result	The majority of children treated with corticosteroids had a favorable outcome	
Authors	Tabarki B, Ponsot G, Prieur AM, Tardieu M	
Publication	*Eur J Paediatr Neurol.* 1998;2(4):205–211	
Follow-up	4.9 years (mean)	
Note	*Outcome parameters (according Bowyer et al.)*:	
	Type 1: Monophasic course of the disease	39%
	Type 2: Polyphasic course	39%
	Type 3: Persistent active disease	8%
	Type 4: Inactive disease with muscular impairment	14%
	Outcome parameters:	
	No functional impairment	78%
	Inactive disease but with persisting disabilities	13.8%
	Active disease despite several years of treatment	8.3%
	Dystrophic calcifications	42%
Adverse events	None reported	

Trial	Azathioprine with prednisone for polymyositis: A controlled, clinical trial
Substance	**Prednisone 15 mg or 60 mg/day** alone (n = 8) **Prednisone plus 2 mg/kg azathioprine/day** (Aza, n = 8) Prednisone dose was adjusted according to clinical criteria, creatinine kinase, manual muscle strength testing *Concomitant medication*: No information was provided Drug changes were permitted
Result	Normalization of the creatinine kinase was not consistent with disease control. Type II fiber atrophy was more marked in women than in men
Patients	16 patients with polymyositis
Authors	Bunch TW, Worthington JW, Combs JJ, Ilstrup DM, Engel AG
Publication	*Ann Intern Med.* 1980;92(3):365–369
Follow-up	3 months
Note	*Outcome parameter:*

	Prednisone	Azathioprine + prednisone
Time to normal CK	53.5 days	69.4 days

Change of:

	Prednisone	Azathioprine + prednisone
Muscle strength score	+1.1	+6.5
Inflammation score	+1.79	+1.65

Adverse events	Prednisone	Azathioprine + prednisone
Nausea	n = 0	n = 1
Diverticulitis	n = 1	n = 0
Pneumonitis	n = 0	n = 1
Leukopenia	n = 0	n = 1

Trial	Prednisone and azathioprine for polymyositis: Long-term follow-up
Substance	**Prednisone alone** (n = 8, doses not listed) **2 mg/kg azathioprine/day (n = 8) plus prednisone** Prednisone dose was adjusted according to clinical criteria, creatinine kinase, manual muscle strength testing *Concomitant medication*: No information was provided Drug changes were permitted
Result	Prednisolone monotherapy in comparison with combination therapy of azathioprine and prednisone of polymyositis showed no significant differences after 3 months. Functional disability improved more in the combination therapy group on long-term follow-up
Patients	16 patients with polymyositis
Authors	Bunch TW
Publication	*Arthritis Rheum*. 1981;24(1):45–48
Follow-up	Approximately 3 years

Note	Clinical follow-up:		
		Prednisone	Azathioprine + prednisone
	Average prednisone dose (mg/day)	11.9	5.4
	CPK (U/L, 1 year)	73.8	49.1
	CPK (U/L, 3 years)	123.3	55.9
	Change of		
		Prednisone	Azathioprine + prednisone
	Functional grade disability (1–6, 1 year)	-0.5	-1.5
	Functional grade disability (1–6, 3 years)	-1.0	-2.4
Adverse events		Prednisone	Azathioprine + prednisone
	CMV infection	n = 0	n = 1
	Death	n = 0	n = 1 (ruptured berry aneurysm)
	Leucocyte count < 3,000/mm³	n = 0	n = 1

Trial	Intravenous cyclophosphamide therapy for progressive interstitial pneumonia in patients with polymyositis/dermatomyositis
Substance	**Cyclophosphamide (CYC, 300–800 mg/m^2), 6 × every 4 weeks Prednisolone oral (0.5–1 mg/kg/day) for 2 weeks and gradually tapered**
	Concomitant medication: Isoniazide as prophylactic treatment for TBC Sulfamethoxazole-trimethoprim as prophylactic treatment for *Pneumocystis jiroveci* pneumonia
Result	Treatment with intravenous cyclophosphamide of polymyositis/ dermatomyositis-associated interstitial pneumonia improved symptoms, pulmonary function tests and HRCT findings
Patients	17 patients with polymyositis/dermatomyositis as defined by the criteria of Bohan and Peter • Or with amyopathic dermatomyositis • With progressive interstitial pneumonia, based on chest X-ray and HRCT
Authors	Yamasaki Y, Yamada H, Yamasaki M, Ohkubo M, Azuma K, Matsuoka S, Kurihara Y, Osada H, Satoh M, Ozaki S
Publication	*Rheumatology (Oxford)*. 2007;46(1):124–130
Follow-up	24 months

Note	*Outcome parameters*:	
	Improvement in their dyspnea	n = 17
	No more dyspnea	n = 11
	Oxygen requirement	n = 6 (before CYC) n = 1 (after CYC)
	≥ 10% improvement of vital capacity	n = 8
	≥ 10% reduction of vital capacity	n = 9
	Flare-up of interstitial pneumonia or myositis	n = 2
	Extent of abnormal lesions in HRCT	−11%
	Vital capacity	+15%
Adverse events	Infection with Mycobacterium avium	n = 1
	Herpes zoster infection	n = 1
	Azoospermia	n = 1

Trial	A controlled trial of high-dose intravenous immune globulin infusions as treatment for dermatomyositis		
Substance	**Immunoglobulins (IVIG, 2 g/kg/month,** n = 8) **Placebo** (n = 7) Patient groups were crossed over after 3 months *Concomitant medication:* 25 mg prednisolone/day DMARDs were continued		
Result	High-dose intravenous immunoglobulin treatment for refractory dermatomyositis was safe and effective		
Patients	15 dermatomyositis patients (age 18–55 years) • Biopsy-proven • Progressive muscle weakness • Unresponsive to corticosteroids or DMARDs for ≥ 6 months		
Authors	Dalakas MC, Illa I, Dambrosia JM, Soueidan SA, Stein DP, Otero C, Dinsmore ST, McCrosky S		
Publication	*N Engl J Med.* 1993;329(27):1993–2000		
Follow-up	6 months		
Note	*Outcome parameters:*		
		IVIG	Placebo
	Major improvement	n = 9	n = 0
	Mild improvement	n = 2	n = 3
	No change	n = 1	n = 3
	Worsening of their condition	n = 0	n = 5
	Change of:		
		IVIG	Placebo
	Improvement in scores of muscle strength	n = 8	n = 0
	Muscle strength scores increased	+10.3	No change or decreased after cross-over
	Neuromuscular symptoms score	+12.4	No change or decreased after cross-over
Adverse events	None reported		

Trial	Results and long-term follow-up of intravenous immunoglobulin infusions in chronic, refractory polymyositis: An open study with 35 adult patients	
Substance	**6 infusions of i. v. immunoglobulins at 1 mg/kg (mean dose 32.7 mg/day) for 2 consecutive 2 days every month** *Concomitant medication*: Corticosteroids were continued DMARDs were continued	
Result	Intravenous immunoglobulin therapy was effective in the majority of patients, even after discontinuation in half of the them	
Patients	35 adult white patients with chronic, refractory polymyositis (20 female and 15 male, mean age 43.5 years), diagnosed according to the criteria of Bohan and Peter	
Authors	Cherin P, Pelletier S, Teixeira A, Laforet P, Genereau T, Simon A, Maisonobe T, Eymard B, Herson S	
Publication	*Arthritis Rheum.* 2002;46(2):467–474	
Follow-up	4 years (mean 51.4 ± 13.1 months)	
Note	*i. v. immunoglobulin responders* (n = 25):	
	British Medical Research Council score	+14.5
	Muscle disability scale score	-12.7
	CK level (U/L)	-1590
	Mean dose of steroids (mg/day)	$32.7 \rightarrow 21.9$
	i. v. immunoglobulin nonresponders (n = 10):	
	British Medical Research Council score	+13.7
	Muscle disability scale score	-7.5
	CK level (U/L)	-940
	Mean dose of steroids (mg/day)	$29.8 \rightarrow 25.8$
Adverse events	Total	n = 29
	Mild headache	n = 4
	Fever with shivering and sweating	n = 3

Trial	Effects of intravenous immunoglobulin therapy in Japanese patients with polymyositis and dermatomyositis resistant to corticosteroids: A randomized double-blind placebo-controlled trial
Substance	**High-dose intravenous immunoglobulin 400 mg (drug code GB-0998) i. v. for 5 days** (IVIG, n = 12) **Placebo** (n = 14) *6-week run-in period*: Corticosteroid resistance was confirmed *Switch over* (*first vs. second period*): After 8 weeks (switch to IVIG n =14, to placebo n = 11) *Previous medication*: 50 mg corticosteroid/day therapy or 1 mg/kg/day ≥ 1 month ≥ 2 methylprednisolone pulse therapies within 6 weeks before the acquisition ≥ 30 mg/day or ≥ 0.6 mg/kg/day
Result	Intravenous immunoglobulin treatment with GB-0998 was safely used with the same precautions as other current IVIG therapy while there was no clear difference between the IVIG and the placebo group in terms of efficacy
Patients	26 patients with corticosteroid-refractory • Polymyositis (PM, n = 16) • Dermatomyositis (DM, n = 10), fulfilling the Bohan and Peter criteria for definite diagnosis
Authors	Miyasaka N, Hara M, Koike T, Saito E, Yamada M, Tanaka Y; Additional Members of the GB-0998 Study Group
Publication	*Mod Rheumatol*. 2012 Jun;22(3):382-93
Follow-up	20 weeks
Note	*Manual muscle test (normal ≥ 90)*:

	IVIG	Placebo
Week 1	33.3	21.4
Week 2	58.3	50.0
Week 4	75.0	64.3
Week 6	91.7	57.1
Week 8	91.7	57.1
First 8 weeks	91.7	57.1
Second 8 weeks	81.8	84.6

Change of:

	IVIG	Placebo
Manual muscle test	+11.8	+9.9
Creatinine kinase	-1.1633	-1.2662
Activities of daily living	+7.3	+4.0

(continued)

Adverse events	Total adverse events	n = 101 n = 99 after initiation of the first period
	Changes in clinical laboratory test results	n = 91
	Mild adverse events	n = 89
	Moderate adverse events	n = 11
	Severe adverse events	n = 1
	Adverse drug reactions	n = 19 (gingivitis, hyperkalemia, disorders of glucose tolerance, diarrhea, dry skin, perspiration disorder, oral herpes, eructation, nausea, increased serum CK, decreased muscle strength, hot sensation, purpura, chest pain, headache, increased serum b-D-glucan, increased blood pressure, bronchitis, and fatigue)
	Serious adverse events	n = 4

Trial	Methotrexate treatment of recalcitrant childhood dermatomyositis	
Substance	**20 mg/m² MTX/week**	
	Concomitant medication:	
	2 mg/kg prednisone/day	
	Additional treatment: 3 weeks of plasmapheresis and 3 months of tolmetin n = 1, 4 weeks of hydroxychloroquine in the other n = 2	
Result	Methotrexate in combination with prednisone was an effective treatment of recalcitrant childhood dermatomyositis	
Patients	16 patients with recalcitrant dermatomyositis	
Authors	Miller LC, Sisson BA, Tucker LB, DeNardo BA, Schaller JG	
Publication	*Arthritis Rheum*. 1992;35(10):1143–1149	
Follow-up	9.5–28 months	
Note	*Outcome parameters*:	
	Regaining muscle strength	n = 12
	Prednisone dosage could eventually be tapered to ≤ 5 mg/day	n = 11
	Normal CK levels	After 2 weeks
	Normal serum aldolase	After 8 weeks
Adverse events	Anemia (hematocrit 23–33%)	19%
	Poor compliance	6%
	Cellulitis	12.5%
	Pneumonia	6%
	Opportunistic infection	6%
	Abdominal pain mild-moderate	69%
	Abdominal pain severe	6%
	Diarrhea	31%
	Nausea and vomiting	6%
	Transient elevations of SGOT and SGPT	50%
	Stomatitis	8%
	Persistent elevation of SGOT and SGPT	8%
	Decreased pulmonary diffusion capacity	8%

Trial	Low-dose methotrexate administered weekly is an effective corticosteroid-sparing agent for the treatment of the cutaneous manifestations of dermatomyositis	
Substance	**Methotrexate oral 2.5–7.5 mg/week, increased as needed (range 2.5–30 mg/week)** Patients needed to avoid the sun *Concomitant medication*: 1% hydrocortisone ointment	
Result	Low-dose oral methotrexate administered weekly was effective in the treatment of the cutaneous manifestations of dermatomyositis and frequently enabled a reduction or discontinuation of corticosteroid therapy	
Patients	13 patients with dermatomyositis according to the criteria of Bohan and Peter	
Authors	Kasteler JS, Callen JP	
Publication	*J Am Acad Dermatol.* 1997;36(1):67–71	
Follow-up	3–22 months	
Note	*Outcome parameters*:	
	Free of all cutaneous manifestations of dermatomyositis	n = 4
	MTX allowed reduction of other therapies	n = 10
Adverse events	Nausea n = 6	

Trial	The effectiveness of treating juvenile dermatomyositis with methotrexate and aggressively tapered corticosteroids
Substance	**Methotrexate 10–20 mg/m²/week** (MTX, max. 25 mg/week, n = 31) **plus 2 mg/kg corticosteroids** (max. 75 mg/day) **2 mg/day corticosteroids only** (n = 22) Corticosteroids tapered aggressively after 6 weeks if possible *Flare*: Dose of prednisone was increased until control was achieved *Additional DMARD treatment*: Azathioprine 3.2% (patients), 0% (controls) Ciclosporin A 3.2% (patients), 0% (controls) Cyclophosphamide 3.2% (patients), 4.6% (controls) Hydroxychloroquine 19.4% (patients), 36.4% (controls) Methotrexate 27.2% (controls)
Result	Methotrexate in conjunction with an aggressively tapered course of prednisone was more effective than a traditional long-term corticosteroid therapy. The cumulative dose of corticosteroids was lower with methotrexate
Patients	31 consecutive children with dermatomyositis (patients) 22 patients with incident cases of juvenile dermatomyositis (controls) who received treatment just before the authors instituted a policy of first-line therapy with MTX
Authors	Ramanan AV, Campbell-Webster N, Ota S, Parker S, Tran D, Tyrrell PN, Cameron B, Spiegel L, Schneider R, Laxer RM, Silverman ED, Feldman BM
Publication	*Arthritis Rheum*. 2005;52(11):3570–3578
Follow-up	48 months
Note	*Outcome parameters*:

	Methotrexate	Control
Time to discontinuation of corticosteroids (months)	10	27

Change of:

	MTX	Control
Increase of BMI (kg/m²)	4.8	2.2
Height velocity (cm/a)	+4.1	+2.8
Rash at 3 years	33%	22%
Rash at 4 years	40%	24%

Adverse events	Methotrexate	Control
Cataract	n = 3	n = 8
Spinal fracture	n = 1	n = 2
Elevated liver enzymes	n = 6	n = 3

Trial	Ciclosporin A versus methotrexate in the treatment of polymyositis and dermatomyositis
Substance	**Prednisone 0.5–1 mg/kg/day** Tapered after week 4 If patients did not respond after 3 weeks **7.5–15 mg methotrexate/week** (MTX, n = 17) **3–3.5 mg/kg/day ciclosporin A** (CsA, n = 19) *Previous medication*: Nonresponsive to 0.5–1 g/kg prednisolone over 3 weeks
Patients	36 patients (20 with dermatomyositis, 16 with polymyositis) • No inclusion body myositis • Manual muscle test grade 3 in ≤ 2 muscle groups • Elevated CK levels
Result	Treatment of polymyositis or dermatomyositis with methotrexate or ciclosporin A added to corticosteroids was associated with an improvement of clinical and laboratory findings
Authors	Vencovský J, Jarosová K, Machácek S, Studýnková J, Kafková J, Bart nková J, Nemcová D, Charvát F
Publication	*Scand J Rheumatol.* 2000;29(2):95–102
Follow-up	6 months
Note	*Outcome parameters*:

	Methotrexate (%)	Ciclosporin A (%)
Muscle endurance and functional test improved	33	47
Muscle endurance and functional test unchanged	60	37
Clinical assessment improved	73	58
Clinical assessment unchanged	20	37
Patient's global assessment improved	67	68
Patient's global assessment unchanged	27	21

Change of:

	Methotrexate	Ciclosporin A
CK (Nkat/L)	-39.53	-13.6
Myoglobulin (mcg/L)	-483	-285
CRP (mg/L)	-7.8	-3.7
ANA positivity	-3%	-10%

(continued)

Adverse events		Methotrexate	Ciclosporin A
	Pancytopenia	n = 1	n = 0
	Gut perforation	n = 1	n = 0
	Acute alveolitis	n = 1	n = 0
	Petechiae	n = 1	n = 0
	Hypertension	n = 1	n = 3
	Rash	n = 1	n = 0
	Creatinine elevation	n = 0	n = 1
	Pneumonia	n = 0	n = 1
	Bronchitis	n = 0	n = 1
	Bronchopneumonia	n = 0	n = 1

Trial	Mycophenolate mofetil as an effective corticosteroid-sparing therapy for recalcitrant dermatomyositis	
Substance	**Mycophenolate mofetil 2 × 500–1´000 mg/day** (max. 3 g/day) *Concomitant medication*: Methotrexate was allowed Prednisone was allowed	
Result	Mycophenolate mofetil treatment of patients with dermatomyositis was effective	
Patients	12 patients with dermatomyositis • Skin lesions recalcitrant to or with toxic effects of traditional therapie	
Authors	Edge JC, Outland JD, Dempsey JR, Callen JP	
Publication	*Arch Dermatol.* 2006;142(1):65–69	
Note	Improvement in both cutaneous and muscular symptoms within 4–8 weeks	n = 10
Adverse events	B-cell lymphoma	n = 1
	Abnormal levels of hepatic enzymes	n = 1
	Leukopenia	n = 2
	Fatigue	n = 1

Trial	Mycophenolate mofetil in juvenile dermatomyositis: A case series
Substance	**800–1'350 mg/m² mycophenolate mofetil/day**
	Concomitant medication:
	0.3–2 mg/kg/day of prednisone-equivalent, mean 1.2 mg/kg/day
Result	Mycophenolate mofetil was safe in juvenile dermatomyositis
Patients	A retrospective chart review of 8 children diagnosed with juvenile dermatomyositis
Authors	Dagher R, Desjonquères M, Duquesne A, Quartier P, Bader-Meunier B, Fischbach M, Guiguonis V, Picherot G, Cimaz R
Publication	*Rheumatol Int.* 2010;32(3):711–716
Follow-up	3 months
Note	*Change of*:	
	Patient improvement in muscle strength	n = 5
	No change in muscle strength	n = 2
	Changes of muscle testing scores	+10.6
	Changes of manual muscle testing scores	+7
	Corticosteroid tapering	-18%
Adverse events	Transient neutropenia	n = 1

Trial	A randomized, pilot trial of etanercept in dermatomyositis
Substance	**Etanercept 50 mg/week** s. c. (n = 11) **Placebo** (n = 5) *Concomitant medication*: Prednisone in a standardized schedule as tolerated over the initial 24 weeks of the study No concurrent cyclophosphamide therapy No azathioprine or mycophenolate *Pervious therapy*: Prednisone for < 12 months Stable dosage of methotrexate ≥ 1 month Intravenous immunoglobulin ≥ 3 months
Result	Treatment of dermatomyositis with etanercept had a steroid-sparing effect and was not associated with any major safety concerns
Patients	16 patients with active dermatomyositis • Symmetric proximal weakness • Characteristic rash • Laboratory evidence of active dermatomyositis with elevated serum creatine kinase (CK) • Electromyography demonstrating myopathic features • Abnormal skeletal muscle magnetic resonance imaging • Or a muscle biopsy demonstrating perifascicular atrophy and perivascular inflammation • No juvenile DM, SLE, cancer, tuberculosis, active infection, chronic hepatitis B or C, other autoimmune neurological disorders
Authors	Amato AA, Tawil R, Kissel J, Barohn R, McDermott MP, Pandya S, King W, Smirnow A, Annis C, Roe K, Tawil R, McDermott MP, Janciuras J, Dilek N, Martens WB, Eastwood E, Amato A, Cochrane T, Donlan M, Chused S, Roe K, Barohn R, Dimachkie M, Aires DJ, Latinis KM, Herbelin L, Michaels H, Cupler E, Deodhar A, Simpson E, Burusnukul P, Edgar E, Serdar A, Brennan T, Gance K, Kissel J, Freimer ML, Hackshaw KV, Lawson V, King WM, Bartlett A, Wolfe G, Nations S, McLin R, Gorham N, Briemberg H, Chapman KM, Dutz JP, Wilson J, Varelas F, Wagner K, Stine LC, Anhalt GJ, Meyerle JH, Swain JO, Brock-Simmons R, Weiss M, Distad BJ, Lin J, Haug JA, Downing S
Publication	*Ann Neurol.* 2011 Sep;70(3):427–436
Follow-up	52 weeks
Note	*Change of (week 24)*:

	Etanercept	Placebo
Average Manual Muscle Testing (MMT) score	0.22	0.27

(continued) ➜

Average standardized Maximum Voluntary Isometric Contraction Testing (MVICT) score	1.58	0.59
Average percentage of predicted normal MVICT score	12.1	4.4
Time to walk 30 ft, s	-3.1	-1.9
Physician global activity assessment	-2.0	-1.0
Patient global activity assessment	-1.7	-2.1
Myositis Disease Activity Assessment Visual Analogue Scales (MYOACT) overall score	-0.029	-0.009
MYOACT muscle disease activity score	-1.14	-0.59
MYOACT cutaneous disease activity score	-0.84	0.07
Cutaneous Disease Activity Score Index (CDASI) score	-4.9	1.5
HAQ score	-0.44	-0.34
SF-36 Physical Component Summary score	7.0	5.7
SF-36 Mental Component Summary score	-7.6	-1.5
INQoL overall quality of life score	0.5	0.4
Log (creatine kinase), U/L	-0.10	0.16

Change of (week 52):

	Etanercept	Placebo
Average MMT score	0.27	0.21
Average standardized MVICT score	1.71	0.47
Average percentage of predicted normal MVICT score	13.0	5.3
Time to walk 30 ft, s	-1.2	-2.3
Physician global activity assessment	-2.4	-1.3
Patient global activity assessment	-2.4	-0.2
MYOACT overall score	-0.054	-0.003
MYOACT muscle disease activity score	-2.2	-0.79
MYOACT cutaneous disease activity score	-1.15	0.71
CDASI score	-3.1	-0.5
HAQ score	-0.34	-0.32
SF-36 Physical Component Summary score	7.5	1.1
SF-36 Mental Component Summary score	0.5	−0.8
INQoL overall quality of life score	-4.0	1.4
Log (creatine kinase), U/L	-0.11	-0.95

End of follow-up

(continued)

		Etanercept	Placebo
	Treatment failure	n = 6	n = 5
	Time to fail treatment (days)	208	125
	Median Prednisolone dosage from weeks 25–52 (mg/day)	1.2	29.2
	Time to walk 30 ft, s	-1.2	-2.3
	Physician global activity assessment	-2.4	-1.3
	Patient global activity assessment	-2.4	-0.2
	MYOACT overall score	-0.054	-0.003
	MYOACT muscle disease activity score	-2.2	-0.79
	MYOACT cutaneous disease activity score	-1.15	0.71
	CDASI score	-3.1	-0.5
	HAQ score	-0.34	-0.32
	SF-36 Physical Component Summary score	7.5	1.1
	SF-36 Mental Component Summary score	0.5	-0.8
	INQoL overall quality of life score	-4.0	1.4
	Log (creatine kinase), U/L	-0.11	-0.95
Adverse events		Etanercept	Placebo
	Serious adverse events	n = 6	n = 3
	New developed ANA	n = 2	n = 1

Trial	A high incidence of disease flares in an open pilot study of infliximab in patients with refractory inflammatory myopathies
Substance	**Infliximab 4 × 5 mg/kg i. v. at weeks 0, 2, 6 and 14** *Previous medication*: Failure to respond to treatment with high doses of glucocorticoids ≥ 6 months in combination with azathioprine and/or methotrexate
Result	Infliximab treatment was not effective in refractory inflammatory myopathies
Patients	13 patients with refractory • Polymyositis n = 5 • Dermatomyositis n = 4 • Inclusion body myositis n = 4 • Diagnosed according to the Bohan and Peter criteria (DM/PM), or Griggs criteria (IBM) • Persisting muscle weakness defined as (80% of muscle strength as measured by functional index) • Active disease was defined as muscle edema observed by MRI, or creatine kinase elevation, or inflammatory cell infiltrates in muscle biopsy
Authors	Dastmalchi M, Grundtman C, Alexanderson H, Mavragani CP, Einarsdottir H, Helmers SB, Elvin K, Crow MK, Nennesmo I, Lundberg IE
Publication	*Ann Rheum Dis*. 2008 Dec;67(12):1670–1677
Follow-up	14 weeks
Note	Improved by ≥ 20%	n = 3
	Improved in muscle strength	n = 0
Adverse events	Discontinued due to adverse events	n = 3
	Discovered malignancy	n = 1
	Developed new autoantibodies	n = 3
	Abdominal pain	n = 3
	Fatigue	n = 4
	Cough	n = 1
	Toxicodermia	n = 1
	Skin affection	n = 1

Trial	Rituximab in the treatment of dermatomyositis: An open-label pilot study
Substance	4 infusions of • **Rituximab 100 mg/m²** (first 3 patients) • **Rituximab 375 mg/m²** (n = 4) Given at weekly intervals Premedication with acetaminophen and diphenhydramine Previous corticosteroid treatment was continued at stable doses or tapered Previous DMARD treatment was continued at stable doses or tapered
Result	Rituximab was effective in patients with dermatomyositis refractory to other immunomodulatory treatment
Patients	7 adult patients with dermatomyositis • Patients had failed to ≤ 1 therapy (corticosteroids, ciclosporin A, methotrexate, IVIG, or other immunosuppressive therapy) • Average muscle strength of < 75%
Authors	Levine TD
Publication	*Arthritis Rheum.* 2005;52(2):601–607
Follow-up	36–52 weeks

Note	*Outcome parameters*:	
	Major clinical improvement	n = 7 (evident n = 1, after min. 4 weeks)
	Muscle strength increased	36–113%
	Return of symptoms	n = 4
	Maintained increased muscle strength at 52 weeks	n = 2
	Creatine kinase levels (range, units/L, range)	128–5'600 → 57–1'168
	FVC improvement	n = 2
	Improvement of hair growth after Alopecia	n = 2
Adverse events	Shortness of breath and hypertension	n = 1
	Cellulitis (grade 3)	n = 1

Trial	A pilot trial of Rituximab in the treatment of patients with dermatomyositis
Substance	**Rituximab (1 g each i. v.) 2 weeks apart**
	Without peri-infusional steroids
	Concomitant medication:
	Continue treatment with topical corticosteroids or immunomodulators
	Continue oral corticosteroids
	Continue antimalarial agents, mycophenolate mofetil, methotrexate, azathioprine at stable doses
Result	Rituximab treatment had modest effects on muscle disease and limited effects on skin disease
Patients	8 adult patients with dermatomyositis, according to the criteria of Bohan and Peter
	≤ 2 of the following criteria:
	• Symmetrical weakness
	• Muscle biopsy features consistent with dermatomyositis
	• Elevation of muscle enzyme levels
	• Electromyographic evidence of muscle inflammation
	• Skin biopsy findings consistent with dermatomyositis
	Mild muscle disease:
	• Modified Medical Research Council
	• Manual Muscle Test (MMT) score < 85
	• Elevation of CPK (> 400 U/L)
	• Aldolase (> 8.0 U/L)
	• Dermatomyositis Skin Severity Index (DSSI) score > 2
	• No cardiac or pulmonary disease, active infection, hepatitis B, hepatitis C, HIV, malignancies
Authors	Chung L, Genovese MC, Fiorentino DF
Publication	*Arch Dermatol.* 2007;143(6):763–767
Follow-up	24 weeks
Note	*Outcome parameters*:

Partial remission	n = 3
DSSI	−9.5%
Subjective assessments changed substantially	n = 0
Creatine kinase levels stable values	n = 3
Creatine kinase levels increasing	n = 1
Change of:	
Creatine kinase level	+17.80%
Aldolase levels	+15.13%

(continued)

Adverse events	Serious infections	n = 0
	Mild infusion reactions (headache, transient hypertension, congestion with facial flushing)	n = 3
	Increase in liver transaminase levels	n = 1 (resolved with the discontinuation of azathioprine)
	Superficial skin infections	n = 2
	Bronchitis	n = 3
	Sinusitis	n = 2
	Urinary tract infection	n = 1
	Otitis media	n = 1
	Death of metastatic cancer	n = 1
	Cellulitis (grade 3)	n = 1

Trial	Rituximab treatment in patients with refractory inflammatory myopathies
Substance	**Rituximab 2 × 1´000 mg i. v., 2 weeks apart** Retreatment with rituximab was conducted if disease activity relapsed *Concomitant medication*: 50 mg methylprednisolone i. v. 2 mg clemastine i. v. *Previous medication*: Immunosuppressive therapy was continued, tapering was permitted Oral corticosteroids were continued, tapering was permitted
Result	Rituximab was an effective treatment in refractory inflammatory myopathies
Patients	13 patients with dermatomyositis or polymyositis, according to the criteria of Bohan and Peter • Typical histological abnormalities in muscle biopsy • Refractory was defined as having failed to respond to at least corticosteroids and one other immunosuppressive drug
Authors	Mahler EA, Blom M, Voermans NC, van Engelen BG, van Riel PL, Vonk MC
Publication	*Rheumatology (Oxford)*. 2011 Dec;50(12):2206–2213
Follow-up	27 months (median)
Note	*Change of*:

Creatinine kinase	-93.2%
Lactate dehydrogenase	-39.8%
Muscle strength (median)	+21.5%
Manual muscle testing at 24 months	+33.3%
ESR (mm/h)	-7.0, -90.1%
HAQ (6 months)	-0.69
SF-36, physical component scale (median, 22.6 months)	+10.9

Adverse events	Hospitalized during rituximab courses	n = 3
	Gastroenteritis	n = 1
	Fever	n = 1
	Heart failure	n = 1

Trial	Controlled trial of plasma exchange and leukapheresis in polymyositis and dermatomyositis
Substance	**Plasma exchange** (replacement of 1–1.5 volume of plasma with 5% albumin in saline, n = 13) **Leukapheresis** (removal of 5–10 × 10^9 lymphocytes, n = 13) **Sham apheresis** (3 × /week, n = 13) 12 treatments given over a 1-month period *Concomitant medication*: Corticosteroid were continued *Previous medication*: Prednisone ≤ 0.25 mg/kg/day for ≤ 1 month Cytotoxic therapy n = 19 (plasma exchange), n = 9 (leukapheresis), n = 10 (Sham apheresis)
Result	Leukapheresis and plasma exchange were no more effective than sham apheresis as treatments of corticosteroid-resistant polymyositis or dermatomyositis
Patients	39 patients with definite polymyositis or dermatomyositis according to the criteria of Bohan and Peter • Biopsy proven • Incomplete response to corticosteroids • No inclusion body myositis • ≤ 16 years of age
Authors	Miller FW, Leitman SF, Cronin ME, Hicks JE, Leff RL, Wesley R, Fraser DD, Dalakas M, Plotz PH
Publication	*N Engl J Med.* 1992;326(21):1380–1384
Follow-up	Mean 3.2 years

Note — *Outcome parameters*:

	Plasma exchange	Leukapheresis	Sham apheresis
Condition improved	n = 3	n = 3	n = 3
Condition deteriorated	n = 1	n = 3	n = 0
No change	n = 9	n = 7	n = 10
Effective tapering of prednisone	n = 1	n = 2	n = 0

No significant differences among the three treatment groups in the final muscle strength or functional capacity of the patients

Adverse events

	Plasma exchange	Leukapheresis	Sham apheresis
Require placement of central venous catheter to maintain venous access	n = 0	n = 9	n = 0
Major vasovagal episodes	n = 0	n = 3	n = 0
Clinical important citrate reactions	n = 0	n = 2	n = 0
Decline of hematocrit	n = 0	n = 0	n = 1

Trial	Efficacy of allogeneic mesenchymal stem cell transplantation in patients with drug-resistant polymyositis and dermatomyositis	
Substance	**1 × 10⁶ cells/kg allogeneic mesenchymal stem cells** Obtained from bone marrow or umbilical cord Prepared by the Stem Cell Center of Jiangsu Province, China, derived from passage 2 to passage 5 *Previous medication*: Incomplete response to moderate-to-high doses of glucocorticoids (prednisone > 15 mg/day or its equivalent) ≥ 1 immunosuppressant drug for > 3 months	
Result	Mesenchymal stem cell transplantation (MSCT) was safe and effective in drug-resistant patients with polymyositis and dermatomyositis	
Patients	10 patients with polymyositis and dermatomyositis meeting the criteria of Bohan and Peter • Refractory to standard treatment, or • Severe systemic involvement	
Authors	Wang D, Zhang H, Cao M, Tang Y, Liang J, Feng X, Wang H, Hua B, Liu B, Sun L	
Publication	*Ann Rheum Dis.* 2011 Jul;70(7):1285–1288	
Follow-up	24 months	
Note	Improvements CK, CK-MB, patient global assessment, and muscle strength	All patients
	Interstitial lung disease	n = 1
	Improvement in chronic nonhealing skin ulcers	n = 1
	Relapse	n = 3, after 6, and 8 months
	CK Level (U/l)	
	Baseline	2´958
	1 month	1´274
	2 months	599
	3 months	109
	4 months	401
Adverse events	Common cold 3 months after the second MSCT leading to deterioration of the disease and death	n = 1

Sjögren's Syndrome

Hydroxychloroquine

Trial	Antimalarials in treatment of Sjögren's syndrome	
Substance	**300 mg/day chloroquine for 3 weeks than 150 mg/day** or **800 mg/day hydroxychloroquine for 3 weeks than 400 mg/day** No information on concomitant medication	
Result	Treatment of Sjögren's syndrome with hydroxychloroquine was effective	
Patients	25 patients with Sjögren's Syndrome • Duration of ocular symptoms 2–20a years	
Authors	Heaton JM	
Publication	*Br Med J.* 1959;1(5136):1512–1513	
Follow-up	4–22 weeks	
Note	*Outcome parameters*:	
	Patients failed to improve	n = 6
	Patients improving	n = 14
	Patients with great improvement	n = 4
	Schirmer's test	No change, subjective amelioration
Adverse events	Stopped because of adverse events	n = 3
	Total patients with adverse events	n = 6
	Nausea	n = 4
	Diarrhea	n = 3
	Malaise	n = 1

R. Müller, J. von Kempis, *Clinical Trials in Rheumatology*,
DOI 10.1007/978-1-4471-2870-0_9, © Springer-Verlag London 2013

Trial	Hydroxychloroquine treatment for primary Sjögren's syndrome: a 2 year double blind cross over trial
Substance	**2 × 200 mg hydroxychloroquine/day** (HCQ → placebo, n = 10) for 1 year
	Placebo (placebo → HCQ, n = 9) for 1 year
	Groups were crossed over after 1 year
	Drug treatment at entry:
	Tear substitutes n = 10
	Salvia substitutes n = 2
	Sedatives n = 6
	NSAIDs n = 4
	Antihypertensive drugs n = 4
	Anticonvulsant drugs n = 2
	L-Thyroxine n = 2
	Insulin n = 2
	Calcium carbonate n = 3
	Lactulose n = 3
	Previous medication:
	No corticosteroids
	No immunosuppressive drugs ≥ 3 months prior study inclusion
Result	Hydroxychloroquine treatment did not show a worthwhile clinical benefit
Patients	19 patients with Sjögren's syndrome
	• Median disease duration 3.0 years
	• No previous immunosuppressive drug treatment
	• No retinitis pigmentosa
	• No RA, SLE, systemic sclerosis, or mixed connective tissue disease
Authors	Kruize AA, Hene RJ, Kallenberg CGM, van Bijsterveld A, van der Heijden A, Kater L, Bijlsma JWJ
Publication	*Ann Rheum Dis*. 1993;52:360–364
Follow-up	2 years

(continued) ➔

Note	Outcome parameters:		
		HCQ → placebo	Placebo → HCQ
	Study not completed	n = 4	n = 4
	Received corticosteroids, because of progressive PNP	n = 1	n = 1
	Burkitt's lymphoma	n = 1	n = 0
	Tears lysozyme concentration (mg/mL):		
		HCQ → placebo	Placebo → HCQ
	Baseline	1´555	1´145
	1 year	1´630	1´345
	2 years	1´590	1´320
	Tear lactoferrin concentration (mm precipitation):		
		HCQ → placebo	Placebo → HCQ
	Baseline	8.1	6.3
	1 year	8.7	8.4
	2 years	10.7	7.2
	Schirmer's test (mm/5 min):		
		HCQ → placebo	Placebo → HCQ
	Baseline	8.4	7.8
	1 year	6.8	8.1
	2 years	8.9	7.0
	Break up time (s):		
		HCQ → placebo	Placebo → HCQ
	Baseline	1.9	4.8
	1 year	2.6	3.5
	2 years	2.5	1.5
	Rose Bengal test (score 0–9):		
		HCQ → placebo	Placebo → HCQ
	Baseline	3.7	3.9
	1 year	5.7	5.4
	2 years	5.7	6.1
	Abnormal/normal scintigraphy (Technecium):		
		HCQ → placebo	Placebo → HCQ
	Baseline	n = 4/1	n = 3/2
	1 year	n = 4/1	n = 3/2
	2 years	n = 4/1	n = 3/2
	Abnormal/normal scintigraphy (Gallium 67):		
		HCQ → placebo	Placebo → HCQ
	Baseline	n = 4/1	n = 4/1
	1 year	n = 4/1	n = 3/2
	2 years	n = 4/1	n = 1/1
	No differences between groups in:		
	Feeling of dryness in the eye, swelling of the salivary gland, fatigue, myalgia, arthralgia, inflammatory reaction of the eye lid		
Adverse events		HCQ	Placebo
	Psychological problems	n = 0	n = 1
	Moderate deterioration of liver function tests	n = 1	n = 0

Trial	Hydroxychloroquine improves dry eye symptoms of patients with primary Sjögren's syndrome		
Substance	**Withdrawal of hydroxychloroquine for 12 weeks** *Previous medication*: HCQ therapy 6.5 mg/kg for at least 2 years *Concomitant medication*: No other medication rather than low dose nonsteroid antiinflammatory drugs or ≤ 10 mg prednisone/day		
Result	Discontinuation of hydroxychloroquine lead to worsening of signs and symptoms of dry eye		
Patients	32 patients with primary Sjögren's syndrome • According to the American/European consensus group • No systemic manifestations other than arthritis or arthralgia		
Authors	Yavuz S, Asfuroğlu E, Bicakcigil M, Toker E		
Publication	*Rheumatol Int.* 2011 Aug;31(8):1045–1049		
Follow-up	12 weeks		
Note	*Change of*:		
		Baseline	12 weeks
	Ocular surface disease index	27.5	29.1
	Symptom severity score	3.1	9.1
	Schirmer's test (mm)	8.0	9.0
	Schirmer's test with anesthesia (mm)	5.0	5.0
	Tear break-up time (s)	7.9	5.9
	Corneal fluorescein in staining score	1.3	1.8
	Oxford score	6.6	13.8
	Average tear drop/day	3.9	4.8
	BAFF levels (ng/mL)	0.8	4.0

Trial	Safety and efficacy of Leflunomide in primary Sjögren's syndrome: a Phase II pilot study
Substance	**20 mg leflunomide/day** (no loading dose) No information on concomitant medication was provided
Result	The efficacy of leflunomide in the treatment of Sjögren's syndrome was modest. The safety profile was acceptable
Patients	15 patients with primary Sjögren's syndrome with early and active disease meeting the European-American Consensus group classification criteria • Sicca complaints ≤ 60 months • Diagnosis established (≤ 36 months) • ESR ≥ 20 mm/h • Serum IgG ≥ 15 mg/L • No hepatic or renal impairment, severe infection or malignancy other than mucosa-associated lymphoid tissue lymphoma
Authors	van Woerkom JM, Kruize AA, Geenen R, van Roon EN, Goldschmeding R, Verstappen SM, van Roon JA, Bijlsma JW
Publication	*Ann Rheum Dis.* 2007;66(8):1026–1032
Follow-up	24 weeks
Note	*Change of*:

VAS general health (0–100 mm)	-7
VAS dry eyes (0–100 mm)	+7
VAS sandy feeling (0–100 mm)	+8
VAS dry mouth (0–100 mm)	-15
VAS sleep disturbance due to dryness (0–100 mm)	-5
Multidimensional fatigue inventory general fatigue	-6
Zung depression score	+4.5
ESR (mm/h)	-6
CRP (g/L)	-1.9
Serum IgA (g/L)	-0.5
Serum IgG (g/L)	-3.4
Serum IgM (g/L)	-0.4
Rheumatoid factor (U/L)	-255
Schirmer's test (mm/5 min)	+3.7
Sialometry (mL/15 min)	+0.1

(continued)

Adverse events	Diarrhea	47%
	GI discomfort	40%
	Anorexia	13%
	Oral ulcers	13%
	Hair loss	47%
	Headache	33%
	Fatigue/lethargy	20%
	Dysesthesia	13%
	Dizziness	26%
	Alcohol intolerance	6%
	Weight loss > 2 kg	33%
	Dyspnea	6%
	Increasing transpiration	6%
	Increasing conjunctivitis	13%
	Pharyngitis	13%
	Decreasing libido	6%
	Mood changes	6%
	Decreasing taste	6%
	ALAT 1–2 × upper normal limits	13%
	ALAT 2 × upper normal limits	13%
	Increase of pre-existing arterial hypertension	13%
	LE skin lesions	33%
	Other skin lesions	20%
	Leukopenia ($3\text{–}4 \times 10^9$/L)	26%
	Leukopenia ($< 3 \times 10^9$/L)	13%
	Anemia < 7.4 mmol/L	33%

Trial	Methotrexate in primary Sjögren's syndrome
Substance	**0.2 mg methotrexate (MTX)/kg/week** *Concomitant medication*: Oral and tear substitution was continued *Previous medication*: 2 months of washout of other therapeutics
Result	Methotrexate improved symptoms of Sjögren's syndrome in a substantial proportion of patients
Patients	18 patients with primary Sjögren's syndrome • Diagnosis according the European community study group criteria • Focus score on salivary gland biopsy > 3/4 mm²
Authors	Skopouli FN, Jagiello P, Tsifetaki N, Moutsopoulos HM
Publication	*Clin Exp Rheumatol.* 1996;14(5):555–558
Follow-up	12 months
Note	*Outcome parameters*:

	6 months	12 months
Subjective symptoms of dry eyes	n = 7	n = 6
Subjective symptoms of dry eyes	n = 7	n = 7
Improvement of dry cough	n = 6	
No improvement of dry cough	n = 5	
Improvement of arthralgia	n = 8	n = 4
Improvement of fatigue	n = 11	n = 6
Improvement of purpura	n = 3	n = 0

Adverse events	Persistent elevation of the hepatic transaminase levels	n = 7 (→ reduction of MTX)
	Anemia and leukopenia	n = 2

Trial	Mycophenolate sodium treatment in patients with primary Sjögren's syndrome: a pilot trial
Substance	**360 mg mycophenolate sodium/day, increased weekly up to 1´440 mg/day** *Previous medication*: No concomitant DMARDs ≤ 8 weeks prior to randomization No prednisolone (or equivalent) ≥ 5 mg/day ≤ 4 weeks prior randomization No secretagogues (pilocarpine and civemeline) or tricyclic antidepressants and anticholinergic drugs
Result	Mycophenolate sodium improved signs and symptoms of patients with shorter disease duration
Patients	11 patients with primary Sjögren's syndrome, active disease, meeting the European-American Consensus criteria • ESR > 25 mm/h • IgG > 1'500 mg/dL • Autoantibodies (anti-SSA, SSB antibodies and/or rheumatoid factor)
Authors	Willeke P, Schlüter B, Becker H, Schotte H, Domschke W, Gaubitz M
Publication	*Arthritis Res Ther.* 2007;9(6):R115
Follow-up	24 weeks
Note	*Change of*:	
	Schirmer's test (mm per 5 min)	+2.4
	Whole saliva (g per 5 min)	+0.07
	Swollen/tender joint count	0.0
	Erythrocyte sedimentation rate (mm/h)	-3.4
	IgG (mg/dL)	-0.134
	IgM (mg/dL)	-47
	IgA (mg/dL)	-70
	Rheumatoid factor IgM (IU/mL)	-96
	Anti-SSA antibodies (U/mL)	+0.029
	Anti-SSB antibodies (U/mL)	+0.103
	VAS sicca syndrome (0–100 mm)	-15.9
	VAS arthralgia (0–100 mm)	-14.6
	VAS fatigue (0–100 mm)	+1.9
	Use of artificial teardrops (times per day)	-2.1
	Health assessment questionnaire score	0.0
Adverse events	Vertigo	n = 1
	Gastrointestinal complaints	n = 4
	Pneumonia	n = 1
	Herpes labialis	n = 1
	Common cold	n = 2

Trial	Pilocarpine tablets for the treatment of dry mouth and dry eye symptoms in patients with Sjögren's syndrome: a randomized, placebo-controlled, fixed dose, multicenter trial. P92-01 Study group
Substance	**Pilocarpine 4 × 2.5 mg/day** (n = 121) **Pilocarpine 4×5 mg/day** (n = 127) **Placebo** tablets 4 times daily (n = 125) *Concomitant medication used*: Analgesic or antiinflammatory drugs (aspirin, ibuprofen, naproxen, acetaminophen, and prednisone) Antirheumatic drugs (HCQ, MTX) Gastrointestinal tract agents (omeprazole) Hormonal replacement drugs (estrogen, medroxyprogesterone) Thyroid preparations (levothyroxine sodium)
Result	Pilocarpine treatment was well-tolerated and lead to a significant improvement of sicca symptoms
Patients	373 Patients with Sjögren's syndrome, fulfilling the European Cooperative Community Classification criteria *With at least one of the following*: • Auto-antibodies against SS-A or SS-B • Rheumatoid factor, or ANA ≥ 1:160 • Positive labial minor salivary gland biopsy sample • Positive lip biopsy samples required a focus score > 1 focus per 4 mm² • Clinically significant dry mouth and dry eye symptoms
Authors	Vivino FB, Al-Hashimi I, Khan Z, LeVeque FG, Salisbury PL III, Tran-Johnson TK, Muscoplat CC, Trivedi M, Goldlust B, Gallagher SC
Publication	*Arch Intern Med*. 1999;159(2):174–181
Follow-up	12 weeks

(continued) ➔

Note	*Salivary flow rates at onset (mL/min):*		
		Placebo	Pilocarpine 5 mg
	Before dosing	0.11	0.11
	30 min after dosing	0.12	0.34
	60 min after dosing	0.13	0.34
	90 min after dosing	0.13	0.27
	60 min after dosing after follow-up:		
		Placebo	Pilocarpine 5 mg
	Week 6	0.15	0.33
	Week 12	0.17	0.38
	Change of:		
		Placebo (%)	Pilocarpine 5 mg (%)
	Dry mouth improvement	31.1	61.3
	Dry eyes, improvement	26.1	42.0

Adverse events		Placebo (%)	Pilocarpine 2.5 mg (%)	Pilocarpine 5 mg (%)
	Sweating	7.2	10.7	43.3
	Headache	24.8	20.7	15.8
	Flu symptoms	8.8	13.2	14.2
	Nausea	8.8	12.4	11.8
	Rhinitis	5.6	7.4	10.2
	Dizziness	8.8	5.0	0.2
	Urinary frequency	1.6	10.7	9.5

Trial	Etanercept in the treatment of patients with primary Sjögren's syndrome: a pilot study
Substance	**2 × 25 mg etanercept/week** s. c. *Concomitant medication*: No concomitant DMARDs No corticosteroids
Result	Treatment with etanercept did not reduce sicca symptoms and other signs of the disease but was beneficial in a small subgroup of patients with severe fatigue
Patients	15 patients with well-defined primary Sjögren's syndrome meeting the European-American Consensus group classification criteria • Evidence of sublabial minor salivary gland biopsy indicated by a lymphocytic focus score > 1 • IgA-containing plasma cells percentage < 70%
Authors	Zandbelt MM, de Wilde P, van Damme P, Hoyng CB, van de Putte L, van den Hoogen F
Publication	*J Rheumatol.* 2004;31(1):96–101
Follow-up	24 weeks
Note	*Change of VAS-Scores*:

	All patients	Responders only
General fatigue	-2.7	-2.1
Physical fatigue	-2.2	-1.2
Reduced activity	-0.9	+0.9
Reduced motivation	-0.9	-0.2
Mental fatigue	-2.5	-3.0
ESR (mm/h)	-4	-4
CRP (mg/L)	-1	+1
Gammaglobulin (g/L)	0	+2
Lymphocytic focus score (week 12)	-0.73	-0.54
IgA% (week 12)	-1.7	-1.4
IgM RF (U/L week 12)	-5	-14

Trial	Etanercept in Sjögren's Syndrome		
Substance	**2 × 25 mg etanercept/week** (n = 14) **Placebo** (n = 14) *Concomitant medication*: Continue long-term medications No tricyclic antidepressants No anticholinergics		
Result	Etanercept was not effective		
Patients	28 patients with Sjögren's syndrome meeting the European-American Consensus group classification criteria • With oral and ocular dryness • Evidence of active Sjögren's Syndrome (elevated ESR or IgG levels)		
Authors	Sankar V, Brennan MT, Kok MR, Leakan RA, Smith JA, Manny J, Baum BJ, Pillemer SR		
Publication	*Arthritis Rheum.* 2004;50(7):2240–2245		
Follow-up	12 weeks		
Note	*Change of*:		
		ETN	Placebo
	Dry mouth (100-mm VAS)	-2	+3
	Dry eyes, by 100-mm VAS	+1	-0.5
	Schirmer I test, mm/5 min	-0.75	-0.50
	van Bijsterveld score	0.0	-0.25
	Total stimulated saliva flow (mL/min)	-0.033	-0.22
	IgG (mg/dL)	+10	-30
	ESR (mm/h)	-5.5	+1.5

Trial	Infliximab in patients with primary Sjögren's syndrome: a pilot study
Substance	**3 × infliximab (3 mg/kg), at 0, 2, and 6 weeks** *Concomitant medication*: No DMARDs ≤ 4 weeks before baseline No corticosteroids ≤ 4 weeks before baseline Continue artificial tears
Patients	16 primary Sjögren's syndrome patients fulfilling the European and the ACR classification criteria • ESR > 25 mm/h • Hypergammaglobulinemia > 1.4 g/L
Result	In patients with active disease, a loading-dose regimen of three infusions of infliximab provided a fast and significant clinical benefit without major adverse reactions
Authors	Steinfeld SD, Demols P, Salmon I, Kiss R, Appelboom T
Publication	*Arthritis Rheum.* 2001;44(10):2371–2375
Follow-up	14 weeks
Note	*Change of*:	
	Patient's global assessment (0–100-mm VAS)	-41.5
	Patient's assessment of pain	-60.5
	Physician's global assessment (0–100-mm VAS)	-26.5
	Tender joint count (0–64 joints)	-5
	Tender point count (0–18 tender points)	-14.5
	Global fatigue (0–100-mm VAS)	-32.5
	Fatigue questionnaire (0–3 scale)	-2
	ESR (mm/h)	-11
	IgG (< 1'000 mg/L)	+0.23
	White blood cell count (× 1'000/mm³)	+0.7
	CD4+ cells/mm³	+37
	CD8+ cells/mm³	+25
	Dry eyes questionnaire (0–2 scale)	-1
	Fluorescein tear film break-up time (seconds/5 min)	+2.5
	Schirmer I test (mm/5 min)	+1.5
	Lissamine green staining (0–9 scale)	-0.5
	Dry mouth questionnaire(0–2 scale)	-0.7
	Speech test ("puttica"/2 min)	+39.5
	Unstimulated salivary flow (mL/min)	+0.59
Adverse events	Facial erythema and dyspnea	n = 1
	Mild respiratory tract infections	n = 2
	Develop any symptoms suggestive of SLE	n = 0 (1 patient with dsDNA antibodies before study entry)

TRIPSS-Trial	Inefficacy of Infliximab in primary Sjögren's syndrome: results of the randomized, controlled Trial of Remicade in Primary Sjögren's Syndrome (TRIPSS) TRIPSS: Trial of Remicade in Primary Sjögren's Syndrome
Substance	**5 mg/kg infliximab (IFX, n = 54) at weeks 0, 2, 6** **Placebo** (n = 49) *Concomitant medication*: No pilocarpine MTX, azathioprine, 6-mercaptopurine, hydroxychloroquine at stable doses Corticosteroids ($\geq$ 15 mg/day) at stable doses
Result	Infliximab in primary Sjögren's syndrome was not effective
Patients	103 patients with primary Sjöegrens' syndrome fulfilling the American-European Consensus group criteria for Sjöegren's syndrome • Positive for anti-Ro/SSA or anti-La/SSB • Active disease as defined by VAS > 50/100 mm for: ∘ Joint pain ∘ Fatigue ∘ The most disturbing buccal, ocular, skin, vaginal, and bronchial dryness
Authors	Mariette X, Ravaud P, Steinfeld S, Baron G, Goetz J, Hachulla E, Combe B, Puéchal X, Pennec Y, Sauvezie B, Perdriger A, Hayem G, Janin A, Sibilia J
Publication	*Arthritis Rheum*. 2004;50(4):1270–1276
Follow-up	22 weeks

(continued) ➔

Note	Outcome parameters (Week 22):		
		Placebo (%)	IFX (%)
	30% decrease in two of three VAS-scores (see inclusion)	20.4	16.7
	30% decrease in pain VAS	26.5	20.4
	30% decrease in fatigue VAS	24.5	24.1
	30% decrease in dryness VAS	16.3	16.7
	Favorable response:		
		Placebo (%)	IFX (%)
	Week 10	26.5	27.8
	Week 22	20.4	16.7
	Change of:		
		Placebo	IFX
	Salivary flow rate (mL/min)	+0.02	+0.03
	Schirmer's test (mm/5 min)	+1.5	+0.9
	Swollen joint count	-0.3	-0.4
	Tender joint count	-2.3	-2.4
	ESR (mm/h)	-0.9	-0.8
	CRP (mg/L)	-0.5	-0.4
	Gamma globulin (g/L)	+0.13	+0.78
	IgG (g/L)	+0.03	+0.74
	IgA (g/L)	+0.09	+0.16
	IgM (g/L)	+0.04	+0.34
Adverse events		Placebo	IFX
	Total	n = 1	n = 6
	Infusion reactions	n = 0	n = 2
	Cutaneous facial eruption	n = 0	n = 1
	Autoimmune hepatitis	n = 0	n = 1
	Pneumococcal septicemia	n = 0	n = 1
	Breast cancer	n = 0	n = 1
	Polyclonal lymph node enlargement	n = 1	n = 0

Trial	Rituximab treatment in patients with primary Sjögren's syndrome: an open label Phase II study
Substance	**Rituximab (4 times once weekly 4 × 375 mg/m²)** *After pretreatment with*: 25 mg prednisone 2 mg clemastine 1 g acetaminophen *Concomitant medication*: No DMARDs No Corticosteroids
Result	Rituximab was effective. A high incidence of human antichimeric antibodies and associated side effects was observed
Patients	15 patients with primary Sjöegren's syndrome (SS), fulfilling the European-American Consensus criteria • B cell hyperactivity (IgG > 15 g/L) • Presence of autoantibodies (IgM rheumatoid factor, anti-SSA/SSB) • Disease duration < 4 years • Treatment with DMARDS (e.g., hydroxychloroquine, methotrexate, ciclosporin), and corticosteroids was not allowed during the study
Authors	Pijpe J, van Imhoff GW, Spijkervet FK, Roodenburg JL, Wolbink GJ, Mansour K, Vissink A, Kallenberg CG, Bootsma H
Publication	*Arthritis Rheum.* 2005;52(9):2740–2750
Follow-up	12 weeks

(continued)

Note	Change of:		
		Primary SS	MALT/SS
	Un-stimulated whole saliva (mL/min)	+0.04	+0.01
	Stimulated whole saliva (mL/min)	+0.2	+0.01
	Parotid stimulated secretion (mL/min)	+0.06	+0.01
	Na^{2+} in parotid saliva (mmol/L)	-11	0
	Schirmer's test (mm/5 min)	+5	+1
	Rose Bengal score	-2	-2
	Tear break-up time (s)	+5	-1
	General fatigue	-9	-3
	Physical fatigue	-7	0
	Reduced activity	-7	+1
	Reduced motivation	-5	0
	Mental fatigue	-2	0
	SF-36 physical functioning	+84	-5
	SF-36 social functioning	+12	+38
	SF-36 role physical	-2	0
	SF-36 role emotional	0	-65
	SF-36 mental health	+4	+8
	SF-36 vitality	+27	+10
	SF-36 bodily pain	+22	0
	SF-36 general health perception	+17	+5
	SF-36 health change	+50	+50
Adverse events		Primary SS	MALT/SS
	Infusion reaction	n = 2	n = 0
	Herpes zoster developed	n = 1	n = 0
	Human antichimeric antibodies	n = 4	n = 0

Trial	Tolerance and efficacy of rituximab and changes in serum B cell biomarkers in patients with systemic complications of primary Sjögren's syndrome	
Substance	**375 mg/m² rituximab (RTX) infusions × 4** (n = 14) **375 mg/m² rituximab infusions × 6** (n =1) **2 × 1 g rituximab infusions** (n = 1) *Concomitant medication*: Pretreatment with immunomodulatory agents n = 9 Concomitant immunosuppressives n = 4	
Result	Rituximab was effective and steroid sparing in patients with severe systemic manifestations in this retrospective study. It achieved complete remissions in four of five patients with lymphoma	
Patients	16 patients with primary Sjögren's syndrome according to the American/European consensus group criteria, with lymphoma or severe systemic complications • Disease duration 16.3 years (mean) • RTX prescribed for lymphoma n = 4 • Refractory pulmonary disease with polysynovitis n = 2 • Severe polysynovitis n = 2 • Mixed cryoglobulinemia n = 5 • Thrombocytopenia n = 1 • Mononeuritis multiplex n = 1	
Authors	Seror R, Sordet C, Guillevin L, Hachulla E, Masson C, Ittah M, Candon S, Le Guern V, Aouba A, Sibilia J, Gottenberg JE, Mariette X	
Publication	*Ann Rheum Dis.* 2007;66(3):351–357	
Follow-up	14.5 months (median)	
Note	*Outcome parameters*:	
	Remission of lymphoma	80%, n = 4
	Relapse of lymphoma	n = 1
	Efficacy for (*examples*):	
	Systemic symptoms	82%
	Cutaneous vasculitis	100%
	Glandular features	100%
	Corticosteroid reduction	n = 7
	Corticosteroid discontinuation	n = 4
	Relapses (non lymphoma)	n = 4
	Time to relapse (median)	8 months
Adverse events	Flue-like syndrome and mild herpetic eruption	n = 1
	Fever, arthralgia, and purpuric lesion	n = 1
	Fever, arthralgia, and urticaria	n = 1

Trial	Improvement of Sjögren's syndrome after two infusions of Rituximab (anti-CD20)	
Substance	**375 mg/m² rituximab infusions** (100 mg/h) weeks 0 and 1 No concomitant corticosteroids No cytotoxic drugs ≥ 4 months	
Result	Low dose rituximab infusions were well-tolerated and improved clinical signs and symptoms	
Patients	16 patients with primary Sjögren's syndrome meeting the European-American Consensus group criteria > 2 out of: • Global disease > 50 (VAS; 100 mm) • Global pain > 50 (VAS; 100 mm) • Global fatigue > 50 (VAS; 100 mm) • Global dryness > 50 (VAS; 100 mm)	
Authors	Devauchelle-Pensec V, Pennec Y, Morvan J, Pers JO, Daridon C, Jousse-Joulin S, Roudaut A, Jamin C, Renaudineau Y, Roué IQ, Cochener B, Youinou P, Saraux A	
Publication	*Arthritis Rheum.* 2007;57(2):310–317	
Follow-up	36 weeks	
Note	*Change of (week 36):*	
	Global disease (VAS, mm)	-16.9
	Pain (VAS, mm)	-27.4
	Fatigue (VAS, mm)	-19.3
	Dryness (VAS, mm)	+44.6
	Tender point count	-2.5
	Tender joint count	-3.3
	Swollen joint count	-1.0
	Salivary flow rate (mL/min)	+0.02
	Schirmer's test (mm)	+0.6
	Focus score (after 12 weeks)	-0.2
	Anti-SSA	-9.5
	ESR (mm/h)	-1.1
	Latex test	-3.1
	IgA-RF (IU)	-0.1
	IgA (mg/L)	+0.2
	IgG (mg/L)	+4.3
	IgM (mg/L)	-0.31
Adverse events	Very moderate hypersensitivity reactions	n = 8
	Transient headache or fatigue	n = 2
	Arthritis	n = 4

Trial	Reduction of fatigue in Sjögren's syndrome with Rituximab: results of a randomized, double-blind, placebo-controlled pilot study
Substance	**2 infusions of rituximab 1 g days 0, 15 (RTX, n = 8)**
	Placebo (n = 9)
	Premedication: 100 mg methylprednisolone 60 mg oral prednisolone/day days 2–14
	30 mg days oral prednisolone/day days 8–14
	Continue with concurrent medication
	No changing or adding of DMARDs
Result	Rituximab was effective in reducing disease activity
Patients	17 patients with primary Sjögren's syndrome, meeting the European-American Consensus criteria
	• Fatigue score (VAS 0–100) > 50
	• Positive for anti-Ro and/or anti-La antibodies
Authors	Dass S, Bowman SJ, Vital EM, Ikeda K, Pease CT, Hamburger J, Richards A, Rauz S, Emery P
Publication	*Ann Rheum Dis.* 2008;67(11):1541–1544
Follow-up	26 weeks

Note	*Outcome parameters:*		
		RTX	Placebo
	20% improvement in fatigue VAS	87.5%	55.6%
	Schimer's test	No significant changes	

Adverse events		RTX	Placebo
	Headache, urticarial rash, fever and meningism	n = 3	n = 0
	Infusion reactions	n = 2	n = 0
	Abdominal pain, eventually diagnosed as gastroenteritis	n = 1	n = 0

Trial	Effectiveness of rituximab treatment in primary Sjögren's syndrome: a randomized, double-blind, placebo-controlled trial
Substance	**1´000 mg rituximab** (n = 20) **Placebo** infusions (n = 10) On days 1 and 15 *Concomitant medication*: Pre-treated with 100 mg i. v. methylprednisolone, 1,000 mg acetaminophen, and 2 mg i. v. clemastine 60 mg oral prednisone on days 1 and 2, 30 mg on days 3 and 4, and 15 mg on day 5 after each infusion Artificial tears and artificial saliva at stable dosage Reliable methods of contraception *Previous medication*: No monoclonal antibodies No prednisone ≤ 1 month No hydroxychloroquine ≤ 1 month No methotrexate, cyclophosphamide, cyclosporine, azathioprine, and other DMARDs ≤ 6 months
Result	Rituximab was an effective and safe treatment strategy
Patients	Patients with active primary Sjögren's syndrome • Meeting the American/European consensus group criteria • Stimulated whole saliva secretion of ≥ 0.15 mL/min • IgM-RF ≥ 10 IU/mL and anti-SSA and/or anti-SSB autoantibody positive • Salivary gland biopsy performed within 12 months before inclusion showing the characteristic features of Sjögren's syndrome
Authors	Meijer JM, Meiners PM, Vissink A, Spijkervet FK, Abdulahad W, Kamminga N, Brouwer E, Kallenberg CG, Bootsma H
Publication	*Arthritis Rheum.* 2010 Apr;62(4):960–968
Follow-up	48 weeks

(continued)

Note	Change of:		
		Placebo	Rituximab
	Whole saliva flow, mL/min unstimulated	-0.01	+0.01
	Whole saliva flow, mL/min stimulated	-0.14	-0.04
	Schirmer's test, mm/5 min	-2	-1
	Lissamine green test	0	-1
	Tear breakup time, seconds	+1	0
	B cells, 109/L	+0.06	-0.04
	IgM-RF, IU/mL	+4	+1
	MFI, general fatigue	0	-1
	SF-36 total score	-2	+3
	VAS score, oral dryness	+10	-5
	VAS score, ocular dryness	+11	-13
Adverse events		Placebo (%)	Rituximab (%)
	Early infusion reaction	0	10
	Late infusion reaction	0	10
	Serum sickness (within 2 weeks after infusion)	0	5
	Upper airway infection (within 2 weeks after infusion)	0	5
	Parvovirus (during 48 weeks of follow-up)	0	5
	Otitis media (during 48 weeks of follow-up)	0	10
	Upper airway infection (during 48 weeks of follow-up)	40	20
	Recurrence of ocular toxoplasmosis (during 48 weeks of follow-up)	0	5
	Parotid gland infection (during 48 weeks of follow-up)	0	15
	Recurrence of herpes zoster (during 48 weeks of follow-up)	10	0
	Epstein-Barr virus (during 48 weeks of follow-up)	10	0
	Rubella (during 48 weeks of follow-up)	10	0

Methotrexate

Trial	Treatment of Glucocorticoid-resistant or relapsing Takayasu arteritis with methotrexate
Substance	Weekly low-dose **0.3 mg/kg/week methotrexate (max. starting dose 15 mg/week)** Dose was increased by 2.5 mg/week to max. 25 mg/week Gradual reduction of MTX dosage if no sign of active vasculitis Discontinuation approximately 1 year after remission MTX+corticosteroids could be resumed in case of reoccurring activity *Concomitant medication*: In case of resistance to glucocorticoids at study entry Increase of dosage to 1 mg/kg/day *After remission at the end of first month*: Glucocorticoids were tapered down by 5 mg every 4 days, on alternate days Further reduction from 20 mg prednisolone/day onward: 2.5 mg every 4 days *Previous treatments*: Glucocorticosteroids (GC) n = 18 (still on GC at study entry: n = 15) Daily cyclophosphamide n = 4 Azathioprine n = 2
Result	Weekly oral low-dose methotrexate was effective in glucocorticoid-resistant disease
Patients	18 patients with Takayasu arteritis *Inclusion criteria*: • Multifocal angiopathic lesions of the aorta or its branches • Failure to respond to glucocorticoid treatment • 1 mg/kg/day for ≥1 month, or inability to taper glucocorticoid treatment within 5 months • Relapse after GC tapering

(continued) ➜

R. Müller, J. von Kempis, *Clinical Trials in Rheumatology*, 1007
DOI 10.1007/978-1-4471-2870-0_10, © Springer-Verlag London 2013

Authors	Hoffman GS, Leavitt RY, Kerr GS, Rottem M, Sneller MC, Fauci AS	
Publication	*Arthritis Rheum.* 1994;37(4):578–582	
Follow-up	2.6 years (mean)	
Note	Remission	81%
	Relapse following remission	54% (re-treatment with second remission 43%)
	Sustained remission	50% (mean 18 months, of them: 50% without GC)
	Remission in absence of GC and MTX	25% (mean duration 11.3 months)
	Progressive disease	19%
	Stable MTX dosage	17.1 mg (mean)
Adverse events	*Pneumocystis carinii* pneumonia	n = 1
	Dose reductions of MTX due to elevation of liver function	n = 5
	Recurrent oral ulcers with MTX >10 mg/ week	n = 1

Trial	Mycophenolate mofetil reduces disease activity and steroid dosage in Takayasu arteritis	
Substance	**2 g/day mycophenolate mofetil (MMF) for 23.3 months (mean)**	
	Previous medication: Corticosteroids	
	Immunosuppressive drugs: Methotrexate n = 4 Azathioprine n = 2 Chlorambucil n = 1	
Result	Mycophenolate mofetil reduced clinical and laboratory parameters of disease activity in patients with resistance to or side-effects of glucocorticosteroids	
Patients	10 consecutive Takayasu arteritis patients • Diagnosed by ≥ 3 ACR criteria • Active disease despite prednisone and/or other immunosuppressive drug or development of side-effects to previous therapy • Disease duration before study 57.5 months (mean)	
Authors	Shinjo SK, Pereira RM, Tizziani VA, Radu AS, Levy-Neto M	
Publication	*Clin Rheumatol.* 2007;26(11):1871–1877	
Follow-up	3 years	
Note		Before MMF	After MMF
	Active disease at	n = 10 (study entry)	n = 1 (end of study)
	Erythrocyte sedimentation rate (mm/h)	24.7	12.8
	C-reactive protein (mg/L)	24.0	11.2
	Prednisone dose (mg/day)	24.5	5.8 (effectively treated patients)
Adverse events	No leukopenia No elevation of serum hepatic enzymes	

Trial	Mycophenolate mofetil in Takayasu's arteritis		
Substance	Retrospective study of case records in patients on **mycophenolate for ≥ 3 months** As initial immunosuppressant n = 11, prior azathioprine n = 10 For active disease n = 19, for steroid tapering n = 2 *Concomitant medication*: Corticosteroids n = 21		
Result	Mycophenolate was safe and clinically and serologically effective in this to date largest case series in Takayasu's arteritis		
Patients	21 consecutive patients with Takayasu's arteritis as diagnosed by the ACR criteria		
Authors	Goel R, Danda D, Mathew J, Edwin N		
Publication	*Clin Rheumatol.* 2010 Mar;29(3):329–332		
Follow-up	3–15 months		
Note		Baseline	Last visit
	Indian Takayasu's arteritis activity score	7 (median, range 0–19)	1 (range 0–7)
	Mean ESR (mm at first hour)	68.0	43.2
	Mean CRP (mg/L)	31.0	17.3
	Steroid dosage (mg/day)	36	19
Adverse events	Patients with adverse drug events	n = 2	
	Rash	n = 1	
	Severe sepsis	n = 1	

Trial	Anti-tumor necrosis factor therapy in patients with difficult-to-treat Takayasu arteritis
Substance	2 × 25 mg etanercept/week s. c. (ETN, n = 7; later changed to infliximab n = 3) **3–5 mg/kg infliximab at weeks 0, 2, and 6, then every 4–8 weeks** (IFX, n = 8) *Previous immunosuppressive drugs*: Methotrexate n = 13 Cyclophosphamide n = 6 Mycophonolate mofetil n = 3 Azathioprine n = 3 Ciclosporin A n = 2 Tacrolimus n = 2 Pretreatment with ≥ two of these agents n = 8 *Concomitant medication*: Azathioprine n = 1 Methotrexate n = 5 Mycophonolate mofetil n = 1 Cyclophosphamide n = 1 Effective glucocorticoid dose before study 20 mg (median)
Result	Anti-TNF therapy resulted in improvement in 14 of 15 patients, with the majority achieving sustained remissions without glucocorticoids
Patients	15 patients with active, relapsing disease Takayasu arteritis • Diagnosed by the ACR-criteria and fulfilling all of the following: ° Previous clinical and imaging (invasive angiography and MRI) ° Required toxic doses of glucocorticoids to maintain remission ° Experienced multiple relapses ° Previous negative screening for tuberculosis by skin test and chest roentgenogram X-ray ° No former complete remission in spite of glucocorticoid treatment n = 3 ° Disease duration before study 6.5 years (mean)
Authors	Hoffman GS, Merkel PA, Brasington RD, Lenschow DJ, Liang P
Publication	*Arthritis Rheum.* 2004;50(7):2296–2304
Follow-up	21.7 months (mean and median)
Note	Improvement	93%
	Glucocorticoid-free, sustained remission	67%
	Partial remission	27%
	Median glucocorticoid dose	20 mg (study entry)
	Median glucocorticoid dose	0 mg (12 months)
	Off additional immunosuppressive drugs at end of study	n = 7
Adverse events	Infusion reaction to infliximab	n = 1(IFX)
	Disseminated histoplasmosis after infliximab	n = 1(IFX)
	Herpes zoster	n = 1 (ETN)

Trial	Anti-tumor necrosis factor therapy in patients with refractory Takayasu arteritis: Long-term follow-up
Substance	**2 × 25 mg s.c etanercept** (ETN, n = 9 later changed to infliximab n = 5) **3–5 mg/kg infliximab at weeks 0, 2, and 6,** then every 4–8 weeks Median stable dose 5 mg, 6 weekly (IFX, n = 21) *Concomitant medication*: Immunosuppressive drugs continued during trial n = 18 *Previous immunosuppressive drugs*: Methotrexate n = 22 Cyclophosphamide n = 10 Azathioprine n = 5 Mycophonolate mofetil n = 3 Ciclosporin A n = 2 Tacrolimus n = 2
Result	In this retrospective study of patients refractory to treatment with glucocorticoids, etanercept and infliximab were effective in inducing clinical remission in a majority of cases and reduction or discontinuation of additional glucocorticoids and immunosuppressive drugs
Patients	25 patients with refractory Takayasu arteritis • Fulfilling the ACR criteria *Refractory defined as stable remission not being achieved despite*: • Prednisone ≤ 10 mg/day • ≥ 1 additional immunosuppressive drug • All patients with prior treatment with glucocorticoid (median dose 19 mg) and 2 (mean) immunosuppressive drugs • No prior remission n = 13 • Median disease duration 9.6 years
Authors	Molloy ES, Langford CA, Clark TM, Gota CE, Hoffman GS
Publication	*Ann Rheum Dis.* 2008;67(11):1567–1569
Follow-up	28 months (median)

Note		ETN	IFX
	Remission and prednisone discontinuation (ETN+IFX)	60%	
	Remission and taper of prednisone to < 10 mg/day (ETN+IFX)	28%	
	Discontinuation of additional immunosuppressive drug	50%	
	Remission	66.6%	85%
	Relapses after initial remission	50%	66.6%
Adverse events	Opportunistic infections	n = 1	
	Breast cancer	n = 1	

Polymyalgia Rheumatica and Giant Cell Arteritis

Giant Cell Arteritis: Corticosteroids

Trial	Daily and alternate-day corticosteroid regimens in treatment of giant cell arteritis: Comparison in a prospective study
Substance	*All groups*: **20 mg prednisone every 8 h for 5 days,** then
	Group A: 15 mg of prednisone every 8 h (n = 20)
	Group B: 45 mg of prednisone every morning (n = 20)
	Group C: 90 mg of prednisone every other morning (n = 20)
	Taper of prednisone after end of study (4 weeks)
	Previous medication:
	No adrenocorticosteroids
Result	Daily doses, but not an alternate day regimen, of corticosteroids effectively suppressed symptoms of temporal arteritis. They were associated with a higher rate of hypercortisolism in this short-term trial
Patients	60 patients with giant cell arteritis
	• Proven by biopsy of temporal artery, without prior steroid therapy
Authors	Hunder GG, Sheps SG, Allen GL, Joyce JW
Publication	*Ann Intern Med.* 1975;82(5):613–618
Follow-up	4 weeks

(continued) ➔

R. Müller, J. von Kempis, *Clinical Trials in Rheumatology*,
DOI 10.1007/978-1-4471-2870-0_11, © Springer-Verlag London 2013

Note	After 4 weeks:			
		Group A	Group B	Group C
	Arteritis clinically completely suppressed	n = 18	n = 16	n = 6
	ESR (mm/h)	-82	-73	-51
Adverse events		Group A	Group B	Group C
	Mild hypercortisolism (after 4 weeks)	n = 9	n = 7	n = 0
	Cushing Syndrome later during the course of the disease	n = 12	n = 0	n = 0
	Mild diabetes	n = 0	n = 1	n = 0
	Insomnia/mild depression (after 4 weeks)	n = 1	n = 0	n = 0
	Lumbar vertebral compression fractures	n = 2	n = 2	n = 0

Trial	Treatment of polymyalgia rheumatica and giant cell arteritis. I. Steroid regimens in the first 2 months
Substance	*High-dose steroid regimen in polymyalgia rheumatica (PMR)*: **Prednisolone 20 mg/day for 4 weeks** Prednisolone 15 mg/day for 2 weeks Prednisolone 10 mg/day for 2 weeks *Low-dose steroid regimen in PMR*: **Prednisolone 10 mg/day for 4 weeks** Prednisolone 7.5 mg/day for 2 weeks Prednisolone 5 mg/day for 2 weeks *High-dose steroid regimen in giant cell arteritis (GCA)*: **Prednisolone 40 mg/day for 5 days** Prednisolone 40 mg/day for 4 weeks Prednisolone 30 mg/day for 2 weeks Prednisolone 20 mg/day for 2 weeks *Low-dose steroid regimen in GCA*: **Prednisolone 40 mg/day for 5 days** Prednisolone 20 mg/day for 4 weeks Prednisolone 15 mg/day for 2 weeks Prednisolone 10 mg/day for 2 weeks
Result	Low-dose regimen was less effective than high dose in patients with both polymyalgia rheumatica or giant cell arteritis
Patients	39 patients with polymyalgia rheumatica and 35 patients with giant cell arteritis • Diagnosed by the criteria of Jones and Hazleman
Authors	Kyle V, Hazleman BL
Publication	*Ann Rheum Dis*. 1989 Aug;48(8):658–661
Follow up	Not described in detail
Note	*Early relapses*:

	Dose increased	Total numbers of patients
PMR, low dose	n = 13	n = 20
PMR, high dose	n = 2	n = 19
GCA, low dose	n = 6	n = 15
GCA, high dose	n = 4	n = 20

Trial	Deflazacort versus Methylprednisolone in polymyalgia rheumatica: Clinical equivalence and relative anti-inflammatory potency of different treatment regimens
Substance	*Group A* (n = 16): *Daily regimen*: **24 mg deflazacort/day** (n = 8) Every-other-day regimen: **48 mg deflazacort every other day** (n = 8) Groups were crossed over after 6 weeks *Group B* (n = 15): *Daily regimen*: **16 mg 6-methylprednisolone daily** (n = 8) Every-other-day regimen: **32 mg 6-methylprednisolone every other day** (n = 7) *Groups were switched after 6 weeks* Total treatment days: 84 First 2 weeks: Fixed dose After week 2: Reduced dose according to physician's expert opinion of disease activity
Result	In this short-term study of polymyalgia rheumatica, neither different dose nor daily nor alternate-day treatment regimens of deflazacort or 6-methylprednisolone showed differences in clinical efficacy. Deflazacort was less potent than presumed
Patients	31 patients with recent onset polymyalgia rheumatica • Pain and stiffness in the proximal muscle groups (shoulder and/or pelvic girdle) • Disease duration > 1 month but < 3 months • ESR > 40 mm/h *Major exclusion criteria*: • Evidence of giant cell arthritis or other inflammatory rheumatic disease • Previous glucocorticoids • Rheumatoid factor
Authors	Di Munno O, Imbimbo B, Mazzantini M, Milani S, Occhipinti G, Pasero G
Publication	*J Rheumatol*. 1995 Aug;22(8):1492–1498
Follow-up	84 days

Note — Change of (*after 42 days*):

	Daily regimen		Every-other-day regimen	
	Group A	Group B	Group A	Group B
Limb pain (VAS)	-4.5	-6.3	-4.6	-6.0
Morning stiffness (min)	-83	-132	-84	-116
ESR (mm/h)	-45	-53	-50	-46
CRP (mg/dL)	-1.6	-1.6	-1.7	-1.4

Adverse events

	Group A	Group B
Moderate gastric pain	n = 1	n = 3
Facial edema and weight increase	n = 0	n = 2

Trial	Efficacy and adverse effects of different corticosteroid dose regimens in temporal arteritis: A retrospective study
Substance	**30–40 mg/day prednisone** (group A, n = 23) **40–60 mg/day prednisone** (group B, n = 45) **> 60 mg/day prednisone** (group C, n = 9) Continuous taper according to clinical activity in all groups
Result	The lowest starting dose of 30–40 mg/day was as effective, less toxic and allowed for equally fast tapering of prednisone, compared to two regimen with higher starting doses in this retrospective analysis of patients with giant cell arteritis, with dosages based on physician's expert opinion
Patients	77 patients with temporal arteritis • Meeting the ACR-criteria • Positive biopsies: group A – 91%, group B – 89%, group C – 89%
Authors	Nesher G, Rubinow A, Sonnenblick M
Publication	*Clin Exp Rheumatol.* 1997;15(3):303–306
Follow-up	3 years

Note — *Mean daily prednisone dose*:

	Group A (mg)	Group B (mg)	Group C (mg)
Month 0	37	59	92
Month 2	21	33	43
Month 6	10	18	22
Month 12	7	10	14
Cumulative prednisone dose (month 12)	5900	8900	11800

Disease exacerbations:

	Group A (%)	Group B (%)	Group C (%)
First year	26	20	11
Second year	5	14	14
Third year	5	4	17

Cumulative cure rate:

	Group A (%)	Group B (%)	Group C (%)
First year	13	13	11
Second year	35	31	29
Third year	50	48	50

Adverse events

	Group A (%)	Group B (%)	Group C (%)
All adverse events	36	78	88
Life-threatening adverse events	14	33	38
Other major adverse events	9	27	37

Trial	An initially double-blind, controlled 96-week trial of depot methylprednisolone against oral prednisolone in the treatment of polymyalgia rheumatica
Substance	*Oral group A* (n = 30): **15 mg oral prednisolone/day** for 3 weeks 12.5 mg prednisolone/day for 3 weeks 10 mg prednisolone/day for 6 weeks Plus placebo i. m. saline every 3 weeks Breakage of code at week 12, no placebo injections from then on After 12 weeks, prednisone 9 mg until week 16 From then 1 mg every 8 weeks *Intramuscular group B* (n = 30): Oral placebo as described above Plus **120 mg i. m. methylprednisolone every 3 weeks** Treatment duration 21 months (group A), 20 months (group B) *Concomitant medication*: No bone modifying treatment No previous steroid therapy
Result	There was no difference in clinical efficacy between intramuscular methylprednisolone or oral prednisolone in this trial of patients with polymyalgia rheumatica. Intramuscular methylprednisolone was associated with fewer fractures and lesser weight gain
Patients	60 patients with polymyalgia rheumatica • With shoulder and pelvic girdle muscular pain in the absence of true muscle weakness • Morning stiffness > 30 min • ESR > 30 mm/h • Absence of rheumatoid or other inflammatory arthritis or malignant disease *Major exclusion criteria*: • Clinical features of giant cell arteritis • Previous steroid therapy
Authors	Dasgupta B, Dolan AL, Panayi GS, Fernandes L
Publication	*Br J Rheumatol.* 1998 Feb;37(2):189–195
Follow-up	96 weeks

(continued) ➔

Note	Outcome parameters:		
		Oral prednisolone	i. m. methylprednisolone
	Study completed	n = 25	n = 24
	Remission (week 12)	60.0%	66.6%
	Remission (week 48)	58%	45%
	Remission (week 96)	30%	33%
	Cumulative mean steroid dose (mg)	3´473	1´978
	Weight gain (kg)	3.42	0.82
	VAS pain at weeks 3 and 6	Lower in group A	
	Early morning stiffness, VAS or ESR at weeks 48 and 96	No difference	
Adverse events		Oral prednisolone	i. m. methylprednisolone
	Fracture	n = 8	n = 1
	Bruising	13.3%	33.3%
	Dyspepsia	9.9%	16.7%
	Chest infections	13.3%	9.9%
	Urinary tract infections	3.3%	0%
	Ankle edema	9.9%	9.9%
	Moon face	9.9%	0%
	Tremor	3.3%	0%
	Depression	3.3%	0%
	Hypertension	6.6%	0%
	Back pain	6.6%	0%
	Cataract	6.6%	0%
	Glaucoma	3.3%	3.3%
	Breathlessness	6.6%	0%

Trial	Corticosteroid injections in polymyalgia rheumatica: A double-blind, prospective, randomized, placebo-controlled study
Substance	*Group A* (n = 10): **Bilateral shoulder injections of 40 mg of 6-methylprednisolone acetate** *Group B* (n = 10): **Placebo** injections *Follow-up*: Responders were treated weekly with the same regimen for a total of 4 bilateral injections and then followed up for 6 months Nonresponders withdrawn from the study and received 16 mg/day prednisolone
Result	Shoulder corticosteroid injections were an effective and safe therapy for polymyalgia rheumatica
Patients	20 consecutive patients with active polymyalgia rheumatica (PMR) • Fulfilling Healey's diagnostic criteria for PMR *Major exclusion criteria*: • Previous treatment with corticosteroids • Peripheral synovitis • Pelvic girdle involvement • Signs and/or symptoms of present giant cell arteritis • Anticoagulant treatment or bleeding disorder
Authors	Salvarani C, Cantini F, Olivieri I, Barozzi L, Macchioni L, Boiardi L, Niccoli L, Padula A, Pulsatelli L, Meliconi R
Publication	*J Rheumatol.* 2000 June;27(6):1470–1476
Duration/follow-up	7/7 months

(continued)

Note	Outcome parameters:		
		Group A	Group B
	Responders	100%	0%
	Response until 6-month follow-up	n = 5	–
	Loss of response after 4 weeks	n = 5	
	MRI showed marked improvement of shoulder lesions 1 week after first injection and an almost complete resolution 1 week after last injection in the responder group		
	Change of:		
		Group A	*Group B*
	Morning stiffness (min)	-183	–
	VAS pain (cm)	-7.4	–
	Patient's global assessment, VAS (cm)	-7.0	–
	Physician's global assessment, VAS (cm)	-6.6	–
	ESR (mm/h)	-69	
	CRP (mg/L)	-6.1	–
	IL-6 (pg/dL)	-22	–
	Systemic symptoms and signs	-50%	–
Adverse events	No side-effects were recorded		

Trial	A randomized, multicenter, controlled trial using intravenous pulses of methylprednisolone in the initial treatment of simple forms of giant cell arteritis: A one-year follow-up study of 164 patients
Substance	*Group A* (n = 61):
	240 mg i. v. pulse of methylprednisolone
	Followed by 0.7 mg/kg/day oral prednisone
	Group B (n = 53):
	0.7 mg/kg/day oral prednisone only
	Group C (n = 50):
	240 mg i. v. pulse of methylprednisolone
	Followed by 0.5 mg/kg prednisone/day
	Administration of oral prednisone b. i. d. in all groups
	Corticosteroids were tapered after normalization of inflammatory variables, with the goal to reach half the initial dose within 1 month for groups A and B, and 20 mg/week for group C
	Taper thereafter of 1 mg every month, not beginning before month 6 of treatment
	Concomitant therapy:
	Anticoagulant therapy: nadroparin or dalteparin during initial study phase 1 g calcium
	8'000 IU ergocalciferol/week for osteoporosis prevention
Result	Methylprednisolone pulses had no corticosteroid sparing effects when added to oral prednisone in patients with giant cell arteritis
Patients	164 patients with giant cell arteritis, either proven by biopsy of the temporal artery or by the ACR-criteria
	Important exclusion criteria:
	• Age > 85 years
	• Ocular or other vascular event within last month
Authors	Chevalet P, Barrier JH, Pottier P, Magadur-Joly G, Pottier MA, Hamidou M, Planchon B, El Kouri D, Connan L, Dupond JL, De Wazieres B, Dien G, Duhamel E, Grosbois B, Jego P, Le Strat A, Capdeville J, Letellier P, Agron L
Publication	*J Rheumatol.* 2000;27(6):1484–1491
Follow-up	1 year

(continued)

Note	Time (mean) to normalization of:			
		Group A	Group B	Group C
	Clinical signs	3.07 days	2.47 days	3.3 days
	CRP	7.39 days	7.77 days	7.69 days
	Time (mean) before:			
		Group A	Group B	Group C
	Obtaining 0.3 mg prednisone/ day	104.8 days	95.0 days	95.2 days
	Obtaining 7 mg/kg prednisone/ day	255.7 days	254.0 days	237.0 day
	Cumulative prednisone dose:			
		Group A	Group B	Group C
	After 1 month	1´084 g	1´146 g	848 g
	After 2 month	1´811 g	1´916 g	1'555 g
	After 6 month	3´973 g	4´065 g	3'530 g
	After 12 month	5´777 g	5´578 g	5'168 g
	Patients taking prednisone after 1 year	85%	77%	89%
	Corticoid dependence in the first 3 months	27%	30%	30%
	Corticoid dependence in the first 4 months	28%	35%	46%
	Corticoid resistance	8%	17%	16%
	Non-corticoid inflammatory therapy	1%	2%	4%
Adverse events		Group A	Group B	Group C
	Infections	n = 15	n = 6	n = 10
	Cushingoid features	n = 7	n = 6	n = 5
	Rheumatic	n = 9	n = 7	n = 2
	Psychiatric	n = 6	n = 2	n = 5
	Cardiovascular	n = 3	n = 3	n = 3
	Diabetic	n = 2	n = 3	n = 2
	Digestive	n = 3	n = 0	n = 4
	Ophthalmologic	n = 3	n = 0	n = 0
	Phlebitis	n = 0	n = 2	n = 2
	Steroid induced myopathy	n = 1	n = 0	n = 1

Trial	Treatment of giant cell arteritis using induction therapy with high-dose glucocorticoids: A double-blind, placebo-controlled, randomized prospective clinical trial
Substance	**15 mg/kg i. v. methylprednisolone** (group A)
	Placebo saline (group B) for 3 days
	Parallel prednisone-tapering therapy (*both groups*):
	40 mg/day prednisone and followed a tapering schedule to control disease activity
	Tapered to 30 mg after 2 weeks
	Tapered by 5 mg/2 weeks until 20 mg
	Tapered by 2.5 mg/2 weeks until 10 mg/day
	Below 10 mg/day, further reduction by 1 mg/2 weeks
	Relapse of disease activity:
	Increase of prednisone dose of 10 mg
	If prednisone $\leq$ 25 mg/day increase by 5 mg
	Tapering was started again after 2 weeks
	Concomitant therapy:
	Calcium (1'200–1'500 mg/day)
	Vitamin D (400–800 IU)
	Bisphosphonates, dependent on bone densitometry measurements
Result	Initial intravenous pulse therapy with methylprednisolone led to a quicker tapering and a higher remission rate, compared to oral prednisone alone, in patients with giant cell arteritis
Patients	77 patients with giant cell arteritis
	• Proven by biopsy and meeting the ACR-criteria
	Major exclusion criteria:
	• Prednisone doses equivalent to > 10 mg/day for > 10 days
	• Recent vision problems or transient ischemic attacks
Authors	Mazlumzadeh M, Hunder GG, Easley KA, Calamia KT, Matteson EL, Griffing WL, Younge BR, Weyand CM, Goronzy JJ
Publication	*Arthritis Rheum.* 2006;54(10):3310–3318
Follow-up	78 weeks

(continued)

Note		Group A	Group B
	< 5 mg/day prednisone at week 36	10/14	2/13
	< 5 mg/day prednisone at week 52	11/14	2/13
	< 5 mg/day prednisone at week 78	12/14	4/12
	Cumulative steroid dose at week 78 (mg)	5'636	7'860
	Total relapses	21/14 patients (1.5/ patient)	37/13 patients (2.8/ patient)
Adverse events		Group A (%)	Group B (%)
	Hypertension	21.1	23.3
	Hyperlipoproteinemia	21.3	23.1
	Coronary artery disease	0	7.7
	Tachycardia	0	15.4
	Upper GI-bleeding	0	0
	Rectal bleeding	0	7.1
	Osteoporosis	21.3	23.1
	Cushingoid habitus	78.6	76.9
	Glucose intolerance	7.1	15.4
	Glaucoma	7.1	0
	Chorioretinopathy	0	7.7
	Subconjunctival hemorrhage	0	7.7
	Varicella zoster virus	7.1	0
	Urinary tract infection	21.3	15.4
	Pneumonia	7.1	15.4
	Candida esophagitis	0	7.7
	Depression	0	7.7
	Dizziness	21.3	0
	Deep venous thrombosis	0	7.7
	Colon cancer	7.1	0
	Sleep apnea	7.1	0

Trial	The correct prednisone starting dose in polymyalgia rheumatica is related to body weight but not to disease severity
Substance	**Prednisone 12.5 mg/day**
Result	12.5 mg prednisone as a starting dose lead to a minimum reduction of 75% of symptoms in three-fourth of patients. The main factor driving response to prednisone was weight
Patients	60 consecutive PMR patients with polymyalgia rheumatica, according to the criteria of Bird et al.
Authors	Cimmino MA, Parodi M, Montecucco C, Caporali R
Publication	*BMC Musculoskeletal Disord.* 2011 May 14;12(1):94
Follow-up	6 months
Note	*Outcome parameters:*

	Responders	Nonresponders
Mean prednisone dose (mg/kg)	0.19±0.03	0.16±0.03

Remission was defined as disappearance of at least 75% of the signs and symptoms:

	Responders	Nonresponders
Number	n = 47 (78.3%)	n = 13 (21.7%)
Gender (women/men)	31/16	4/9
Age (years)	71.3	71.5
Weight (kg)	67.4	78.5
Disease duration (days)	90	86
Morning stiffness (min)	100.7	89.0
Fatigue	55.3%	76.9%
Fever	21.3%	30.0%
Weight loss	34.0%	15.4%
Peripheral arthritis	27.7%	30.8%
Carpal tunnel syndrome	34.0%	15.4%
RS3PE	17%	15.4%
Tenosynovitis	8.5%	7.7%
ESR (mm/h)	63.8	62.5%
CRP (mg/L)	30	30

Trial	Azathioprine in giant cell arteritis/polymyalgia rheumatica: A double-blind study
Substance	**Azathioprine 2×50 mg/day** (n = 16)
	Placebo (n = 15)
	Concomitant therapy:
	Previous steroid had been reduced to a minimum sufficient to control symptoms
	5 mg metoclopramide in case of nausea
	Previous medication:
	Corticosteroids (all patients)
Result	The mean prednisolone after one year was lower in the azathioprine treatment than the placebo treatment group in this mixed study population of patients with giant cell arteritis or polymyalgia rheumatica
Patients	31 patients with polymyalgia rheumatica, or giant cell arteritis, diagnosed on the basis of the criteria proposed by Jones and Hazelmann
	• Disease duration (azathioprine/placebo group, mean): 2.3/2.5 years
	• Pretreatment with steroids in all cases
Authors	De Silva M, Hazleman BL
Publication	*Ann Rheum Dis*. 1986;45(2):136–138
Follow-up	52 weeks

Note	*Prednisolone dose:*	Azathioprine (mg/day)	Placebo (mg/day)
	Week 0	8.1	7.4
	Week 12	5.1	4.8
	Week 24	3.6	3.7
	Week 36	2.8	3.3
	Week 52, at end of study	1.9	4.2

Adverse events		Azathioprine	Placebo
	Nausea	n = 4	n = 2
	Vomiting	n = 2	n = 0
	Diarrhea	n = 1	n = 1
	Collapse	n = 1	n = 0

Trial	No additional steroid-sparing effect of Ciclosporin A in giant cell arteritis
Substance	*Group A* (n = 30): **Prednisone** monotherapy, starting dose **40 mg/day** *Group B* (n = 30): **Ciclosporin A 2 mg/kg/day** (dose could be increased to 3.5 mg/kg/day or decreased) Plus prednisone
Result	In this study of giant cell arteritis, ciclosporin A had no steroid-sparing effect, at least partly due to a high drop-out rate because of side-effects
Patients	60 consecutive patients with biopsy-proven giant cell arteritis, meeting the ACR-criteria *Major exclusion criteria*: • > 1 month corticosteroid therapy • Combination with other immunosuppressive drug • Uncontrolled hypertension • Signs of threatening vascular ischemia
Authors	Schaufelberger C, Möllby H, Uddhammar A, Bratt J, Nordborg E
Publication	*Scand J Rheumatol.* 2006;35(4):327–329
Duration	12 months
Note	

	Group A	Group B
Premature termination	n = 1	n = 11
Termination because of side-effects	n = 0	n = 9
No steroid-sparing effect by addition of ciclosporin A		

Trial	Can methotrexate be used as a steroid-sparing agent in the treatment of polymyalgia rheumatica and giant cell arteritis?
Substance	*Corticosteroid therapy* (*both groups*): **Prednisone 20 mg/day** Tapered by 2.5 mg every 3 weeks if ESR ≥ 15 mm/h or CRP≥ 0.6 mg% After reaching 7.5 mg, further tapered by 2.5 mg every 6 weeks *MTX group* (n = 20): **Methotrexate 7.5 mg/week** Stop after prednisone discontinuation *Placebo group* (n = 20): **Placebo** *Concomitant therapy*: Calcium supplements Stop of NSAIDs at study entry
Result	A low-dose and rapidly tapered prednisone regimen was effective in this study population of predominantly polymyalgia rheumatica rather than giant cell arteritis patients. Methotrexate at 7.5 mg/week did not show additional efficacy or result in a lower cumulative dose of prednisone
Patients	40 patients with active, untreated polymyalgia rheumatica (PMR) six of whom also had clinical symptoms of giant cell arteritis (GCA) Positive temporal artery biopsies PMR n = 3, GCA n = 3 *Inclusion criteria PMR*: • Age ≥ 50 years • ESR ≥ 40 mm/h • Pain/stiffness shoulders ± hips *Inclusion criteria GCA*: • New onset temporal headache, jaw claudication, temporal artery tenderness on palpation or decreased pulsation, abnormal temporal artery biopsy specimen • Age ≥ 50 years, ESR ≥ 50 mm/h *Major exclusion criteria PMR and GCA*: • Signs (clinical or laboratory) of polyarthritis, polymyositis, Parkinson's disease • AST or ALT> twice normal value, serum creatinine > 150 mmol/L
Authors	van der Veen MJ, Dinant HJ, van Booma-Frankfort C, van Albada-Kuipers GA, Bijlsma JW
Publication	*Ann Rheum Dis*. 1996 Apr;55(4):218–223
Follow-up	2 years

(continued) ➜

Note	Outcome parameters:		
		MTX	Placebo
	Remissions	n = 11	n = 9
	Median duration of remission (weeks)	7	35
	Median cumulative prednisone dose (mg) after 2 years	2´400	2´947
	Number of relapses	n = 18	n = 15
	Median time to reach remission+stop of prednisone (weeks)	48	45
Adverse events		MTX	Placebo
	Gastrointestinal disorder	n = 5	n = 5
	Hair loss	n = 1	n = 0
	Oral ulcerations	n = 3	n = 3
	Rash	n = 0	n = 1
	Increased blood pressure	n = 11	n = 8
	Hypertension	n = 9	n = 5
	Increase in body weight	n = 14	n = 11
	Cardiac insufficiency	n = 2	n = 1
	Osteoporotic fractures	n = 1	n = 2
	Infections	n = 5	n = 2
	Thrombocytopenia	n = 0	n = 1
	Increase AST/ALT	n = 15	n = 8
	Increase in serum creatinine	n = 7	n = 10
	Hyperglycemia	n = 5	n = 7

Trial	Methotrexate in polymyalgia rheumatica: Preliminary results of an open, randomized study
Substance	*Group A* (n = 12):
	Prednisone (Pdn)15 mg/day every week for 3 months
	Tapered to 10 mg Pdn/day for the 4 months
	Tapered to 5 mg Pdn/day for the 5 months
	Finally tapered to 2.5 mg Pdn/day for the 6 months
	Group B (n = 12):
	Methotrexate 10 mg/week plus
	25 mg Pdn/day for 4 weeks
	12.5 mg Pdn/day for the 2 months
	10 mg Pdn/day for the 3 months
	6.25 mg Pdn/day for the 4 months
	5 mg Pdn/day for the 5 months
	Finally 2.5 mg Pdn/day for the 6 months
	Previous medication:
	No calcium supplements
	No calcitonin, other bone mass affect in medications
Result	Additional methotrexate treatment of polymyalgia rheumatica reduced the cumulative prednisone dose and prevented loss of bone mass over one year, in comparison with prednisone alone
Patients	24 patients with recent onset polymyalgia rheumatica, diagnosed on the basis of the Goodwin-criteria
	• Duration of symptoms (mean) 2.3 months (group A), 1.8 months (group B)
	• Failed treatment with NSAIDs
	Major exclusion criteria:
	• RA
	• SLE
Authors	Ferraccioli G, Salaffi F, De Vita S, Casatta L, Bartoli E
Publication	*J Rheumatol.* 1996 Apr;23(4):624–628
Follow-up	12 months

(continued)

Note	Outcome parameters:		
		Group A	Group B
	Remissions at month 12	n = 12	n = 12
	No longer taking prednisone at month 12	n = 0	n = 6
	Change of:		
		Group A	Group B
	ESR (mm/h)	-60	-56
	CRP (mg/L)	-85	-70
	Total prednisone dose (g)	3.2	1.84
	Bone mineral density	-4.78	-2.12
	OH-Pro/creatinine (mg/L)	+32.8	-18
	Alkaline phosphatase (mg/L)	-0.9	-14
	Ca/creatinine (mg/L)	+2.9	-3.9
Adverse events		Group A	Group B
	Abnormal liver function tests	n = 0	n = 4
	Vertebral fracture	n = 1	n = 0
	Hypertension	n = 2	n = 0
	Hyperglycemia	n = 2	n = 0
	Cataract	n = 2	n = 0
	Nausea	n = 0	n = 2

Trial	Combined treatment of giant-cell arteritis with methotrexate and prednisone. A randomized, double-blind, placebo-controlled trial
Substance	**10 mg methotrexate/week** p. o. for 24 months (group A, n = 21)
	Placebo (group B, n = 21)
	Prednisone therapy:
	Prednisolone 20mg t. i. d. for 1 week
	Prednisolone 20 mg/day (from second week: 60 mg q. d.)
	Tapered in steps of 10 mg/week to 40 mg/day
	Tapered by 5 mg steps to 20 mg
	Tapered by 2.5 mg every 2 weeks until withdrawal
	Concomitant therapy:
	Calcium (1'000 mg/day)
	Vitamin D3 (600 IU/day)
	Folic acid (5 mg/day)
	Isoniazid (600 mg/day for 6 months) when signs of tuberculosis visible on chest radiography
	Previous medication:
	No immunosuppressive drugs
Result	Treatment with methotrexate plus prednisolone in patients with giant cell arteritis was safe, more effective and resulted in a reduced cumulative prednisolone dose, in comparison with prednisolone monotherapy
Patients	42 patients with new-onset giant cell arteritis diagnosed by biopsy
	• ≤ 2 weeks of treatment with high-dose corticosteroid (prednisone > 10 mg/day)
	Major exclusion criteria:
	• Serum creatinine > 2 mg/dL
	• Low-dose prednisone equivalent ≤ 10 mg/day for > 3 months
	• Previous immunosuppressive drugs
Authors	Jover JA, Hernández-García C, Morado IC, Vargas E, Bañares A, Fernández-Gutiérrez B
Publication	*Ann Intern Med.* 2001;134(2):106–114
Follow-up	24 months

(continued) ➜

Note	*After 24 months*:		
		Group A	Group B
	Relapse rate	45%	84.2%
	Cumulative steroid dose	4´187 mg	5´489.5 mg
	Completion of follow-up analysis (n = 39; including drop-outs):		
		Group A	Group B
	Patients without relapse	n = 11	n = 3
	Patients with one relapse	n = 7	n = 7
	Patients with two relapses	n = 1	n = 8
	Patients with three relapses	n = 1	n = 1
	Total patients with relapse	n = 9	n = 16
	Total relapses	n = 12	n = 26
	Patients with cranial relapse	n = 2	n = 7
	Patients with noncranial relapse	n = 7	n = 9
	Completion of treatment analysis (n = 33):		
		Group A	Group B
	Patients without relapse	n = 8	n = 3
	Patients with one relapse	n = 6	n = 7
	Patients with two relapses	n = 1	n = 7
	Patients with three relapses	n = 0	n = 1
	Total patients with relapse	n = 7	n = 15
	Total relapses	n = 8	n = 24
	Patients with cranial relapse	n = 1	n = 6
	Patients with noncranial relapse	n = 6	n = 9

(continued) →

Adverse events	Group A (%)	Group B (%)
Fracture	20	10.5
Neuropsychiatric disorder	50	42.1
Diabetes	15	36.8
Glucose intolerance	10	10.5
Arterial hypertension	60	84.2
Cushingoid appearance	15	31.8
Weight gain	35	47.3
Myopathy	10	5.2
Cataract	10	5.2
Hypercholesterinemia	0	10.5
Increase liver enzymes	35	31.8
Nausea and vomiting	0	5.2
Thrombocytopenia	15	5.2
Oral ulcers	0	5.2
Alopecia	5	10.5
Infections	40	52.5
Peptic disease	5	15.7
Diarrhea	5	15.7

Trial	A prospective, double-blind, randomized, placebo-controlled trial of methotrexate in the treatment of giant cell arteritis (GCA)
Substance	**Prednisone** *therapy*:
	Recommended starting dose **1 mg/kg/day** or 1 g, but lower doses possible
	Tapered by 10 mg/week based on the clinical course
	After reaching 40 mg/day tapering by 5 mg/week until 20 mg
	Then tapering by 2.5 mg/week until withdrawal
	Randomized trial:
	After reaching **30 mg prednisone/day**
	Group A (n = 12):
	7.5 mg MTX/week
	Dosage was increased by 2.5–20 mg/week
	Monthly taper to 0 by 2.5 mg every 4 weeks after discontinuation of prednisone
	Group B (n = 9):
	Placebo
	Concomitant therapy:
	Folic acid 1 mg/day
	Calcium carbonate (1′500 mg/day), vitamin D3 (800 IU/day)
	Previous medication:
	No immunosuppressive therapy
Result	Addition of methotrexate to prednisone, compared to prednisone alone, did not result in a steroid-sparing effect or in faster control of giant cell arteritis in this study
Patients	21 patients with newly diagnosed temporal arteritis
	Proven by biopsy or one of the following:
	• Ischemic optic neuropathy with WSR > 50 mm/h and the presence of polymyalgia rheumatica (PMR)
	• Stenotic disease of the aorta, or cranial symptoms including visual loss, together with ESR > 50 mm/h
	• ESR > 50 mm/h and cranial symptoms or PMR
	• No evidence of other disease plus favorable clinical response to high-dose steroids
	Major exclusion criteria:
	• Serum creatinine > 2 mg/dL
Authors	Spiera RF, Mitnick HJ, Kupersmith M, Richmond M, Spiera H, Peterson MG, Paget SA
Publication	*Clin Exp Rheumatol.* 2001;19(5):495–501
Follow-up	≤ 68 weeks (no detailed information provided)

(continued) ➜

Note		Group A	Group B
	Cumulative corticosteroid dose	6´469 mg	5´908 mg
	Time to complete steroid treatment	68 weeks	60 weeks
	Time to reach prednisone ≤ 10 mg/day	23 weeks	25 weeks
Adverse events		Group A	Group B
	Musculoskeletal weakness	n = 12	n = 8
	Vertebral fracture	n = 1	n = 3
	Mood changes	n = 12	n = 9
	Tired/insomnia	n = 10	n = 7
	Back pain	n = 5	n = 3
	Tremor	n = 6	n = 2
	Loss of balance/dizziness	n = 3	n = 5
	Memory loss	n = 3	n = 0
	Gastrointestinal discomfort	n = 10	n = 6
	Diarrhea	n = 1	n = 0
	Skin fragility	n = 4	n = 1
	Alopecia	n = 6	n = 5
	Hirsutism	n = 1	n = 1
	Rash	n = 1	n = 2
	Acne	n = 0	n = 1
	Cushingoid habitus	n = 3	n = 3
	Hyperglycemia	n = 1	n = 1
	Cellulitis	n = 1	n = 1
	Herpes zoster infection	n = 2	n = 1
	Fungal skin infection	n = 2	n = 0
	Urinary tract infection	n = 1	n = 1
	Pneumonia	n = 0	n = 1
	Adenocarcinoma	n = 1	n = 0
	Squamous cell carcinoma	n = 0	n = 1
	Basal cell carcinoma	n = 1	n = 0

INSSYS-Trial	A multicenter, randomized, double-blind, placebo-controlled trial of adjuvant methotrexate treatment for giant cell arteritis (GCA) INSSYS: International Network for the Study of Systemic Vasculitides
Substance	*Group A* (n = 51): **Methotrexate (MTX) 0.15 mg/kg/week with** **Increase to 0.25 mg/kg/week, max.15 mg/week** *Group B* (n = 47): **Placebo** *Parallel corticosteroid therapy*: Prednisone 1 mg/kg/day, max. 60 mg/day) After 4 weeks prednisone was reduced by 5 mg every 4 days on alternate days reaching 60 mg every other day after 3 months Then reduction by 5 mg/week until discontinuation Total duration of prednisone = 6 months *Concomitant therapy*: Folic acid 5 mg/week (24 h after MTX) Calcium (1´000 mg/day) and 0.5 mg 1.25 vitamin D twice a week
Result	Methotrexate, added to prednisone, was not superior to prednisone alone in controlling disease activity or decreasing the cumulative dose and toxicity of corticosteroids in this trial of patients with giant cell arteritis
Patients	98 patients with giant cell arteritis • Age > 50 years • ESR ≥ 40 mm/h • Onset of giant cell arteritis (GCA) symptoms ≤ 6 months *± at least 1 of the following*: • Positive temporal artery biopsy • Unequivocal symptoms of GCA • Angiographic abnormalities • Symptoms of polymyalgia rheumatica (PMR) plus cranial symptoms *Major exclusion criteria*: • Prednisone initiated > 21 days prior to study serum creatinine ≥ 2 mg/dL • Prior diagnosis of GCA or PMR • Lack of response to prednisone therapy within 5 days (because suggestive for other form of vasculitis)

(continued) ➔

Authors	Hoffman GS, Cid MC, Hellmann DB, Guillevin L, Stone JH, Schousboe J, Cohen P, Calabrese LH, Dickler H, Merkel PA, Fortin P, Flynn JA, Locker GA, Easley KA, Schned E, Hunder GG, Sneller MC, Tuggle C, Swanson H, Hernández-Rodríguez J, Lopez-Soto A, Bork D, Hoffman DB, Kalunian K, Klashman D, Wilke WS, Scheetz RJ, Mandell BF, Fessler BJ, Kosmorsky G, Prayson R, Luqmani RA, Nuki G, McRorie E, Sherrer Y, Baca S, Walsh B, Ferland D, Soubrier M, Choi HK, Gross W, Segal AM, Ludivico C, Puechal X; International Network for the Study of Systemic Vasculitides		
Publication	*Arthritis Rheum.* 2002;46(5):1309–1318		
Follow-up	12 months		
Note		MTX	Placebo
	Treatment failure in 6 months	24.4%	35.4%
	First relapse in 6 months	68.9%	66.1%
	Treatment failure in 12 months	57.5%	77.3%
	First relapse in 12 months	74.8%	91.3%
	Total dose of prednisone	5´375 mg	5´275 mg
	Median duration of corticosteroid treatment	5.6 months	5.4 months
Adverse events		MTX	Placebo
	Headache or scalp pain	48.7%	55.2%
	Tongue or jaw pain	20.0%	4.8%
	Polymyalgia rheumatica	39.9%	73.7%
	Vision loss	10.2%	19.7%
	Sustained fever	3.9%	18.1%
	ESR increase	61.7%	76.1%
	Death	n = 2	n = 1

Trial	Prednisone plus methotrexate for polymyalgia rheumatica: A randomized, double-blind, placebo-controlled trial
Substance	*Corticosteroid therapy*: **Prednisone (Pdn) 25 mg/day** Pdn/day tapered to 17.5 mg after 4 weeks Then for 4 weeks each: 12.5, 7.5, 5, and 2.5 mg/day, then discontinuation *Clinical trial*: Plus **methotrexate 10 mg/week** p. o. (MTX, n = 36) Plus **placebo** (n = 36) Both groups for 48 weeks *Concomitant medication*: Folic acid 7.5 mg (single dose), 24 h after MTX or placebo Oral calcium (1 g/day) Vitamin D3 (800 IU/day)
Result	Addition of methotrexate to standard treatment with prednisone, as compared to placebo, was associated with shorter prednisone treatment, fewer relapses and had a steroid-sparing effect
Patients	72 patients with newly diagnosed polymyalgia rheumatica (PMR) *Inclusion criteria*: • Age ≥ 50 years • ESR ≥ 40 mm/h • Aching and stiffness at shoulder, hip girdle, or both for more than 1 month *Major exclusion criteria*: • Other musculoskeletal or connective tissue diseases • Chronic liver disease, AST > normal value • No elevated serum creatinine kinase • Osteoporotic fractures • Steroid medication within the last month • Previous methotrexate or other immunosuppressive agent • Concomitant analgesic medications • Duration of symptoms (months, mean): 3.2 (group A) 2.6 (group B)
Authors	Caporali R, Cimmino MA, Ferraccioli G, Gerli R, Klersy C, Salvarani C, Montecucco C; Systemic Vasculitis Study group of the Italian Society for Rheumatology
Publication	***Ann** Intern Med.* 2004 Oct 5;141(7):493–500
Follow-up	76 weeks

(continued) ➜

Note	Outcome parameters (weeks 0–24):		
		Methotrexate	Placebo
	Patients no longer taking prednisone	n = 16	n = 15
	Relapses	n = 8	n = 8
	Recurrences	n = 0	n = 0
	Patients with ≥ 1 relapse or recurrence	n = 7	n = 8
	Outcome parameters (weeks 24–48):		
		Methotrexate	Placebo
	Patients no longer taking prednisone	n = 26	n = 14
	Relapses	n = 12	n = 18
	Recurrences	n = 3	n = 11
	Patients with ≥ 1 relapse or recurrence	n = 10	n = 19
	Outcome parameters (weeks 48–76):		
		Methotrexate	Placebo
	Patients no longer taking prednisone	n = 28	n = 16
	Relapses	n = 0	n = 7
	Recurrences	n = 4	n = 6
	Patients with ≥ 1 relapse or recurrence	n = 4	n = 10
	Duration of prednisone therapy (weeks)	5.1	14.4
	Median duration of prednisone therapy (weeks)	0	18
	Total prednisone dose (g)	0.19	0.62
	Median prednisone dose (1st to 3rd quartiles, g)	0	0.56
Adverse events		Methotrexate (%)	Placebo (%)
	Weight gain	11.2	5.6
	Urinary tract infection	19.6	16.8
	Hypertension	14	8.4
	Tachycardia	0	5.6
	Fracture	5.6	2.8
	Neuropathic disorder	8.4	14
	Dyspepsia	16.7	5.6
	Nausea	2.8	2.8
	Diarrhea	5.6	0
	Stomatitis	2.8	0
	Alopecia	2.8	0
	Diabetes	0	5.6
	Cataract	0	5.6

Trial	Treatment of refractory polymyalgia rheumatica with Etanercept: An open pilot study
Substance	**Etanercept 2×25 mg/week** for 24 weeks
	Corticosteroid therapy:
	Prednisone 12.5 mg/day
	Tapered to 10 mg after 1 month of remission
	Further reduction by 2.5 mg every 4 weeks until lowest effective dose
	Discontinuation after 24 weeks in case of complete remission, otherwise kept at 2.5 mg/day
Result	Etanercept was safe and effective. The cumulative dose of prednisone reached during the study was lower than in the same period of time before its start
Patients	6 patients with polymyalgia rheumatica (PMR), diagnosed according to the Healey criteria
	Inclusion criteria:
	• Relapsing PMR
	• Inability to reduce prednisone dosage below 7.5–10 mg/day
	• Presence of corticosteroid adverse events
	Major exclusion criteria:
	• Evidence of giant cell arteritis
	• Fulfillment of the ACR-criteria for RA
	• Presence of latent tuberculosis
	• Disease duration 45 months (mean)
	• Previous relapses n = 3.33 (mean)
	• Corticosteroid adverse events: one n = 6, two n = 5
Authors	Catanoso MG, Macchioni P, Boiardi L, Pipitone N, Salvarani C
Publication	*Arthritis Rheum.* 2007 Dec 15;57(8):1514–1519
Follow-up	9 months
Note	*Outcome parameters:*

	Outcome parameters	
	Sustained EULAR-PMR response ≥ 70%	n = 4
	Sustained EULAR-PMR response ≥ 50%	n = 2
	Leeb-DAS Score < 7	n = 5
	Change of Leeb-DAS Score	-79
	Decrease of prednisone dose (mg/day)	-6.875
	Cumulative prednisone dose during 9 months before vs. 9 months after study start (mg)	-1037
	Improvements at month 6 in ultrasounds of the shoulders	n = 6
	Change of ESR (mm/h)	-7.5
	Change of CRP (mg/dL)	-25.3
Adverse events	Influenca	n = 1
	Bacterial cystitis	n = 2

Trial	A double-blind, placebo-controlled trial of Etanercept in patients with giant cell arteritis and corticosteroid side-effects
Substance	**Etanercept 2 × 25 mg/week** (n = 8)
	Placebo (n = 9)
	After 1 month of stable corticosteroids
	Corticosteroid therapy:
	1 month of stable corticosteroids (no dose named):
	Then tapered by 10 mg/week to 30 mg
	Then tapered by 5 mg/week to 15 mg
	Then tapered by 2.5 mg/week until discontinuation
	Screening for TBC (PPD skin test ± chest X-rays), if suspicious:
	300 mg isoniazid/day for 9 months, or
	600 mg rifampicin/day for 4 months – in case of toxicity
	Previous medication:
	Pretreatment with corticosteroids 10 months (mean), mean dose 15 mg/day at start of study
	≥ 10 mg prednisone during previous 4 weeks
Result	Disease was controlled in more patients treated with etanercept than with placebo, the cumulative corticosteroid dose was lower in the etanercept group in this study of giantcell arteritis
Patients	17 patients with biopsy-proven giant cell arteritis, with side-effects secondary to corticosteroids (at least one):
	• Steroid-induced diabetes mellitus
	• Osteoporosis
	• High blood pressure
Authors	Martinez Taboada VM, Rodríguez-Valverde V, Carreño L, Lopez-Longo J, Figueroa M, Belzunegui J, Martín-Mola E, Bonilla G
Publication	*Ann Rheum Dis.* 2008;67(5):625–630
Follow-up	15 months

Note		Etanercept	Placebo
	Controlled disease activity	50%	22.2%
	Accumulated dose of prednisone	1.5 g	3 g
	Patients with relapses	50%	77.8%

Adverse events		Etanercept (%)	Placebo (%)
	Infections	50	44
	Injection-site reaction	12.5	22
	Cardiac failure	12.5	0
	Abnormal liver function	25	11

Trial	Effect of etanercept in polymyalgia rheumatica: A randomized controlled trial		
Substance	**Etanercept 2 × 25 mg/week** (n = 10)		
	Placebo (n = 10)		
	For 14 days		
	Previous medication:		
	No glucocorticosteroids		
	No DMARDs		
	Concomitant medication:		
	No NSAIDs		
	Tramadol was permitted		
Result	Etanercept monotherapy modestly reduced disease activity in glucocorticosteroid naïve patients in this short-term trial		
Patients	20 newly diagnosed, glucocorticoid naïve patients with polymyalgia rheumatica (PMR)		
	20 matched patients without PMR (control)		
Authors	Kreiner F, Galbo H		
Publication	*Arthritis Res Ther.* 2010;12(5):R176		
Follow-up	14 days		
Note	*Change of*:		
		Etanercept	Placebo
	PMR activity score	-24% (patients)	No change (patients)
		No change controls	
	Cumulative tramadol intake	-17% (patients)	No change (patients)
Adverse events		Etanercept	Placebo
	Minor local injection-site reactions	n = 1 (control)	n = 0
		n = 2 (PMR)	
	Unsuspected feeling of fatigue	n = 0	n = 1 (control)

Trial	Infliximab for maintenance of Glucocorticosteroid-induced remission of giant cell arteritis (GCA): A randomized trial
Substance	**Infliximab (IFX, 5 mg/kg,** n = 28)
	Placebo (n = 16)
	Started after 1 week of 40–60 mg prednisolone
	Corticosteroid therapy:
	Glucocorticosteroid starting dose was between 40 and 60 mg/day
	Tapered in steps of 10 mg/week to 20 mg/day
	Tapered by 2.5 mg steps to 10 mg every 2 weeks until 10 mg/week
	Tapered by 1 mg/week until withdrawal after 23 weeks at the latest
	Previous medication:
	No methylprednisolone > 1´000 mg/day for > 3 days
	No DMARDs
	No biologic agents
Result	Infliximab as maintenance therapy of giant cell arteritis in glucosteroid-induced remission, using a rapidly tapered glucocorticosteroid regimen, did not improve clinical results, i. e. the rate of relapses and remissions, in comparison with placebo, and was associated with more infections
Patients	44 patients with newly diagnosed giant cell arteritis on the basis of the ACR-criteria
	• Diagnosis of giant cell arteritis within 4 weeks of enrollment
	• ESR ≥ 40 mm/h at the time of diagnosis
	• Achieved clinical remission before randomization
	• Prednisone or prednisolone 40–60 mg/day for ≥ 1 week before randomization
	• ESR < 40 mm/h
	• Symptoms or signs of active giant cell arteritis
	Major exclusion criteria:
	• Diagnosis of GCA or polymyalgia rheumatica > 4 weeks before screening
	• No response to glucocorticosteroid therapy within 5 days
	• Prior immunosuppressive therapy or biological agents
Authors	Hoffman GS, Cid MC, Rendt-Zagar KE, Merkel PA, Weyand CM, Stone JH, Salvarani C, Xu W, Visvanathan S, Rahman MU; Infliximab-GCA Study Group
Publication	*Ann Intern Med*. 2007 1;146(9):621–630
Follow-up	54 weeks, study was ended after an interim analysis at week 22

(continued) ➔

Note	*Week 22 (study ended at this point after this analysis by steering committee and sponsor)*:		
		Placebo (%)	IFX (%)
	Patients without relapse	50	43
	< 10 mg corticosteroid	75	61
	Complete remission	44	39
Adverse events		Placebo	IFX
	Infection	56%	71%
	≥ 1 adverse event	94%	93%
	≥ 1 serious adverse event	25%	29%
	Discontinuation due to an adverse event	13%	11%
	All infections	n = 23	n = 47
	Patients with ≥ 1 infection	56%	71%
	Patients with ≥ 1 infection requiring oral or parenteral antimicrobial treatment	50%	57%
	Patients with ≥ 1 serious infections	6%	11%
	Infusion reactions	0%	5%
	Patients with ≥ 1 infusion reactions	0%	21%
	Antinuclear antibodies (newly positive)	33%	52%
	Antibodies to double-stranded DNA	0%	16%

Trial	Infliximab plus prednisone or placebo plus prednisone for the initial treatment of polymyalgia rheumatica: A randomized trial
Substance	**Infliximab, 3 mg/kg** (n = 23)
	Placebo infusions (n = 28)
	at weeks 0, 2, 6, 14, and 22
	Corticosteroid therapy:
	Prednisone 15 mg/day
	Tapered in 4 week periods to 10, 5, and 2.5 mg
	Then discontinued (after 16 weeks), if possible
	Previous medication:
	No steroids
	No biological agents
	No immunosuppressive agents
Result	Infliximab was not superior to placebo as an induction treatment regimen additional to prednisone in this trial of glucocorticosteroid-naive polymyalgia rheumatica. There was a high rate of relapses on the background of a low-dose and rapidly tapered regimen of prednisone
Patients	51 patients with newly diagnosed polymyalgia rheumatica according to the Healey-criteria
	Inclusion criteria:
	• > 50 years of age
	• ESR > 40 mm/h
	• Persistent pain (≥ 1 month)
	• Involving two of 3 areas (neck, shoulders, or pelvic girdle)
	• Morning stiffness lasting > 1 h
	• Rapid response to prednisone, 20 mg/day or less
	Major exclusion criteria:
	• Clinical or histologic evidence of giant cell arteritis
	• RA, signs and symptoms of SLE or other connective tissue disease, myositis, latent or active tuberculosis
	• Duration of symptoms (months, mean): 11 (group A), 10 (group B)
Authors	Salvarani C, Macchioni P, Manzini C, Paolazzi G, Trotta A, Manganelli P, Cimmino M, Gerli R, Catanoso MG, Boiardi L, Cantini F, Klersy C, Hunder GG
Publication	*Ann Intern Med.* 2007 May 1;146(9):631–639
Follow-up	52 weeks

(continued) ➜

Note	*Outcome parameters*:		
		Infliximab	Placebo
	Patients without relapse or recurrence	30%	37%
	Patients not receiving prednisone	50%	54%
	Total relapses and recurrences	n = 22	n = 32
	Median cumulative dose of prednisone (week 52, g)	17.1	12.2
Adverse events		Infliximab	Placebo
	Diabetes mellitus	n = 1	n = 0
	Infusion reaction	n = 4	n = 0
	System. infection	n = 1	n = 0
	Pancreatitis	n = 1	n = 0
	Cataract	n = 0	n = 1
	Dyspepsia	n = 0	n = 1
	Hypertension	n = 0	n = 2
	Bladder cancer	n = 0	n = 1

Trial	Rapid induction of remission in large vessel vasculitis by IL-6 blockade: A case series	
Substance	**Tocilizumab (TCZ) 8 mg/kg infusions every 4 weeks**	
	Concomitant medication:	
	Prednisone in n = 5 (mean doses at first tocilizumab application – 29.5 mg)	
	Tapered to 2.5 mg over 12 weeks	
Result	Tocilizumab was as effective in inducing rapid remission in this case series of large vessel vasculitides	
Patients	5 consecutive patients with giant-cell arteritis (GCA), 2 biopsy proven, 2 with Takayasu arteritis	
Authors	Seitz M, Reichenbach S, Bonel HM, Adler S, Wermelinger F, Villiger PM	
Publication	*Swiss Med Wkly*. 2011 Jan 17;141:w13156	
Follow-up	4.3 months (mean, range 3–7 months)	
Note	Complete clinical response	All patients
	Normalization of the acute phase proteins	All patients
	After 8.3 months still on monthly TCZ infusions	n = 3 (GCA)
	TCZ stopped after 7 months	n = 2 (GCA)
Adverse events	No adverse events were observed	

ANCA-Associated Vasculitis and combination trials of Churg-Strauss Syndrome and Polyarteritis Nodosa

Churg-Strauss Syndrome, Azathioprine

Trial	Treatment of Churg-Strauss syndrome without poor prognosis factors: a multicenter, prospective, randomized, open-label study of 72 patients

Substance	Corticosteroid therapy:
	I. v. pulse methylprednisolone (15 mg/kg, n = 72)
	Followed by oral prednisone (1 mg/kg/day) for 3 weeks
	Tapered by 5 mg every 10 days to 0.5 mg/kg/day
	Then by 2.5 mg every 10 days to a dosage of 15 mg/day
	Finally by 1 mg every 10 days to the minimal effective dosage or withdrawal
	
	Patients in whom prednisone doses could not be tapered below 20 mg:
	Azathioprine arm (n = 10):
	6 months of oral **2 mg/kg/day azathioprine**
	
	Cyclophosphamide arm (n = 9):
	6 i. v. pulses of **600 mg/m² cyclophosphamide** (CYC) every 2 weeks for 1 month
	Then every 4 weeks thereafter
	
	Concomitant medication:
	Uromitexan together with CYC (compulsory):
	    Potassium
	    Calcium
	    Vitamin D3
	    Bisphosphonates
	400 mg trimethoprim/day plus 80 mg sulfamethoxazole/day (CD4 count < 300/mm³)
	
	Previous medication:
	None for Churg-Strauss syndrome

(continued)

R. Müller, J. von Kempis, *Clinical Trials in Rheumatology*, 1051
DOI 10.1007/978-1-4471-2870-0_12, © Springer-Verlag London 2013

Result	Remission was achieved by prednisone alone in most patients, with common relapses and requirement of additional immunosuppressive therapy in one-third of them. Azathioprine or pulse cyclophosphamide both had additional effects in a significant proportion of patients with prednisone-resistant disease or major relapse
Patients	72 patients with Churg-Strauss syndrome
	Five Factor Score (FFS) for poor prognostic criteria = 0
	FFS:
	• Serum creatinine > 140 mmol/L (1.58 mg/dL)
	• Proteinuria > 1 g/day
	• Presence of severe gastrointestinal tract involvement
	• Cardiomyopathy and/or
	• Central nervous system involvement
Authors	Ribi C, Cohen P, Pagnoux C, Mahr A, Arène JP, Lauque D, Puéchal X, Letellier P, Delaval P, Cordier JF, Guillevin L; French Vasculitis Study Group
Publication	*Arthritis Rheum.* 2008;58(2):586–594
Follow-up	56.2 months
Note	*Outcome parameters (all patients):*

Remission achieved with prednisone therapy alone	93%
Long-term remission	79%
Patients in remission still taking corticosteroids	n = 52 out of 66
Relapse rate	42%
	n = 5 (non-responders to corticosteroids)
	n = 25 (relapse during tapering)
Time to relapse	18.3 months
Survival rates in all patients (year 1)	100%
Survival rates in all patients (year 5)	97%

Randomized patients:

	Azathioprine	Cyclophosphamide
Remission	n = 5	n = 7

(continued)

Adverse events	Subclinical osteoporosis	$n = 10$
	Infection requiring hospitalization	$n = 8$
	Osteoporotic fractures	$n = 7$
	Arterial hypertension	$n = 7$
	Thromboembolic events	$n = 7$
	Diabetes mellitus	$n = 5$
	Adrenal insufficiency	$n = 5$
	Ophthalmologic complications	$n = 4$
	Osteonecrosis of the femoral head	$n = 3$
	Cardiovascular damage	$n = 3$
	Glycosteroid-induced myopathy	$n = 2$
	Malignancy	$n = 2$
	Hepatotoxicity	$n = 2$
	Drug eruption	$n = 2$
	Tendon rupture	$n = 2$
	Sleep apnea syndrome	$n = 2$
	Esophageal candidiasis	$n = 2$
	Gastrointestinal ulcers	$n = 1$
	Hematologic toxicity	$n = 1$
	Azoospermia	$n = 1$
	Cyclophosphamide-induced cystitis	$n = 1$

Trial	Trimethoprim–sulfamethoxazole (Co-trimoxazole) for the prevention of relapses of Wegener's granulomatosis. Dutch Co-Trimoxazole Wegener Study Group
Substance	**Co-trimoxazole (2 × 800 mg sulfamethoxazole plus 160 mg trimethoprim, n = 41)** **Placebo** (n = 40) *Concomitant medication*: Prednisolone n = 23 (co-trimoxazole), n = 19 (placebo) Cyclophosphamide n = 21 (co-trimoxazole), n = 20 (placebo) *Previous medication*: Cyclophosphamide was permitted Prednisolone was permitted
Result	There was a difference in the incidence of relapses between placebo and co-trimoxazole, favoring co-trimoxazole, in patients in remission in this trial of patients with Wegener's granulomatosis under or after treatment with cyclophosphamide
Patients	81 patients with Wegener's granulomatosis in complete remission *Further inclusion criteria*: • Biopsy-proven glomerulonephritis, or • Biopsy-proven airway involvement, or • Fulfilling the ACR criteria and positive for ANCA *Major exclusion criteria*: • No history of adverse reaction to co-trimoxazole • No impaired renal function (24-h creatinine clearance of ≤ 30 mL/min) • Long-term therapy with antibiotics or co-trimoxazole *Disease duration*: • 30 months (median) • ANCA positive n = 52
Authors	Stegeman CA, Tervaert JW, de Jong PE, Kallenberg CG
Publication	*N Engl J Med*. 1996;335(1):16–20
Follow-up	24 months

(continued)

Note	Outcome parameters:		
		Co-trimoxazole	Placebo
	Patients in remission at 24 months	n = 31	n = 23
	Relapses	n = 7	n = 16
	Progressive glomerulonephritis	n = 4	n = 7
	Pulmonary lesions	n = 3	n = 2
	Nasal/upper airway lesions	n = 1	n = 11
	Scleritis	n = 1	n = 4
	Mononeuritis multiplex	n = 2	n = 0
	Dermal granulomatous vasculitis	n = 2	n = 4
Adverse events		Co-trimoxazole	Placebo
	Catomegalo virus infections	n = 0	n = 1
	Anorexia and nausea	n = 4	n = 0
	Rash	n = 2	n = 0
	Presumed interstitial nephritis with fever and eosinophilia	n = 1	n = 0
	Asymptomatic hepatotoxic effects	n = 1	n = 0
	Macrocytic anemia	n = 1	n = 0
	Recurrent urinary tract infections	n = 0	n = 1
	Myocardial infarction and death	n = 0	n = 1
	Herpes zoster	n = 2	n = 3

Trial	Co-trimoxazole and prevention of relapses of PR3-ANCA positive vasculitis with pulmonary involvement		
Substance	**960 mg co-trimoxazole 3×/week** (n = 16) **Placebo** (n = 15) *Previous medication*: Cyclophosphamide and prednisolone		
Result	Treatment with co-trimoxazole reduced the incidence of relapses in patients with Wegener's granulomatosis in remission		

Patients	31 patients with Wegener's granulomatosis
	In remission as assessed:
	  • Clinical scoring
	  • Laboratory variables
	  • Imaging		

Authors	Zycinska K, Wardyn KA, Zielonka TM, Krupa R, Lukas W		
Publication	*Eur J Med Res.* 2009 Dec 7;14 (Suppl 4):265–267		
Follow-up	18 months		
Note	*Patients in remission*:		
		Co-trimoxazole	Placebo
	Month 0	n = 16	n = 15
	Month 12	n = 14	n = 11
	Month 18	n = 12	n = 8
Adverse events		Co-trimoxazole	Placebo
	Infections/year (median)	0.0	4.0
	Herpes zoster	n = 3	n = 3
	CMV infection	n = 0	n = 2

Trial	Cyclophosphamide therapy of severe systemic necrotizing vasculitis	
Substance	**2 mg/kg cyclophosphamide/day**	
	Concomitant medication:	
	Corticosteroids (mean starting dose 62.6 mg, range 50–175 mg) Tapered to alternate-day administration of minimal dose after 2 weeks azathioprine n = 1 Prednisolone n = 23 (co-trimoxazole), n = 19 (placebo) Cyclophosphamide n = 21 (co-trimoxazole), n = 20 (placebo)	
	Previous medication:	
	Corticosteroids in n = 16 (mean duration 22 months) Azathioprine n = 2	
Result	Historically decisive systematic description of the usefulness of cyclophosphamide in the induction of remission after insufficient corticosteroid therapy in a heterogeneous population of patients with necrotizing vasculitis	
Patients	17 patients with necrotizing vasculitis <ul><li>With or without skin involvement</li><li>Proven by organ biopsy (n = 15) and/or by angiogram</li><li>All progressive despite treatment</li><li>HB-antigen positive n = 7</li><li>Cryoglobulinemia n = 6</li></ul>	
Authors	Fauci SF, Patz P, Haynes BF, Wolff SM	
Publication	*N Engl J Med*. 1979;301(5):235–238	
Follow-up	11 years	
Note	*Outcome parameters*:	
	Remissions	n = 14
		• n = 1 treated with azathioprine instead of CYC
	Mean duration of remission	22 months
Adverse events	Deaths	n = 3
		• Due to vasculitis n = 2
		• Unknown cause n = 1

Trial	Long-term follow-up after treatment of polyarteritis nodosa and Churg-Strauss angiitis with comparison of steroids, plasma exchange, and cyclophosphamide to steroids and plasma exchange. A prospective randomized trial of 71 patients. The Cooperative Study Group for Polyarteritis Nodosa
Substance	*Group A*: **13 × plasma exchanges** (60 mL/kg/session, 3 × in the first week, 2 ×/s week, then after 10, 15, 21, and 30 days and for another 4 months, 1/month, n = 39) *Group B*: **13 × plasma exchanges** **Cyclophosphamide 2 mg/kg/day** (n = 32) *Concomitant medication*: Replacement fluids for plasma exchange: 500 mL fluid gelatin, 4% albumin, fresh-frozen plasma Prednisone 1 mg/kg/day for 2 months Maintained for 3 weeks Tapered by 2.5 mg every 10 days to half of the initial level Then tapered by 2.5 mg every week to 20 mg/day Further tapered by 1 mg every week to 10 mg/day Maintained at 10 mg for 3 weeks, finally tapered to 5 mg/day by 1 mg *Previous medication*: No previous high-dose corticosteroids Low-dose corticosteroid predescribed for asthma ≤ 10 mg/day were permitted
Result	Reduced incidence of relapses by prednisone and plasma exchanges plus cyclophosphamide, without additional effect on long-term survival or increased treatment-associated mortality, as compared to prednisone and plasma exchange alone
Patients	71 patients with vasculitis according to the *Fauci classification*: • Polyarteritis nodosa (PAN) or Churg-Strauss angiitis • Clinical, histological, and/or arteriographic evidence of vasculitis • Sufficient disease activity to justify immunosuppressive treatment
Authors	Guillevin L, Jarrousse B, Lok C, Lhote F, Jais JP, Le Thi Huong Du D, Bussel A
Publication	*J Rheumatol.* 1991;18(4):567–574
Follow-up	10 years

(continued) ➔

Note	Outcome parameters:		
		Group A	Group B
	Treatment stopped because of ineffectiveness	n = 9	n = 1
	Relapses	38.5%	9.4%
	Higher doses of corticosteroids for relapse	n = 13	n = 1
	Introduction of CYC/reinstallation of plasma exchange for active disease	n = 4/3	n = 1
	Control of disease activity after 6 months	90%	93.5%
	10-year cumulative survival rates	72%	75%
Adverse events		Group A	Group B
	Treatment was stopped because of side effects	n = 1	n = 8
	Death related to vasculitis (total)	n = 3	n = 2
	Death due to bowel perforation	n = 2	n = 0
	Death due to cardiac insufficiency	n = 1	n = 0
	Multivisceral involvement	n = 0	n = 2
	Infectious adverse events of treatment (total)	n = 3	n = 2
	Bacterial pneumonia/septicemia	n = 3	n = 1
	Tuberculosis	n = 0	n = 1
	Death not related to systemic vasculitis (total)	n = 5	n = 4
	Sudden death	n = 2	n = 0
	Suicide	n = 0	n = 1
	Traffic accident	n = 1	n = 0
	Cancer	n = 1	n = 1
	Liver cirrhosis (post-HBV)	n = 0	n = 2
	Pulmonary embolism	n = 1	n = 0

Trial	Corticosteroids plus pulse cyclophosphamide and plasma exchanges versus corticosteroids plus pulse cyclophosphamide alone in the treatment of polyarteritis nodosa and Churg-Strauss syndrome patients with factors predicting poor prognosis. A prospective, randomized trial in 62 patients
Substance	*Both groups*: **Methylprednisone 15 mg/kg/day** for 3 days **Prednisone 1 mg/kg/day** for 1 month Tapered to 0 during the follow-up **Plus cyclophosphamide 0.6 g/m²** (CYC, i. v. bolus every 4 weeks over 12 months) *Group A (n = 28)*: **Prednisone plus CYC** (i. v. bolus) *Group B (n = 34)*: **Prednisone plus CYC** (i. v. bolus) **Plus plasma exchanges** (60 mL/kg, 9 × during 3 weeks) Replacement fluids for plasma exchange: 500 mL fluid gelatin, 4% albumin, fresh-frozen plasma *Concomitant medication*: Prednisone 5–10 mg/day (CSS patients with asthma) CD4 count < 300/mm³ ⇒ 1 Tbl. co-trimoxazole/day
Result	Treatment with prednisone, cyclophosphamide, and plasma exchanges was not superior over treatment with prednisone and cyclophosphamide alone

Patients	62 patients with severe polyarteritis nodosa
	  • Polyarteritis nodosa (PAN, n = 48), Churg-Strauss syndrome (CSS, n = 14)
	  • Typical biopsies n = 42
	  • Positive angiograms n = 30
	
	Inclusion criteria:
	  • Systemic PAN diagnosed by the presence of multiple system involvement
	  • ≥ 1 criteria for poor prognosis according to Five Factor Score
	  • Histological evidence of vascular lesion
	  • If no histological evidence: arteriographic evidence
	Or:
	  • Fulfillment or the ACR criteria for PAN
	Or:
	  • Fulfillment or the ACR criteria for CSS
	
	Major exclusion criteria:
	HBsAG/HBeAG-positivity
	Cutaneous or other limited forms of PAN or other systemic vasculitides

(continued) ➜

Authors	Guillevin L, Lhote F, Cohen P, Jarrousse B, Lortholary O, Généreau T, Léon A, Bussel A		
Publication	*Arthritis Rheum*. 1995;38(11):1638–1645		
Follow-up	5 years		
Note	*Outcome parameters*:		
		Group A	Group B
	Relapse	n = 4	n = 3
	Remission	n = 16	n = 22
	Remission without treatment	n = 3	n = 2
	Clinical remission requiring a maintenance of low-dose corticosteroids	n = 2	n = 2
Adverse events		Group A	Group B
	Death (total)	n = 7	n = 4
	Death due to vasculitis	n = 2	n = 2
	Death due to septicemia	n = 1	n = 0
	Unknown death	n = 3	n = 0
	Death due to shock	n = 1	n = 1
	Death due to lymphoma	n = 0	n = 1
	Pulmonary tuberculosis	n = 0	n = 3
	Pneumonia	n = 0	n = 3
	Sigmoiditis	n = 0	n = 1
	Septicemia	n = 0	n = 2
	Osteoporosis	n = 5	n = 5
	Vertebral fractures	n = 2	n = 2
	Cataract	n = 1	n = 1
	Diabetes	n = 2	n = 2
	Nervous breakdown	n = 1	n = 1

Trial	Controlled trial of pulse versus continuous prednisolone and cyclophosphamide in the treatment of systemic vasculitis
Substance	*PCYP arm (n = 24)*: **Pulse i. v. cyclophosphamide and prednisolone** After remission expanding oral pulse intervals *CCAZP arm (n = 30)*: **Continuous oral cyclophosphamide plus prednisolone** Followed by azathioprine at 3 months *Escalation of treatment*: Additional plasma exchange n = 8 (PCYP), n = 1 (CCAZP) I. v. prednisolone n = 12 (PCYP), n = 8 (CCAZP) I. v. immunoglobulins n = 8 (PCYP), n = 3 (CCAZP) Continuous oral prednisolone n = 13 (PCYP), n = 0 (CCAZP)
Result	No difference was observed in the frequency of remissions, relapses, or treatment failures between the two treatment arms. There was a tendency toward increased toxicity in patients treated with the continuous oral cyclophosphamide regimen
Patients	54 patients with systemic vasculitis • Classical polyarteritis n = 8 • Microscopic polyarteritis n = 17 • Wegener's granulomatosis n = 29 All diagnosed according to categories resembling the CHC definitions plus histologic or arteriographic evidence
Authors	Adu D, Pall A, Luqmani RA, Richards NT, Howie AJ, Emery P, Michael J, Savage CO, Bacon PA
Publication	*QJM.* 1997;90(6):401–409
Follow-up	40.4 months (median)

Note	*Outcome parameters*:	PCYP	CCAZP
	Partial remission	n = 12	n = 19
	Complete remission	n = 8	n = 7
	Treatment failure	n = 4	n = 4
	Death	n = 5	n = 4
	Relapse	n = 7	n = 8
	Chronic dialysis	n = 2	n = 3
Adverse events		PCYP	CCAZP
	Leukopenia	n = 7	n = 13
	Infective episodes	1.7/pat.	1.66/pat.
	Chest infection	n = 9	n = 9
	Ear-nose -throat infection	n = 6	n = 3
	Conjunctivitis	n = 1	n = 2
	Urine	n = 8	n = 10
	Septicemia	n = 3	n = 2
	Cellulitis	n = 2	n = 4
	Peritonitis	n = 1	n = 2
	Herpes zoster	n = 0	n = 1
	Herpes simplex	n = 1	n = 3
	Gastroenteritis	n = 2	n = 1

Trial	Treatment of good-prognosis Polyarteritis nodosa and Churg-Strauss syndrome: comparison of steroids and oral or pulse cyclophosphamide in 25 patients. French Cooperative Study Group for Vasculitides
Substance	*Group oral (n = 12)*: **Oral 2 mg/kg cyclophosphamide/day** for 12 months *Group i. v. (n = 13)*: **Monthly i. v. 0.6 g/m² cyclophosphamide** pulses *Flair*: Increase of prednisone dose *Concomitant medication*: 1 mg/kg prednisone/day Daily dose was tapered by 2.5 mg every week until 10 mg/day Daily dose was tapered by 1 mg every week until withdrawal Prophylactic antiemetic treatment was not systematically prescribed 500 mg calcium/day was recommended 800 IU vitamin D/day was recommended *Previous medication*: Low-dose corticosteroids to control asthma No cytotoxic agents
Result	No difference of efficacy was observed between the two regimens; more toxicity in patients treated with oral cyclophosphamide
Patients	25 patients suffering from systemic vasculitis with recent onset of symptoms: 　• Churg-Strauss vasculitis (n = 8) 　• Polyarteritis nodosa (n = 17), all fulfilling the ACR criteria *Inclusion criteria*: 　• Systemic PAN or CSS diagnosed by the presence of multiple system involvement 　• Absence of ≥ 1 criteria for poor prognosis according to Five Factor Score 　• Histologic evidence of vascular lesion 　• If no histologic evidence: arteriographic evidence
Authors	Gayraud M, Guillevin L, Cohen P, Lhote F, Cacoub P, Deblois P, Godeau B, Ruel M, Vidal E, Piontud M, Ducroix JP, Lassoued S, Christoforov B, Babinet P
Publication	*Br J Rheumatol.* 1997;36(12):1290–1297
Follow-up	60.8 months

(continued) ➜

Note	*Outcome parameters*:		
		Oral Cyc	i. v. Cyc
	Complete recovery	n = 9	n = 10
	Relapse	n = 2	n = 2
	Treatment failure	n = 1	n = 1
Adverse events		Oral Cyc	i. v. Cyc
	Toxic side effects	n = 27 in 10 patients (%)	n = 14 in 8 patients (%)
	Osteopenia	33	0
	Cushing's syndrome	17	23
	Amenorrhea	25	15
	Weight gain	8	15
	Malaise during infusion	0	23
	Alopecia	17	0
	Hemorrhagic cystitis	17	0
	Neutropenia	17	0
	Hypertension	17	0
	Skin folliculitis	17	0
	Urinary tract infection	0	8
	Hepatitis	8	0
	Herpes keratitis	8	0
	Osteonecrosis	8	0
	Cataract	8	0
	Digestive candidiasis	8	0
	Sinusitis	8	0
	Gastric ulcers	8	0
	Pulmonary infections	0	8
	Infectious bronchitis	0	8
	Acne	0	8

Trial	A prospective, multicenter, randomized trial comparing steroids and pulse cyclophosphamide versus steroids and oral cyclophosphamide in the treatment of generalized Wegener's granulomatosis
Substance	*Initial regimen*: **Methylprednisolone 15 mg/kg/day** i. v. for 3 days Followed by oral 1 mg/kg prednisone/day Tapering every 10 days by 2.5 mg until the half the initial dose Dose maintained stable for 3 weeks Tapered every 10 days by 2.5–20 mg/day Then tapered every 2 weeks by 1 mg until discontinuation On the day after the third methylprednisolone: 1 pulse 0.7 g/m² pulse of cyclophosphamide CYC *Randomization phase*: ***I. v. CYC group A*** (*i. v.*, *n* = 27): **0.7 g/m² pulse of CYC**, every 3 weeks until complete remission and 1 year thereafter Intervals between pulse treatments were then increased to 4 weeks for a 4-month period, then to 5 weeks for another 4-month period, and finally, to 6 weeks until discontinuation after 2 years *After 2 years of treatment*: **Oral CYC group** (*p. o.*, *n* = 23): **Oral 2 mg/kg CYC/day** starting day 10 until complete remission and 1 year thereafter *Concomitant medication*: 400 mg trimethoprim–sulfamethoxazole/day
Result	Pulse and oral cyclophosphamide were equally effective in achieving initial remission, with fewer side effects for pulse cyclophosphamide. In the long term, pulse cyclophosphamide was inferior with respect to maintenance of remission or prevention of relapses, but was associated with higher survival
Patients	50 patients with systemic Wegener's granulomatosis (WG) *Inclusion criteria*: • Systemic WG diagnosed by multiorgan or severe monovisceral involvement • Characteristic histology Positive immunofluorescence for ANCA n = 42
Authors	Guillevin L, Cordier JF, Lhote F, Cohen P, Jarrousse B, Royer I, Lesavre P, Jacquot C, Bindi P, Bielefeld P, Desson JF, Détrée F, Dubois A, Hachulla E, Hoen B, Jacomy D, Seigneuric C, Lauque D, Stern M, Longy-Boursier M
Publication	*Arthritis Rheum.* 1997;40(12):2187–2198
Follow-up	60 months

(continued) ➔

Note	Outcome parameters (6 months):		
		i. v. CYC (%)	oral CYC (%)
	Remission	88.9	78.3
	Complete remission	59.3	65.2
	Partial remission	29.6	13.0
	Treatment failure	11.1	21.7
	Death	14.8	26.1
	Long-term outcome:		
		i. v. CYC (%)	oral CYC (%)
	Sustained remission	47.8	70.6
	Relapse	52.2	17.6
	Death	21.7	23.5
	Final outcome:		
		i. v. CYC (%)	oral CYC (%)
	Remission	66.7	56.5
	Death rate	33.3	43.5
	Survived without relapse	37	48
	Relapse rate	59.2	13
Adverse events		i. v. CYC (%)	oral CYC (%)
	Infectious side effects	66.7	69.6
	Pneumocystis carinii pneumonia	11.1	30.4
	Oesophageal candidiasis	3.7	4.3
	Bacterial pneumonia	3.7	8.7
	Septicemia (other)	3.7	4.3
	Septicemia linked to dialysis catheter	3.7	0
	Septic arthritis	3.7	0
	Herpes zoster/CMV pneumonia	3.7	4.3
	Herpes zoster/CMV retinitis	0	4.3
	Papovavirus multifocal leukoencephalitis	0	3.7
	Patients with ≥ 1 side effect	66.7	69.6
	No. of side effects	n = 21	n = 23
	Death related to treatment side effects	11.1	26.1
	Hemorrhagic cystitis	3.7	8.7
	Transient aplasia	7.4	4.3
	Amenorrea	50	20
	Nausea	3.7	0
	Dysmyelopoesis	0	4.3
	Corticosteroid-related side effects	7.4	8.7
	Diabetes	3.7	4.3
	Glaucoma	3.7	0
	Osteoporosis with fractures	0	4.3
	Infections	40.7	69.6
	Psychiatric disorders	3.7	0
	Atherosclerosis	3.7	0

Trial	Intravenous pulse administration of cyclophosphamide versus daily oral treatment in patients with antineutrophil cytoplasmic antibody-associated vasculitis and renal involvement: a prospective, randomized study
Substance	*I. v. cyclophosphamide group (n = 22):* **0.75 g/m² cyclophosphamide** (CYC) i. v. every 4 weeks for 1 year *Oral cyclophosphamide group (n = 25):* **Oral 2 mg/kg CYC/day** for 1 year *Concomitant medication:* I. v. methylprednisolone 0.5 g on days 1–3 Oral p. o. 1 mg/kg prednisolone day 4–day 14 Tapered by 10 mg/week to 30 mg/day Tapered by 5 mg/week to 15 mg/day Tapered by 2.5 mg/week to 30 mg/day Stop of treatment after 1 year Treatment continued if remission not achieved for at least 6 months and ANCA titers not below 1:64 *Concomitant medication (only i. v. CYC):* Antiemetic drugs; alizapride or ondansetron 3 L of fluid was administered on the day of CYC treatment No prophylaxis for infectious complications such as *Pneumocystis carinii* pneumonia, tuberculosis, or fungal infections
Result	Intravenous and oral cyclophosphamide administration were equally effective, intravenous cyclophosphamide with lower toxicity concerning rate of leukopenia, severe infections, and gonadal function
Patients	47 patients with systemic vasculitis with first manifestations of: • Wegener's disease (WG, n = 22) • Microscopic polyangiitis (MPA, n = 25) • Diagnosed by the ACR criteria for WG or the presence of necrotizing pauci-immune vasculitis or glomerulonephritis without granuloma for MPA Further inclusion criteria: • Renal involvement (proteinuria, erythrocyturia) • Positive cANCA (WG) • Positive c- or pANCA (MPA) • Granulomatous inflammation evident on histology (WG) *Major exclusion criterion:* Creatinine > 200 µmol/L
Authors	Haubitz M, Schellong S, Göbel U, Schurek HJ, Schaumann D, Koch KM, Brunkhorst R
Publication	*Arthritis Rheum.* 1998;41(10):1835–1844
Follow-up	12 months

(continued) ➔

Note	Prednisolone dose not different between the two groups after 3, 6, 9, and 12 months
	Gonadal toxicity, leukopenia, and severe infections significantly reduced in the i. v. group compared with the p. o.-treated group

Outcome parameters:

	Oral CYC	i. v. CYC
Remission	n = 21	n = 22
Outcome complete remission	n = 3	n = 4
Partial remission	n = 1	n = 0
Oral prednisolone dose at 12 months	3 mg/day	4 mg/day
Time to remission (months)	1.5–12	2–9
Improvement of renal function	64%	59%
Renal survival after 2–3 years	64%	59%
Relapse during CYC	n = 3	n = 5

Organ manifestation at relapse:

	Oral CYC	i. v. CYC
Kidney	n = 3	n = 1
Eye	n = 1	n = 1
Arthralgia	n = 1	n = 1
Ear-nose-throat	n = 1	n = 0
B symptoms	n = 2	n = 3

Adverse events	Oral CYC	i. v. CYC
Nausea, partly with vomiting	n = 5	n = 11
FSH (IU/L)	+29.0	+12.6
Death	n = 3	n = 0
Leukopenia	60%	18%
Lymphopenia	86%	47%

CHUSPAN-Trial	Treatment of polyarteritis nodosa and microscopic polyangiitis with poor prognosis factors: a prospective trial comparing glucocorticoids and 6 or 12 i. v. cyclophosphamide pulses in 65 patients CHUSPAN: Churg-Strauss and Polyarteritis nodosa
Substance	*All patients*: **Glucocorticoids 15 mg/kg** for 3 days Then 1 mg/kg/day glucocorticoids orally for 3 weeks Glucocorticoids tapered by 5 mg every 10 days until 0.5 mg/kg Then tapered by 2.5 mg every 10 days until 15 mg/day Glucocorticoids < 10 mg, reduced by 1 mg every 10 days until being definitively stopped *Cyclophosphamide*: **3 × 0.6 g/m² cyclophosphamide** every 2 weeks, subsequently administered monthly **6 pulses** (n = 31) **12 pulses** (n = 34) *Concomitant medication*: CD 4 T cells < 300/mm³ ⇒ co-trimoxazole Uromitexan Bisphosphonates for osteoporosis
Result	A lower relapse probability and higher event-free survival for the 12-versus the 6-pulses cyclophosphamide pulse group was demonstrated

Patients	65 patients with
	  • Polyarteritis nodosa (PAN, n = 18)
	  • Microscopic polyangiitis (MPA, n = 47)
	Histologically proven or
	Meeting the ACR classification criteria and the CHC nomenclature for MPA
	
	Inclusion with ≥ 1 criteria of poor prognosis according to Five Factor Score:
	  • Serum creatinine > 1.58 mg/dL
	  • Proteinuria > 1 g/day
	  • Presence of severe gastrointestinal tract involvement
	  • Cardiomyopathy and/or
	  • Central nervous system involvement ANCA positive n = 37

Authors	Guillevin L, Cohen P, Mahr A, Arène JP, Mouthon L, Puéchal X, Pertuiset E, Gilson B, Hamidou M, Lanoux P, Bruet A, Ruivard M, Vanhille P, Cordier JF
Publication	*Arthritis Rheum*. 2003;49(1):93–100
Follow-up	36 months

(continued)

Note	Outcome parameters:				
		MPA, 12 pulses (%)	PAN, 12 pulses (%)	MPA, 6 pulses (%)	PAN, 6 pulses (%)
	Complete remission	86	100	74	100
	Death	21	0	26	17
	Relapses	21	17	37	50
	Events (relapse and/or death)	39	17	68	58
	Event occurring after the end of the study	22	17	67	58
Adverse events		6 pulses	12 pulses		
	Non-insulin-dependent diabetes	n = 1	n = 2		
	Insulin-dependent diabetes	n = 1	n = 0		
	Femoral osteonecrosis	n = 3	n = 1		
	Vertebral fracture	n = 3	n = 1		
	Cushing's syndrome	n = 1	n = 3		
	Obesity	n = 1	n = 2		
	Cataract	n = 1	n = 0		
	Esophagitis	n = 1	n = 1		
	Myopathy	n = 2	n = 0		
	Arterial hypertension	n = 0	n = 1		
	Amenorrhea	n = 0	n = 1		
	Leukopenia	n = 0	n = 1		
	Cardiomyopathy	n = 0	n = 1		
	Skin allergy to Mesna	n = 0	n = 1		
	Adrenal insufficiency	n = 0	n = 1		
	Mild thrombocytopenia	n = 1	n = 0		
	Abdominal abscess (S. aureus)	n = 0	n = 1		
	Cellulitis	n = 1	n = 0		
	Bacterial sacroiliitis	n = 1	n = 0		
	Cytomegalovirus pancreatitis	n = 0	n = 1		
	Herpes zoster	n = 1	n = 3		
	Septicemia on indwelling catheter	n = 0	n = 1		
	Bacterial pneumonia	n = 1	n = 0		
	Fungal infection	n = 1 (death)	n = 0		
	Pneumonia	n = 1	n = 0		
	Sinusitis	n = 1	n = 0		
	Methotrexate pneumonia	n = 1	n = 0		
	Skin allergy to i. v. immunoglobulins	n = 1	n = 0		
	Lymphoma	n = 1 (death)	n = 0		
	Prostate cancer	n = 1 (death)	n = 0		
	Malabsorption (small bowel resection)	n = 3	n = 1		
	Pulmonary embolism	n = 1	n = 0		
	Thrombosis	n = 1	n = 0		

CYCAZAREM-Trial	A randomized trial of maintenance therapy for vasculitis associated with antineutrophil cytoplasmic autoantibodies CYCAZAREM: Cyclophosphamide versus Azathioprine as Remission Maintenance Therapy for ANCA-associated Vasculitis Study
Substance	*Induction of remission*: 3 months of **2 mg/kg cyclophosphamide/day p. o. plus 1 mg/kg prednisolone/day** Tapered to 0.25 mg/kg/day by 12 weeks *Maintenance therapy (after begin of remission)*: **Cyclophosphamide 1.5 mg/kg/day** (n = 71) or **Azathioprine 2 mg/kg/day** (n = 73) *After 12 months (both groups)*: Azathioprine 1.5 mg/kg/day Plus 7.5 mg prednisolone/day *Concomitant medication*: Prednisolone 10 mg/day Prophylaxis against corticosteroid-induced gastritis, fungal infection, and *Pneumocystis carinii* pneumonia was recommended but not mandatory *Previous medication*: No cytotoxic drug within previous year
Result	In patients with generalized ANCA-associated vasculitis the substitution of cyclophosphamide by azathioprine after remission was clinically equivalent to the continuation with cyclophosphamide and did not increase the rate of relapse
Patients	Patients with a new diagnosis of generalized vasculitis, according to CHC definitions modified earlier by the authors • Wegener's granulomatosis n = 95 • Microscopic polyangiitis n = 60 • Renal involvement and/or threatened loss of function of other vital organ • Presence of ANCA • Serum creatinine $\leq$ 5.7 mg/dL • Patients without ANCA only in case of histologically proven vasculitis (n = 10) • DEI/BVAS at study start: 6.1/18.9 (means)
Authors	Jayne D, Rasmussen N, Andrassy K, Bacon P, Tervaert JW, Dadoniené J, Ekstrand A, Gaskin G, Gregorini G, de Groot K, Gross W, Hagen EC, Mirapeix E, Pettersson E, Siegert C, Sinico A, Tesar V, Westman K, Pusey C; European Vasculitis Study Group
Publication	*N Engl J Med.* 2003;349(1):36–44
Follow-up	18 months

(continued) ➔

Note	*Outcome parameters*:		
		Azathioprine	Cyclophosphamide
	Relapse rate	15.5%	13.7%
	Increase of glomerular filtration rate	7.5 mL/min	23.5 mL/min
Adverse events		Induction (%)	Azathioprine (%)	Cyclophosphamide (%)

	Induction (%)	Azathioprine (%)	Cyclophosphamide (%)
Leukopenia mild	30	21	32
Leukopenia severe	7	1	3
Anemia mild	0	2	1
Anemia severe	0	0	0
Diabetes mild	3	2	2
Diabetes severe	2	1	0
Infection mild	3	9	10
Infection severe	4	4	3
Bone fracture mild	0	0	0
Bone fracture severe	0	2	2
Gastrointestinal events mild	3	3	2
Gastrointestinal events severe	0	0	3
Cardiovascular events mild	0	1	1
Cardiovascular events severe	4	2	2
Cystitis mild	0	1	3
Cystitis severe	0	0	0
Allergy mild	3	4	2
Allergy severe	0	1	0
Amenorrhea mild	0	0	0
Amenorrhea severe	0	1	2
Alopecia mild	3	0	2
Alopecia severe	0	0	0
Psychiatric events	3	0	0

NORAM-Trial	Randomized trial of Cyclophosphamide versus Methotrexate for induction of remission in early systemic antineutrophil cytoplasmic antibody-associated vasculitis NORAM: Treatment of Non-Renal Wagener's granulomatosis
Substance	*Methotrexate group (n = 51)*: **Methotrexate 15 mg/week** p. o. Escalation to a maximum of 20–25 mg/week by 12 weeks Month 10: tapered and discontinued by month 12 *Cyclophosphamide group (n = 49)*: **Cyclophosphamide 2 mg/kg/day** p. o. (max. 150 mg/day) until remission (minimum 3, maximum 6 months) Then reduction to 1.5 mg/kg/day *Concomitant medication*: Prednisone 1 mg/kg Tapered to 7.5 mg by 6 months Discontinued after 12 months Antimicrobial prophylaxis optional
Result	Methotrexate was as effective as cyclophosphamide in the induction of remission of early ANCA-associated vasculitis, but less effective in patients with extensive disease and pulmonary involvement. More relapses were observed with methotrexate than with cyclophosphamide after termination of treatment. High relapse rates in both treatment arms after end of treatment at 12 months
Patients	100 patients with newly diagnosed ANCA-associated vasculitis • Wegener's granulomatosis (n = 89) or • Microscopic polyangiitis (n = 6), according to the CHC definitions • Involvement of one or more organ systems • Serum creatinine levels < 150 μmol/L Additional inclusion criteria: • ESR > 45 mm/h and/or • CRP > 2 × the upper limit of normal values, or ANCA positivity • Histologic confirmation of WG or MPA n = 51 • c- or p-ANCA positive n = 86 • PR3- or MPO-ANCA positive n = 82 • DEI (median) 11 • BVAS (median) 15 • VDI (median) 0
Authors	De Groot K, Rasmussen N, Bacon PA, Tervaert JW, Feighery C, Gregorini G, Gross WL, Luqmani R, Jayne DR
Publication	*Arthritis Rheum.* 2005;52(8):2461–2469
Follow-up	18 months

(continued)

Note	*Outcome parameters*:		
		Methotrexate	Cyclophosphamide
	Remission at 6 months	89.8%	93.5%
	Relapse rate/18 months	69.5%	46.5%
	Time remission–relapse (median)	13 months	15 months
	Death	n = 2	n = 2
	MTX median remission delayed in patients with entry disease extent index (DEI) above median of 10 and lower respiratory tract involvement		
Adverse events		Methotrexate	Cyclophosphamide
	Allergy	n = 1	n = 0
	Thrombocytopenia	n = 0	n = 1
	Mild infections	n = 5	n = 5
	Severe infections	n = 4	n = 4
	Leukopenia	n = 3	n = 14
	Multiple leukopenia	n = 0	n = 6
	Alopecia	n = 0	n = 1
	Cataract	n = 0	n = 1
	Osteoporosis	n = 0	n = 1
	Avascular necrosis	n = 1	n = 0
	Diabetes	n = 0	n = 3
	Infertility	n = 1	n = 0
	Hypertension	n = 3	n = 1
	Liver dysfunction	n = 7	n = 1
	Nausea	n = 1	n = 0
	Hypersensitivity	n = 0	n = 1

CYCLOPS-Trial	Pulse versus daily oral cyclophosphamide for induction of remission in antineutrophil cytoplasmic antibody-associated vasculitis
Substance	*Pulse cyclophosphamide (n = 76)*: **Cyclophosphamide, 3 pulses at 15 mg/kg** (CYC) i. v. given 2 weeks apart After that, pulses in 3 weeks intervals at 15 mg/kg i. v. or 5 mg/orally on 3 consecutive days, until remission Then for another 3 months Maximum CYC dose 1.2 g/pulse Or *Daily oral cyclophosphamide group (n = 73)*: **2 mg/kg Cyc/day,** until remission Then 1.5 mg/kg cyc/day for another 3 months Maximum daily oral dose 200 mg. Age- and leukocyte nadir-adapted reductions applied *Both groups*: CYC continuation for 3 months after remission, then change to azathioprine, 2 mg/kg/day, maximum daily dose 200 mg *Concomitant therapy*: Prednisolone 1 mg/kg/day Tapered to 12.5 mg at the end of month 3 Tapered to 5 mg at the end of 18 months *Pneumocystis jiroveci* prophylaxis recommended for all patients calcium and vitamin D supplementation for patients > 50 years
Result	No difference in the pulse or oral cyclophosphamide therapy groups with respect to induced remissions. Pulse therapy with a lower cumulative cyclophosphamide dose and lower incidence of leucopenia, with no difference in other adverse events during the observation period
Patients	149 patients with systemic vasculitis, diagnosed according to the CHC definitions, modified earlier by the authors • Wegener's granulomatosis (n = 56) • Microscopic polyangiitis (n = 71) • Renal limited vasculitis (n = 22) *Renal involvement of active vasculitis with at least one of the following*: • Serum creatinine 1.7–5.7 mg/dL • Biopsy of necrotizing glomerulonephritis • Erythrocyte casts • Hematuria • Proteinuria • Plus confirmatory histology or ANCA negative n = 3 • Confirmatory biopsy n = 117 • BVAS at study start: 20 (i. v.), 21 (oral) • DEI at study start: 2.2 (i. v.), 2.2 (oral)

(continued) ➔

Authors	de Groot K, Harper L, Jayne DR, Flores Suarez LF, Gregorini G, Gross WL, Luqmani R, Pusey CD, Rasmussen N, Sinico RA, Tesar V, Vanhille P, Westman K, Savage CO; EUVAS (European Vasculitis Study Group)
Publication	*Ann Intern Med.* 2009;150(10):670–680
Follow-up	18 months (median)
Note	*Clinical outcome parameters (both groups)*

Patients with achieved remission	n = 131
Time to remission (median)	3 months
Time to remission: no difference between groups, hazard ratio	1.098
Prompt and sustained reduction of BVAS to 1–2 (estimated according to Figure 4, no detailed numbers provided)	Both groups

Remission:

	i. v. CYC	oral CYC
At 3 months	n = 49	n = 43
At 6 months	n = 61	n = 55
At 9 months	n = 61	n = 58
At 12 months	n = 61	n = 55
At 15 months	n = 61	n = 54
At 18 months	n = 61	n = 54

Outcome parameters:

	i. v. CYC	oral CYC
Major relapses within 9 months	n = 7	n = 3
Minor relapses within 9 months	n = 6	n = 3
Improvement of glomerular filtration rate (median, estimated, mL/min per 1.73 m^2)	32 ⇒ 45	29 ⇒ 45
Absolute CYC-dose (median)	15.9	8.2

End-stage renal disease:

	i. v. CYC	oral CYC
At 3 months	n = 1	n = 0
At 6 months	n = 4	n = 0
At 9 months	n = 4	n = 0
At 12 months	n = 4	n = 1
At 15 months	n = 4	n = 1
At 18 months	n = 5	n = 1

(continued)

Adverse events		i. v. CYC	oral CYC
	Any adverse events	n = 58	n = 56
	Mild or moderate episodes	n = 77	n = 101
	Severe or life threatening	n = 19	n = 31
	Death (total)	n = 5	n = 6
	Death associated to active vasculitis	n = 3	n = 7
	Leukopenia	n = 20	n = 33
	Patients with ≥ 2 episodes	n = 4	n = 15
	Episodes (total)	n = 28	n = 59
	Infection	n = 20	n = 21
	Mild or moderate	n = 15	n = 19
	Severe or life threatening	n = 7	n = 10
	New or worsening diabetes	n = 8	n = 4
	Liver dysfunction	n = 2	n = 3
	Alopecia	n = 0	n = 2
	Hypersensitivity reaction to azathioprine	n = 10	n = 5
	Osteoporosis	n = 2	n = 0
	Cancer	n = 1	n = 0
	Hemorrhagic cystitis	n = 2	n = 1
	Amenorrea	n = 1	n = 0
	Cataract	n = 0	n = 3
	Hypertension	n = 0	n = 2
	Cardiovascular events	n = 3	n = 2
	Pulmonary embolism/deep venous thrombosis	n = 2	n = 4
	Other	n = 15	n = 18

Trial	Churg-Strauss syndrome with poor-prognosis factors: a prospective multicenter trial comparing glucocorticoids and 6 or 12 cyclophosphamide pulses in 48 patients
Substance	*Initial corticosteroid therapy*:
	3 consecutive i. v. pulses **15 mg/kg methylprednisolone** on days 1–3
	Then oral prednisone (GC, 1 mg/kg/day) for 3 weeks
	Tapered by 5 mg every 10 days to 0.5 mg/kg/day
	Then further tapered by 2.5 mg every 10 days to 15 mg/day
	Finally tapered by 1 mg every 10 days to the minimal effective dose
	1 g calcium/day
	After randomization:
	Cyclophosphamide 6 pulses 0.6 g/m² (n = 23)
	Or
	Cyclophosphamide 12 pulses 0.6 g/m² (n = 25)
	Pulses every 2 weeks for 1 month
	Then cyclophosphamide pulses (0.6 g/m²) every 4 weeks
	Concomitant medication:
	Vitamin D3 400 IU
	Bisphosphonates oral daily or weekly
	Mesna at the same dose as cyclophosphamide
	Co-trimoxazole (400/80 mg) was strongly recommended if CD 4 T cell count ≤ 300/mm³
Result	Twelve cyclophosphamide pulses resulted in fewer relapses in severe Churg-Strauss syndrome than a six-pulse regimen
Patients	48 patients with recently diagnosed, untreated Churg-Strauss syndrome, satisfying the CHC definitions
	• Biopsy-proven necrotizing vasculitis
	• Eosinophilia > 1'500/mm³ or > 10%
	• Asthma and clinical manifestations of systemic vasculitis
	• Fulfilled ≥ 4 ACR criteria: n = 38
	At least one factor associated with poor outcome according to Five Factor Score:
	• Creatinine > 140 mmol/L (1.58 mg/dL)
	• Proteinuria > 1 g/day
	• Central nervous system
	• Gastrointestinal or myocardial involvement
Authors	Cohen P, Pagnoux C, Mahr A, Arène JP, Mouthon L, Le Guern V, André MH, Gayraud M, Jayne D, Blöckmans D, Cordier JF, Guillevin L; French Vasculitis Study Group
Publication	*Arthritis Rheum.* 2007;57(4):686–693
Follow-up	36 months

(continued) ➔

Note	Outcome parameters:		
		6 pulses (%)	12 pulses (%)
	Clinical remission	91.3	84
	Failure	8.7	16
	Patients who relapsed	78.2	52
	Major relapses	55.5	61.5
	Minor relapses	77.7	46.1
	Patients with severe side effect	47.8	52
	Death	8.7	8
Adverse events		6 pulses	12 pulses
	Infections	n = 11	n = 10
	GC-induced osteoporotic fractures	n = 3	n = 5
	GC-induced diabetes mellitus	n = 2	n = 1
	Venous thromboembolism	n = 1	n = 1
	GC-induced osteonecrosis	n = 1	n = 1
	Amenorrhea	n = 1	n = 2
	Glaucoma	n = 1	n = 1
	GC-induced cataract	n = 1	n = 1
	Neutropenia < $1,000/mm^3$	n = 1	n = 1
	Miscellaneous	n = 1	n = 6

Trial	Treatment of polyarteritis nodosa and microscopic polyangiitis without poor-prognosis factors: a prospective randomized study of 124 patients
Substance	*Corticosteroid therapy*: **Methylprednisolone i. v. pulse (15 mg/kg,** n = 124) Followed by oral prednisone (1 mg/kg/day) for 3 weeks Tapered by 5 mg every 10 days to 0.5 mg/kg/day Then by 2.5 mg every 10 days to a dosage of 15 mg/day Finally by 1 mg every 10 days to the minimal effective dosage or withdrawal *Azathioprine (AZA, n = 19)*: **Azathioprine 2 mg/kg/day** for 6 months *Cyclophosphamide (n = 20)*: **Cyclophosphamide 6 i. v. pulses of 600 mg/m^2** (CYC) every 2 weeks for 1 month Then every 4 weeks *Concomitant medication*: Uromitexan together with Cyc (compulsory): Potassium Calcium Vitamin D3 Bisphosphonates 400 mg trimethoprim/day plus 80 mg sulfamethoxazole/day (CD 4 T cell count < 300/mm^3)
Result	First-line corticosteroid treatment was able to achieve and maintain remission in only about half of the patients. Azathioprine or pulse cyclophosphamide therapy was fairly effective for treating corticosteroid-resistant disease or major relapses
Patients	124 patients with newly diagnosed polyarteritis nodosa (n = 58) or microscopic polyangiitis (n = 66) • Five Factor Score = 0 • No other systemic vasculitides, e.g., Wegener's granulomatosis, rheumatoid vasculitis, Henoch-Schönlein purpura, or cryoglobulinemia
Authors	Ribi C, Cohen P, Pagnoux C, Mahr A, Arène JP, Puéchal X, Carli P, Kyndt X, Le Hello C, Letellier P, Cordier JF, Guillevin L; French Vasculitis Study Group
Publication	*Arthritis Rheum.* 2010 Apr;62(4):1186–1197
Follow-up	62 ± 33 months

(continued) ➜

Note	Treatment with corticosteroids alone induced remission n = 98		
	Sustained disease remission n = 50		
	Relapse n = 46		
	Failed treatment with corticosteroids alone n = 26		
	Required additional immunosuppression n = 49		
		CYC	AZA
	Remission	n = 13	n = 14
	1-year survival rates	99%	
	5-year survival rates	92%	
Adverse events		CYC	AZA
	Death	n = 6	n = 2
	Infection	n = 4	n = 5
	Ophthalmologic complications	n = 5	n = 2
	Hypertension	n = 1	n = 1
	Osteoporotic fractures	n = 2	n = 3
	Diabetes mellitus	n = 1	n = 1
	CS-induced myopathy	n = 0	n = 2
	Thromboembolic events	n = 2	n = 0
	Malignancy	n = 0	n = 0
	Subclinical osteoporosis	n = 0	n = 1
	Cardiovascular damage	n = 0	n = 1
	Cerebrovascular damage	n = 1	n = 1
	Hematologic toxicity	n = 1	n = 2
	Adrenal insufficiency	n = 0	n = 1
	CS-induced psychiatric disorder	n = 0	n = 0
	Osteonecrosis of the femoral head	n = 0	n = 0
	Hepatotoxicity	n = 0	n = 1
	Iatrogenic aneurysm	n = 0	n = 0
	Cyc-induced cystitis	n = 1	n = 0

Trial	Methotrexate plus leflunomide for the treatment of relapsing Wegener's granulomatosis. A retrospective uncontrolled study
Substance	**Methotrexate 18.9 ± 6.8 mg/week** (MTX, n = 36) **Leflunomide 21.0 ± 7.8 mg/day** (Lef, n = 15) *Concomitant medication*: 7.2 ± 4.8 mg/day prednisolone *Previous medication*: Relapsing patients were subsequently treated with a combination therapy of MTX plus Lef.
Result	The combination of methotrexate and leflunomide combination therapy in patients not requiring cyclophosphamide, if tolerated well, was effective in this retrospective study

Patients	51 Wegener's granulomatosis patients
	With non-life-threatening relapses despite MTX or leflunomide monotherapy
	   • Generalized disease n = 41
	   • Early systemic disease n = 8
	   • Localized disease n = 2
	   • ANCA positive n = 46

Authors	Bremer JP, Ullrich S, Laudien M, Gross WL, Lamprecht P
Publication	*Clin Exp Rheumatol.* 2010 Jan-Feb;28(1 Suppl 57):67–71
Follow-up	26.0 months (mean)
Note	*Outcome parameters*:

Controlled relapsing disease	84%
BVAS = 0	54.9%
No response	15.7%
Minor relapse	27.5%
Major relapse	3.9%
Decrease of the BVAS	-3.4

Rates of discontinuation:

	Year 1 (%)	Year 2 (%)	Year 3 (%)
Because of relapse	88.5	84.9	80.7
Because of adverse event	77.1	71.7	71.7

(continued)

Adverse events	Hypertension	n = 11
	Bronchitis	n = 5
	Nausea	n = 5
	Diarrhea	n = 4
	ASAT/ALAT > 3×	n = 3
	Psychic	n = 3
	Neoplasia	n = 2
	Skin infection	n = 2
	Pneumonia	n = 2
	Wound healing disorder	n = 2
	Leukopenia	n = 1
	Erysipelas	n = 1
	Allergic reaction	n = 1
	Skin nodule	n = 1
	Conjunctivitis	n = 1
	MTX pneumopathy	n = 1
	CMV reactivation	n = 1
	PJ pneumonia	n = 1
	Lethal myocardial infarction	n = 1
	Bacterial sinusitis	n = 1
	Polyneuropathy	n = 1
	Total	n = 50

Trial	The treatment of Wegener's granulomatosis with glucocorticoids and methotrexate	
Substance	**Methotrexate 0.3 mg/kg/week** (max. 15 mg, increased to max. 25 mg/week) Increased every 1–2 week to max. 25 mg/week *Concomitant medication*: Oral prednisolone 1 mg/kg/day Tapered down in case of significant improvement, after 1 month, eventually to alternate day schedule *Previous medication*: Various medical therapies Cyclophosphamide n = 2	
Result	Weekly low-dose methotrexate was an effective alternative to cyclophosphamide in patients without immediately life-threatening disease or with ineffective or seriously toxic prior cyclophosphamide treatment	
Patients	29 patients with Wegener's granulomatosis • With current of past evidence of upper and/or lower airway disease • And/or other organ involvement • Without immediately life-threatening disease	
Authors	Hoffman GS, Leavitt RY, Kerr GS, Fauci AS	
Publication	*Arthritis Rheum.* 1992;35(11):1322–1329	
Follow-up	25 months	
Note	*Outcome parameters*:	
	Remission	69%, n = 20
	Marked improvement	76%, n = 22
	Disease progression	n = 5
	Sustained remission after discontinuation of prednisolone	n = 13
	Relapse after discontinuation of prednisolone	n = 2
Adverse events	Abnormal liver function tests	10%
	Pneumocystis carinii pneumonia	10%
	MTX pneumonitis	7%
	Oral ulcers and rash	3%

Trial	An analysis of 42 Wegener's granulomatosis patients treated with methotrexate and prednisone	
Substance	**Methotrexate low-dose 0.3 mg/kg/week** (MTX, max. 15 mg at start, increased to 20–25 mg/week) Maintained at this dose for 1 year in the case of remission Then taper of 2.5 mg/month until discontinuation, if possible plus approximately 1 mg/kg prednisone/day Begin of taper after 4 weeks, to 0, if possible	
	Previous medication: No increase in immunosuppressive drugs ≤ 4 weeks No therapy 16% Prednisone alone 33% Prednisone plus trimethoprim/sulfamethoxazole 10% Prednisone plus cyclophosphamide 10% Azathioprine 10%	
Result	Weekly low-dose methotrexate was an effective alternative in patients with Wegener's granulomatosis without immediately life-threatening disease or with prior serious cyclophosphamide-associated toxicity	
Patients	42 patients with biopsy-proven active Wegener's granulomatosis (i. e., necrotizing vasculitis, granulomatous inflammation) • No immediately life-threatening disease • Patients with ineffective pretreatment 62% (n = 26) • Patients without therapy immediately before study entry 38% (*n* = 16) • No renal failure/insufficiency	
Authors	Sneller MC, Hoffman GS, Talar-Williams C, Kerr GS, Hallahan CW, Fauci AS	
Publication	*Arthritis Rheum.* 1995;38(5):608–613	
Follow-up	38 months	
Note	*Outcome parameters*:	
	Patients surviving	93%
	Remission of disease	71%
	Relapses after achieving remission	36%
	Medan time to remission (months)	4.2
	Median time to relapse in patients achieving remission (months)	29
	Induced remission after second course of MTX plus prednisone	75%
	Discontinuation of prednisolone (months, median)	7
Adverse events	Elevated transaminase levels	24%
	Leukopenia	7%
	Opportunistic infections	9.5%
	MTX pneumonitis	7%
	Stomatitis	2%

Trial	Therapy for the maintenance of remission in 65 patients with generalized Wegener's granulomatosis. Methotrexate versus trimethoprim/sulfamethoxazole
Substance	*Induction of remission*: **Cyclophosphamide 2 mg/kg/day** p. o. or **I. v. cyclophosphamide 650 mg/m²** pulse plus **1 mg/kg prednisone/day** Until *Maintenance of remission (after beginning of complete or partial remission)*: **0.3 mg/kg methotrexate/week** i. v., alone (group A; n = 22) **Trimethoprim/sulfamethoxazole, 160/800 mg, alone** (group B; n = 24) **Methotrexate plus concomitant prednisone** (median dose 3 mg/day, group C; n = 11) **Trimethoprim/sulfamethoxazole plus prednisone** (median dose 10 mg/day, group D; n = 8)
Result	Low-dose methotrexate, with or without concomitant prednisone, was effective in most patients and more effective than trimethoprim/sulfamethoxazole for the maintenance of remission in patients with generalized disease after induction of remission with cyclophosphamide
Patients	65 patients with generalized Wegener's granulomatosis • Diagnosis according to ACR criteria and CHC definitions • Histologically proven disease n = 58 • Serum creatinine ≤ 150 mmol/L • cANCA positivity in n = 61; in all 7 patients without histologic prove of disease
Authors	de Groot K, Reinhold-Keller E, Tatsis E, Paulsen J, Heller M, Nölle B, Gross WL
Publication	*Arthritis Rheum.* 1996;39(12):2052–2061
Follow-up	33 months

(continued)

Note	Outcome parameters:				
		Group A	Group B	Group C	Group D
	Partial or complete remission	86% (n = 19)	58% (n = 14)	91% (n = 10)	0% (n = 8)
	Median time of remission	16 months	36.5 months	22 months	–
	Change of:				
		Group A	Group B	Group C	Group D
	DEI	-2.0	0	-1.5	+2.5
Adverse events				Groups A plus C	Groups B plus D
	Nausea			n = 6	n = 0
	Leukopenia			n = 5	n = 5
	Rise in transaminase levels			n = 2	n = 0
	Mucositis			n = 1	n = 0
	Rise in creatinine levels			n = 0	n = 4
	MTX pneumopathy			n = 1	n = 0
	Additional folinic acids			n = 11	n = 0
	Opportunistic infections			n = 0	n = 0
	Dosage reduction due to adverse events			n = 6	n = 0
	Withdrawal due to adverse events			n = 2	n = 3
	Pancytopenia			n = 1	n = 0

Trial	Induction of remission in Wegener's granulomatosis with low-dose methotrexate	
Substance	**0.3 mg/kg methotrexate/weekly** i. v. Plus low-dose **prednisone 10 mg/day**	
	Previous medication: Previous untreated disease n = 11 Oral cyclophosphamide plus prednisone n = 4 Azathioprine plus prednisone n = 1 Dapsone plus prednisone n = 1	
Result	Weekly low-dose methotrexate in combination with low-dose corticosteroids lead to remission in almost 60% without significant side effects	
Patients	17 patients with non-life-threatening, generalized Wegener's granulomatosis • Serum creatinine ≤ 150 mmol/L	
Authors	de Groot K, Mühler M, Reinhold-Keller E, Paulsen J, Gross WL	
Publication	*J Rheumatol.* 1998;25(3):492–495	
Follow-up	24.5 months (median)	
Note	*Outcome parameters*:	
	Complete remission	n = 6 (median 24.5 months)
	Partial remission	n = 4
	Minor relapse	n = 2
	Major relapse	n = 0
	Non-responders	n = 7
	Median prednisone dose	1.75 mg/day (7.5 mg in non-responders; high concomitant)
	Median time to discontinuation of prednisone	7.5 months
	Median DEI at study start	5.5
	Median DEI at study end	0 (responders)
	De novo glomerulonephritis	n = 5 (high likelihood in patients with need for higher concomitant prednisone)
	Relapse after initial response	n = 2 (need for higher concomitant prednisone at risk for nonresponse)
	Progressive disease despite MTX treatment	n = 5
Adverse events	Nausea	n = 1
	Oral mucositis	n = 1

Trial	A staged approach to the treatment of Wegener's granulomatosis: induction of remission with glucocorticoid and daily cyclophosphamide switching to methotrexate for remission maintenance
Substance	*Induction of remission*: **Cyclophosphamide 2 mg/kg/day** plus **prednisone 1 mg/kg/day** *Maintenance of remission (after achieving remission)*: **Prednisone tapered** by 5 mg every other day in 1-week intervals until 60 mg every other day Then tapered by 2.5–5 mg/week until discontinuation Cyclophosphamide was discontinued at remission **3 mg/kg methotrexate/week** (max. 15 mg/week and increased to 25 mg/week)
Result	Methotrexate-mediated maintenance of remission after cyclophosphamide- and glucocorticoid-induced remission was effective
Patients	31 Wegener's granulomatosis patients • 28 patients with biopsy-proven Wegener's granulomatosis (necrotizing vasculitis, granulomatous inflammation) • Three Wegener's granulomatosis patients without biopsy-proven disease, diagnosed by all of: pos. cANCA, upper airways disease, active glomerulonephritis, ≥ 1 other major organ system, after exclusion of infection • All patients ANCA positive, cANCA n = 27, pANCA/MPO n = 4 • No evidence of chronic renal insufficiency (serum creatinine > 2.5 mg/dL at remission)
Authors	Langford CA, Talar-Williams C, Barron KS, Sneller MC
Publication	*Arthritis Rheum.* 1999;42(12):2666–2673
Follow-up	16 months (median)

(continued) ➔

Note	Outcome parameters:	
	Deaths	n = 0
	Drop out because of toxicity	n = 2 (both survived)
	Achieving remission	100%
	Relapse after achieving remission	16%
	Months to remission (median)	3
	Time to taper to alternate-day prednisone (median)	4 months
	Time to discontinuation of prednisone (median)	8 months
	Time from remission to relapse for five patients (median)	13 months
	Prednisone discontinued before relapse for five patients (median)	8 months
Adverse events	Leukopenia requiring dosage reduction of cyclophosphamide	10%
	Leukopenia requiring dosage reduction of methotrexate	13%
	Methotrexate pneumonitis	6%
	Cystitis	6%
	Avascular necrosis	3%
	Cataracts	3%
	Diabetes mellitus	3%
	Cutaneous herpes zoster	13%
	Bacterial pneumonia	6%

Trial	Use of methotrexate and glucocorticoids in the treatment of Wegener's granulomatosis Long-term renal outcome in patients with glomerulonephritis
Substance	**Methotrexate low-dose 0.3 mg/kg/week** (max. 15 mg at start, increased to 20–25 mg/week) Maintained at this dose for 1 year in the case of remission Then taper of 2.5 mg/month until discontinuation, if possible Plus prednisone 1 mg/kg/day Tapered after 4 weeks to 0, if possible
Result	The combination of methotrexate and prednisone was effective as initial therapy for patients with active glomerulonephritis
Patients	42 patients with Wegener's granulomatosis (WG), fulfilling the ACR criteria <ul><li>21 with active glomerulonephritis (GN)</li><li>All 42 patients with biopsy-proven WG</li><li>With necrotizing vasculitis</li><li>Granulomatous inflammatory changes or both in a typical organ system</li><li>All with active disease requiring therapy</li></ul> *Important exclusion criteria*: <ul><li>Life-threatening disease:<ul><li>Acute renal failure with serum creatinine < 2.5 mg/dL</li><li>Acute pulmonary hemorrhage with an arterial PO_2 < 70 mmHg and/or DLCO < 70% of predicted</li><li>Presence of chronic liver disease</li></ul></li><li>Recent increase in immunosuppressive medication</li></ul>
Authors	Langford CA, Talar-Williams C, Sneller MC
Publication	*Arthritis Rheum.* 2000;43(8):1836–1840
Follow-up	76 months (median)

Note	*Outcome parameters*:	
	Renal remission	n = 20 of 21 patients with GN
	Stable creatinine levels at 1 and 6 months after study entry	n = 6
	Improved creatinine levels at 1 and 6 months after study entry (> 0.2 mg/dL)	n = 12

Adverse events	*Stable or improved creatinine levels in 18 patients*	
	Death	n = 1 (week 14, opportunistic infection)
	Relapse	n = 11
	Remission after retreatment with MTX	n = 7
	Long-term decline of renal function	n = 2

Trial	High rate of renal relapse in 71 patients with Wegener's granulomatosis under maintenance of remission with low-dose methotrexate
Substance	*Induction of remission*: **Cyclophosphamide 2 mg/kg/day** (CYC) p. o. With equivalent dose of uromitexan, in 3–4 doses per day Plus **glucocorticosteroid 1 mg/kg/day** Tapered weekly by 10–20 mg Tapered further by 2.5 mg/3 weeks to 5 mg/day In stable remission, further reduction by 1 mg/month until discontinuation *Maintenance of remission*: At ≤ 7.5 mg glucocorticosteroid and persistent complete or partial remission for ≥ 3 months Methotrexate 7.5 mg (MTX)/week i. v. with escalation to 0.3 mg/kg/week (mean dosage of 22.5 mg) Seven patients with glucocorticosteroid dose of ≥ 7.5 included because of persistent leukopenia under Cyc MTX tapered by 2.5 mg/month in case of persistent complete remission for 6 months and no glucocorticosteroids
Result	Efficacy of methotrexate in the long-term maintenance of remission was limited by relapses during ongoing treatment in 36.6% of patients. No additive protective effect with regard to maintenance of remission of glucocorticosteroids was observed
Patients	71 patients, fulfilling the ACR criteria for Wegener's granulomatosis (WG) • Biopsy: necrotizing vasculitis, granuloma, or both n = 58 • In the patients with no histologic confirmation, the diagnosis was made on the basis of the typical history, characteristic clinical findings, and a positive cANCA on immunofluorescence, with anti-PR3 specificity • Positive c/PR3-ANCA n = 69 • Enrollment within first WG episode n = 53 • Enrollment after relapse already n = 18 • DEI at diagnosis/start of study 10.1/2.1
Authors	Reinhold-Keller E, Fink CO, Herlyn K, Gross WL, De Groot K
Publication	*Arthritis Rheum.* 2002;47(3):326–332
Follow-up	77 months

(continued) ➔

Note	Outcome parameters:	
	Media duration of prior CYC	10 months
	Patients with concomitant glucocorticosteroid therapy during induction therapy with CYC	n = 70 out of 71
	At study start low-dose glucocorticosteroids (5.9 mg/day)	n = 55
	Relapse	36.6% (n = 26)
	Time to relapse	19.4 months within mean observation period of 25.2 months
	Relapses classified as major	n = 18
		n = 16 of them with switch to CYC
	Terminated glucocorticosteroid therapy at the time of relapse	65.4% (n = 17)
	Relapses mainly in the initially involved organ systems:	
	Significant increase in ANCA titer prior or parallel to relapse	15/26
	Initial manifestation in the ear, nose, throat tract	18/26
	Initial manifestation in the kidney	16/26
	MTX cessation because of persistent leukopenia	n = 2
Adverse events	Leukopenia	n = 9
	• Leading to MTX dose reduction	n = 7
	• Leading to MTX cessation	n = 2
	Leukopenia with infection	n = 7 (bacterial n = 5)
	Segemental herpes zoster	n = 2

Trial	Churg-Strauss syndrome—successful induction of remission with methotrexate and unexpected high cardiac and pulmonary relapse ratio during maintenance treatment

Substance	*Induction of remission (n = 11)*:
	Methotrexate 0.3 mg/kg (MTX)/week i. v.
	Folinic acid given on the next day (induction, n = 11)
	Initial MTX dosage 7.5 mg/week
	Increased by 2.5 mg every week to 0.3 mg/kg/day
	
	Maintenance of remission (n = 25):
	Methotrexate 0.3 mg/kg/week
	
	After induction of remission:
	  • With successful MTX induction therapy n = 8 out of 11 patients (induction of remission)
	  • With p. o. cyclophosphamide (n = 11)
	  • With pulse Cyclophosphamide n = 3
	  • With azathioprine n = 1
	  • With prednisolone alone n = 2
	
	If BVAS ≥10 or DEI ≥6:
	Plus individual doses of prednisolone, increased to 1 mg/kg/day in
	Taper: 10 mg every 3 days until 20 mg/day
	Then 2.5 mg/week until 5 mg, then 1 mg/month
	
	Concomitant medication:
	Prednisolone (median) at start: 10 mg/day (induction) 8 mg/day (maintenance)

Result	Methotrexate was safe and effective for the induction of remission in non-life-threatening disease. Limited efficacy of methotrexate to prevent cardiac and pulmonary relapses within the observation period

Patients	28 consecutive patients with Churg-Strauss syndrome
	Diagnosed according to the ACR criteria and the CHC definition
	Major exclusion criteria:
	  • Life-threatening disease
	  • Serum creatinine > 1.5 mg/dL
	  • Leukopenia < 4,000 mL
	  • Thrombocytopenia < 100,000 mL
	  • Hemoglobin < 10 g/dL
	  • Biopsy-proven patients (*n*, positive/negative): 7/4 (induction), 16/7 (maintenance)
	  • ANCA-positive patients (*n*, positive/negative): 0/11 (induction), 4/19 (maintenance)
	  • Median DEI/BVAS/FFS at start of study 7/6/0

Authors	Metzler C, Hellmich B, Gause A, Gross WL, de Groot K
Publication	*Clin Exp Rheumatol.* 2004;22(6 Suppl 36):S52–S61
Follow-up	48 months (median)

(continued) ➜

Note	Outcome parameters:	
	Induction of remission after MTX treatment	n = 8
	Complete remission after MTX treatment	n = 6
	Median time to remission (months)	5
	Remission maintained	n = 12
	Major relapses	n = 8
		Cardiac n = 6
		Pulmonary events n = 5
	Minor relapses	n = 3
	Cumulative prednisone dose (during MTX induction, g)	6.2
	Reduction of prednisone dose during MTX maintenance	53%
Adverse events	Pneumonitis	n = 1
	Upper respiratory tract infections	n = 8
	Urinary tract infection	n = 1
	Cystitis	n = 1
	Leukopenia	n = 2
	Diarrhea	n = 1

Trial	Elevated relapse rate under oral methotrexate versus leflunomide for maintenance of remission in Wegener's granulomatosis
Substance	*Induction of remission*:
	Cyclophosphamide 2 mg/kg p. o.
	Plus **prednisone 1 mg/kg/day** for 6 months
	Prednisone tapered by 10 mg every 3 days until 20 mg/day
	Followed by a 2.5-mg reduction/week until 5 mg/day and then of 1 mg/month
	Maintenance of remission:
	Leflunomide (Lef): After complete or stable partial remission ≥ 3 months
	20 mg/day (100 mg for the first 3 days) until week 4
	Then 30 mg/day 4, n = 26
	Or
	Methotrexate (MTX): 7.5 mg/week p. o. for 4 weeks 15 mg methotrexate/week p. o. for 4 weeks
	20 mg methotrexate/week p. o. (n = 28)
	Concomitant medication:
	Folic acid once weekly at 10 mg, 24 h after MTX
	Concomitant prednisone ≤ 10 mg/day
	Tapered by 2.5 mg/month until 5 mg
	Then tapered by 1 mg/month
	Calcium 1 g/day and vitamin D 1'000 I.E./day
Result	Leflunomide decreased the relapse rate. It was associated with an increased frequency of adverse events. Higher incidence of major relapses were observed in the methotrexate group
Patients	44 patients with Wegener's granulomatosis
	Diagnosed according to the ACR criteria and CHC definitions
	Major exclusion criteria:
	• Leukopenia < 4,000/mL
	• Hemoglobin < 10 day/dL
	• Thrombocytopenia < 100,000/mL
	• Serum creatinine > 1.3 mg/dL
	Confirmative biopsy (*positive/negative*):
	• 18/8 in the Lef, 18/10 in the MTX group
	ANCA (*positive/negative*):
	• 23/3 in the Lef, 25/3 in the MTX group
	• Median DEI at randomization: 0 in both groups
Authors	Metzler C, Miehle N, Manger K, Iking-Konert C, de Groot K, Hellmich B, Gross WL, Reinhold-Keller E; German Network of Rheumatic Diseases
Publication	*Rheumatology (Oxford)*. 2007;46(7):1087–1091
Follow-up	25 months

(continued) →

Note	Outcome parameters:		
		Lef	MTX
	Withdrawal	n = 6	n = 2
	Relapse rate	n = 6 (major n = 1)	n = 13 (major n = 7)
	Time point of relapse	7 months	6 months
	Premature termination of study because of higher incidence of major relapses in MTX group		
Adverse events		Lef (%)	MTX (%)
	CNS granuloma	n = 0	n = 1
	Cold/fever	12	7
	Cough/bronchitis	8	0
	Chronic obstructive pulmonary disease	4	15
	Gastroenteritis/diarrhea/ abdominal pain	4	4
	Urinary tract infection	4	7
	Sinusitis	4	4
	Pneumonia	4	0
	Herpes zoster	4	0
	Erysipel	4	0
	Lumbalgia/disc protrusion	4	1
	Arthralgia/myalgia	15	4
	Edema	4	1
	Cardiac insufficiency	4	0
	Tachycardia	4	0
	Weakness/nausea	4	0
	Dry skin	0	4
	Thrombophlebitis	4	0
	Hypertension	8	0
	Leukopenia	8	0
	Cholecystectomy	0	4
	Removal of osteosynthetic material	4	0
	Peripheral neuropathy	4	0
	Leiomyosarcoma	4	0

WEGENT-Trial	Azathioprine or methotrexate maintenance for ANCA-associated vasculitis WEGENT: Wegener's Granulomatosis Entretien
Substance	*Induction of remission*: **Methylprednisolone 15 mg/kg** for 3 days Followed by oral **1 mg/kg prednisone** for 3 weeks Tapered to a daily dose of 12.5 mg at 6 months and 5 mg/day at 18 months Complete discontinuation after the 24th month **Cyclophosphamide, 3 pulses of 0.6 g/m^2** every 2 weeks Then every 3 weeks 0.7 g/m^2 cyclophosphamide until remission Followed by three additional consolidation pulses 0.7 g/m^2 cyclophosphamide (n = 201) *Concomitant medication*: Mesna and trimethoprim–sulfamethoxazole 80/400 or 160/800 mg, or (in case of intolerance) aerosolized pentamidine (300 mg every 3–4 weeks) *Maintenance of remission (after achieving remission)*: **Azathioprine (AZA, 2.0 mg/kg/day,** n = 63) Or **Methotrexate 0.3 mg/kg (MTX)/day** p. o. (increased every week by 2.5 mg, to 25 mg per week, n = 63) Starting 2–3 weeks after the last pulse 12 months of maintenance therapy Then withdrawal of MTX or AZA over a period of 3 months
Result	The primary hypothesis that methotrexate is less toxic than azathioprine was not supported. Both agents had similar efficacy and safety in patients with Wegener's granulomatosis and microscopic polyangiitis after initial remission

Patients	159 eligible patients with active Wegener's granulomatosis (WG) or microscopic polyangiitis (MPA)
	  • Patients with WG meeting either ACR criteria or CHC definition and renal disease
	  • Involvement of ≥ 2 organs or 1 organ plus general symptoms e.g. fever > 38°C
	  • Patients with MPA meeting the CHC definition and at least one item of the FFS
	  • Remission after induction therapy and subsequent randomization n = 126
	  • Biopsy-proven WG with necrotizing vasculitis, granulomatous inflammation
	
	Important exclusion criterion:
	  • Use of corticosteroids for > 1 month before induction therapy

(continued)

Authors	Pagnoux C, Mahr A, Hamidou MA, Boffa JJ, Ruivard M, Ducroix JP, Kyndt X, Lifermann F, Papo T, Lambert M, Le Noach J, Khellaf M, Merrien D, Puéchal X, Vinzio S, Cohen P, Mouthon L, Cordier JF, Guillevin L; French Vasculitis Study Group				
Publication	*N Engl J Med.* 2008;359(26):2790–2803				
Follow-up	36 months				
Note	Primary hypothesis: MTX less toxic than AZA (see also "adverse events")				

		AZA	MTX		
	Outcome parameters:				
	Relapse rate	n = 23	n = 21		
	Event-free survival	69.9%	60.8%		
	Death	n = 1	n = 0		

		Any AE		Severe AE	
Adverse events		AZA	MTX	AZA	MTX
	Adverse events (total)	n = 29	n = 35	n = 5	n = 11
	Adverse event requiring study-drug withdrawal or causing death	–	–	n = 7	n = 12
	Cutaneous eruption	n = 1	n = 1	n = 0	n = 0
	Lymphopenia	n = 10	n = 14	n = 1	n = 3
	Anemia	n = 2	n = 2	n = 0	n = 1
	Neutropenia	n = 2	n = 3	n = 0	n = 3
	Thrombocytopenia	n = 1	n = 3	n = 0	n = 1
	Mucosal toxicity	n = 0	n = 7	n = 0	n = 4
	Gastrointestinal event any	n = 8	n = 11	n = 0	n = 0
	Liver toxicity any	n = 4	n = 4	n = 4	n = 2
	Infection	n = 12	n = 15	n = 1	n = 5
	Cumulative no. of infections	n = 19	n = 25	–	–
	Respiratory event	n = 1	n = 3	n = 0	n = 2
	Bone fracture	n = 1	n = 3	n = 0	n = 0
	Cystitis	n = 0	n = 0	–	–
	Psychiatric event any	n = 1	n = 2	n = 0	n = 0
	Cancer	–	–	n = 2	n = 1
	Venous thrombotic event	–	–	n = 1	n = 2

Trial	Mycophenolate mofetil for maintenance therapy of Wegener's granulomatosis and microscopic polyangiitis: a pilot study in 11 patients with renal involvement
Substance	*Induction of remission*: **Cyclophosphamide 2 mg/kg/day** of plus oral corticosteroids 1 mg/kg/day for at least 3 months or longer until remission was achieved *Maintenance of remission*: **Mycophenolate mofetil 2 g/day** Taper of oral corticosteroids to ≤ 7.5 mg/day at the end of the study
Result	Mycophenolate mofetil in combination with low-dose corticosteroids was safe and effective for the maintenance of remission in patients with Wegener's granulomatosis and microscopic polyangiitis
Patients	Newly detected or untreated patients with Wegener's granulomatosis (WG, n = 9, all c-ANCA/PR3 positive) or microscopic polyangiitis n = 2 (all p-ANCA/MPO positive) • Diagnosed based on clinical presentation, serology, and/or histology • Renal involvement and/or severe involvement of other organs required • BVAS 2 of 5 = grumbling disease still present at start of maintenance therapy
Authors	Nowack R, Göbel U, Klooker P, Hergesell O, Andrassy K, van der Woude FJ
Publication	*J Am Soc Nephrol.* 1999;10(9):1965–1971
Follow-up	15 months

Note	*Outcome parameters*:	
	Relapse	n = 1 (WG)
	Stable remission at the end of the study	n = 10
	BVAS2 negative	n = 6
	Oral glucocorticoids could be reduced to a median daily dose of 5 mg and discontinued	n = 3
	Proteinuria at baseline	0.5 g/day
	Proteinuria end of study	0.2 g/day
	No further decline of renal function during maintenance therapy	
Adverse events	Abdominal pain	n = 3
	Diarrhea	n = 2
	Respiratory infection	n = 2
	Leukopenia (< 3,000/mL)	n = 2

Trial	Mycophenolate mofetil for remission maintenance in the treatment of Wegener's granulomatosis
Substance	*Induction of remission*: **Cyclophosphamide (Cyc) 2 mg/kg/day** Plus **1 mg/kg prednisone/day** Tapering after 1 month Change to alternate day regime and subsequent discontinuation (during therapy for maintenance), if clinically possible *Maintenance of remission*: **Mycophenolate mofetil (MMF) 2 g/day** (initiated 1–2 days after the last application of CYC) *Concomitant medication*: Trimethoprim/sulfamethoxazole (160/800 mg; one tablet three times weekly) and Calcium carbonate/calcitriol or calcium carbonate/etidronate
Result	Mycophenolate mofetil plus prednisone for maintenance of remission was safe, with limited efficacy with regard to the frequency of relapses
Patients	• 14 patients with active Wegener's granulomatosis • 13 patients with biopsy-proven Wegener's granulomatosis with necrotizing vasculitis, granulomatous inflammation or both in a typical organ system • 1 patient diagnosed on the basis of upper airway and lower airway disease—where infection had been ruled out and by the presence of PR3-ANCA • 13 patients with cANCA, 1 with p/MPO-ANCA
Authors	Langford CA, Talar-Williams C, Sneller MC
Publication	*Arthritis Rheum.* 2004;51(2):278–283
Follow-up	18 months (median)

(continued)

Note	*Outcome parameters:*	
	Deaths	n = 0
	Remission	n = 14
	Time to remission (months, median)	3
	Relapse after achieving remission	n = 6
	Time from remission to relapse (months, median)	10
	Discontinuation of prednisone	n = 12
	Time to tapering to alternate-day prednisone (months, median)	4
	Time discontinuation of prednisone (months, median)	8
	Time from remission to relapse in six patients (months, median)	10
	Time off prednisone before relapse in six patients (months, median)	5
Adverse events	Bone marrow toxicity requiring dosage reduction	n = 4 (Cyc) n = 2 (MMF)
	Cataracts	n = 1
	Diabetes mellitus	n = 2
	Dermatomal cutaneous herpes zoster	n = 4
	Bacterial pneumonia	n = 2
	Pneumocystis carinii pneumonia	n = 2

Trial	A pilot study using Mycophenolate mofetil in relapsing or resistant ANCA small vessel vasculitis
Substance	Mycophenolate mofetil (MMF) 2 × 500 mg/day
	Then increased to 2 × 1'000–1'500/day, for a maximum of 24 weeks, the decision about continuation of MMF or change to different medication
	Patients with relapse:
	Begin of **corticosteroids at 1 mg/kg/day** for ≤ 30 days, then taper by 25% of initial dose per week for 1 month, discontinuation after 3 months
	Rapid loss of renal function: initial i. v. pulses of methylprednisolone
	Patients with resistance to cyclophosphamide (CYC): no increase of corticosteroids allowed
	Concomitant therapy:
	With corticosteroids allowed
	Vitamin D and calcium for all patients on corticosteroids
Result	Mycophenolate mofetil was safe and adequately efficient in the treatment of non-life-threatening vasculitis which was either relapsing or resistant to therapy with cyclophosphamide or showed toxicity to cyclophosphamide or azathioprine
Patients	12 patients with active, either therapy resistant (n = 6) to CYC or relapsing (n = 6) disease
	• Wegener's granulomatosis n = 7
	• Polyangiitis n = 2
	• Isolated renal vasculitis n = 2
	• Churg-Strauss syndrome n = 1
	Major inclusion criteria:
	• Treatment resistance or relapse plus one of the following:
	• Two prior courses of 6 monthly CYC (intravenous or daily oral); toxicity of CYC or azathioprine; patient's refusal of further treatment after one course; current disease activity despite a full course of CYC
	Major exclusion criteria:
	• Glomerulonephritis only, i.e., no extrarenal manifestation of vasculitis, with advanced renal failure
	• Total BVAS at start of study: 9.1 (mean) PR3-ANCA n = 9
	• MPO-ANCA n = 3
Authors	Joy MS, Hogan SL, Jennette JC, Falk RJ, Nachman PH
Publication	*Nephrol Dial Transplant.* 2005;20(12):2725–2732
Follow-up	52 weeks

(continued) ➔

Note	*Outcome parameters*:			
		Baseline	Week 24	Week 52
	Total BVAS	9.1	2.8	2.8
	ANCA titers	57	43.3	50.7
	Prednisone dose	42 mg	12.5 mg	
	One patient with significant increase of activity after initial 24 weeks			
	Two patients with minor increase of activity after initial 24 weeks			
	Two patients withdrawn early because of worsening of vasculitis and/or signs of infection			
Adverse events	Upper respiratory tract infection events	n = 5		
	Urinary tract infection symptoms	n = 1		
	Herpes zoster infection	n = 1		
	Diarrhea/loose stools	n = 4		
	Abdominal cramping	n = 3		
	Nausea/vomiting	n = 2		
	Constipation	n = 1		
	Leukopenia	n = 2		
	Insomnia	n = 2		
	Mid-epigastric pain	n = 1		
	Increased serum amylase	n = 1		
	Adverse events were all transient			

IMPROVE-Trial	Mycophenolate mofetil versus azathioprine for remission maintenance in antineutrophil cytoplasmic antibody-associated vasculitis: a randomized controlled trial IMPROVE: International Mycophenolate Mofetil Protocol to Reduce Outbreaks of Vasculitides
Substance	*For induction of remission* (n = *175*): **Cyclophosphamide (daily oral or pulse)** (0–3 (up to 6) months) **Prednisolone 1 g/day** for 3 days, afterwards taper until withdrawal after 24 months *For maintenance of remission*: **Azathioprine 2 mg/kg/day** (AZA, n = 80) **Mycophenolate mofetil 2 g/day** (MMF, n = 76) *Previous medication*: No previous exposure to cytotoxic drugs
Result	Mycophenolate mofetil was almost as effective as azathioprine for maintaining disease remission after induction of remission with cyclophosphamide in ANCA-associated vasculitis patients. Both treatments had similar adverse event rates
Patients	156 patients with a new diagnosis of Wegener's granulomatosis or microscopic polyangiitis • According to the 1992 Chapel Hill Consensus Conference
Authors	Hiemstra TF, Walsh M, Mahr A, Savage CO, de Groot K, Harper L, Hauser T, Neumann I, Tesar V, Wissing KM, Pagnoux C, Schmitt W, Jayne DR; European Vasculitis Study Group (EUVAS)
Publication	*JAMA.* 2010 Dec 1;304(21):2381–2388
Follow-up	39 months (range 0.66–53.6 months)

Note		AZA	MMF
	Relapse	n = 30	n = 42
	Crossed to the other drug because of intolerability	n = 6	n = 2
	Prednisolone dose (mg)	8´411	8´535
	Median estimated glomerular filtration (mL/min/1.73 m^2)	59.2	52.8
	Proteinuria (g/day)	0.53	0.82
	Median increase of vasculitis damage index	+2	+2
Adverse events		AZA	MMF
	Severe adverse events	n = 22	n = 8
	Severe infection	n = 8	n = 3
	Any adverse events	n = 97	n = 75
	Any infection	n = 37	n = 29
	Cardiovascular	n = 4	n = 4
	Neoplasia	n = 5	n = 1
	Gastrointestinal tract	n = 10	n = 10
	Drug intolerance	n = 6	n = 2
	Hepatic dysfunction	n = 3	n = 0
	Leukopenia	n = 11	n = 5
	Other	n = 21	n = 24
	Death	n = 1	n = 1

SOLUTION-Trial	Treatment of refractory Wegener's granulomatosis with anti-thymocyte globulin (ATG): an open study in 15 patients SOLUTION: Name of study, not an acronym
Substance	*Individual amount of infusions*: Anti-human rabbit anti-Thymocyte globulin (ATG) each 2.5 mg/kg over 10 days (IMIX SangStat n = 14: mean of 2.2 infusions, mean total dose 300 mg; AQTG-Fresenius n = 1: 5 infusions, total 1'050 mg) Further doses adjusted according to lymphocyte count (SOLUTION protocol) *Concomitant medication*: Methylprednisolone 100 mg before the first administration of ATG Azathioprine 2 mg/kg throughout ATG treatment to prevent serum sickness Co-trimoxazole was permitted Amphotericin-B was permitted *Previous medication*: Glucocorticosteroids (all patients) Oral cyclophosphamide (all patients) Plasma exchange n = 5 Mycophenolate mofetil n = 4 Intravenous immunoglobulins n = 3 Cyclosporine A n = 2 15-deoxyspergualine n = 2
Result	Anti-T-cell-directed treatment with anti-thymocyte globulin was effective in most treated cases of severe refractory Wegener's granulomatosis despite limited safety due to bacterial infections and pulmonary hemorrhage
Patients	15 patients with active, severely refractory Wegener's granulomatosis • Histologically proven; all c/PR3-ANCA positive • Unresponsive to cyclophosphamide n = 7, intolerant n = 8 • Cumulative DEI 8.7 (mean) • Number of previous therapeutics 5.2 (mean) • Cumulative dose of cyclophosphamide 56.5 g (mean) • Disease duration before study entry 63.2 (mean) • Number of relapses before study entry 2.8 (mean)
Authors	Schmitt WH, Hagen EC, Neumann I, Nowack R, Flores-Suárez LF, van der Woude FJ; European Vasculitis Study Group
Publication	*Kidney Int*. 2004;65(4):1440–1448
Follow-up	21.8 (range 6–68)

(continued) ➔

Note	Outcome parameters:	
	Favorable response	n = 13
	Partial remission	n = 9
	Complete remission	n = 4
	Relapsed after a mean of 8.4 months	n = 7
	Death	n = 2
Adverse events	Fever and chills	n = 10
	Serum sickness	n = 2
	Serious bacterial infections	n = 5
	Death of a pulmonary bacterial infection	n = 1
	Death of pulmonary hemorrhage	n = 1

Trial	Etanercept combined with conventional treatment in Wegener's granulomatosis: a 6-month open-label trial to evaluate safety	
Substance	**Etanercept 2 × 25 mg/week** s. c.	
	Concomitant medication:	
	Added to standard therapies for Wegener's granulomatosis (glucocorticoids, methotrexate, cyclophosphamide, azathioprine, ciclosporin) plus	
	Trimethoprim-sulfamethoxazole, double-strength three times a week one tablet	
Result	Etanercept used in combination with standard treatments was well tolerated with few adverse events. There were intermittent flares in most cases, severe flares in a minority. Activity was reduced in the majority of patients after 6 months	
Patients	20 patients with Wegener's granulomatosis	
	• Diagnosed clinically and on the basis of ≥ 2 of modified ACR criteria (1990 criteria plus PR3-ANCA)	
	Major inclusion criteria:	
	• BVAS ≥ 1	
	• Time since diagnosis: 63.6 months (mean)	
	• BVAS/WG at study entry: 3.6 (mean)	
Authors	Stone JH, Uhlfelder ML, Hellmann DB, Crook S, Bedocs NM, Hoffman GS	
Publication	*Arthritis Rheum.* 2001;44(5):1149–1154	
Follow-up	6 months	
Note	*Outcome parameters*:	
	Still taking etanercept at 6 months	n = 16
	BVAS/WG = 0 (6 months)	n = 12
	Some increase in BVAS/WG within study period	n = 12 (75%)
	Minor increase	n = 10
	Major flares	n = 3
		Glomerulonephritis plus mesenteric vasculitis n = 1
		Recurrent orbital disease n = 2
	Change of:	
	BVAS/WG	-3
	Physicians global assessment (mm)	-25.3
	Mean daily prednisone dose (mg)	-11.6
Adverse events	Injection-site reactions	n = 8
	Hospitalization needed	n = 5
	Herpes zoster infection	n = 1
	Infections	n = 2
	Elevated liver transaminases	n = 1
	Cytopenia	n = 5
	Sleep disturbances	n = 1

WGET-Trial	Etanercept plus Standard Therapy for Wegener's Granulomatosis WGET: Wegener's Granulomatosis Etanercept Trial
Substance	*Additional immunosuppressive therapy* (*begin before randomization*): <u>Severe disease</u>: **Cyclophosphamide 2 mg/kg/day** for at least 3–6 months Exchanged for Methotrexate at remission or when reclassified as limited disease or **Azathioprine,** if serum creatinine > 2 mg/dL Plus glucocorticoids <u>Limited disease</u>: **Methotrexate 0.25 mg/kg/week** (for 12 months after remission, increased to max. 25 mg/week) plus glucocorticoids *Randomized phase*: **Etanercept 2 × 25 mg (ETN)/week** (group A, n = 89) Or **Placebo** (group B, n = 92) <u>Both groups</u>: Glucocorticoids at start with i. v. pulse methylprednisolone 1 g for 3 days or 0.5–1 mg/kg/day (max. 80 mg), taper with aim to reach 20 mg/day after 2 months and to discontinue within 6 months *Concomitant therapy*: All patients trimethoprim/sulfamethoxazole (80/400 mg) Folic acid (1 mg/day, MTX-treated patients) Prophylactic treatment for pneumocystis infection and for osteoporosis More details on therapy regimen in: *Control Clin Trials.* 2002;23:450–468
Result	Etanercept was not effective for the maintenance of remission in patients with severe or limited disease, respectively. There was a high rate of treatment-related complications with all six reported solid cancers occurring in the etanercept group

(continued)

Patients	180 patients with severe Wegener's granulomatosis
	• Diagnosed clinically and on the basis of ≥ 2 of modified ACR criteria (1990 criteria plus PR3-ANCA)
	• Both patients with a new diagnosis or with flares of previously quiescent existing disease
	Biopsy results:
	• Granulomatous inflammation 54.9%
	• Vasculitis/glomerulonephritis 63.4%
	Inclusion criteria:
	• Without immediate threat to either the patient's life or vital organ function
	• Serum creatinine ≤ 1.4 mg/dL plus no change to patient's baseline over 25%.
	• No more than circumscribed pulmonary involvement
	• Active for the previous 28 days, either under first course of treatment or with flare
	• BVAS/WG ≥ 3
	• Further details on inclusion/exclusion and baseline cohort data in: *Control Clin Trials*. 2002;23:450–468 and *Arthritis Rheum*. 2003;48(8):2299–2309
	• Severe disease n = 128, limited disease n = 52 BVAS/WG (mean) 6.5 (group A), 7.5 (group B)
	• ANCA-IF positive (%): 87.1
	• PR3/MPO positive (%): 72.6/11.9
Authors	Wegener's Granulomatosis Etanercept Trial (WGET) Research Group
Publication	*N Engl J Med*. 2005;352(4):351–361
Follow-up	25 months (group A), 19 months (group B; mean)

Note	*Outcome parameters*:		
		Group A (%)	Group B (%)
	Completed study	60.7	63.0
	Sustained remission	69.7	75.3
	Remission at any time during trial	89.9	92.3
	Remained in remission	49.4	not shown
	Sustained low level of disease activity	86.5	90.6
	All disease flares	66.3	74.1
	Severe disease flares	14.9	12.8
	No difference between group A and group B with respect to time to sustained remission		
	Overall also no difference in severe and limited or new and existing disease in all outcome parameters		
	No details on previous immunosuppressive therapies provided in all three publications		

(continued)

Adverse events	At least 1 event of:		
		Group A	Group B
	Grade 3 plus grade 4 plus Grade 5 adverse events	56.2%	57.1%
	Grade 5 events	n = 4	n = 2
		Cholangiocarcinoma n = 1	Cardiac arrest n = 1
		Sepsis n = 1	Sepsis n = 1
		Cardiac arrest n = 2	
	Cancers during trial period	n = 11	n = 4
		Prostate cancer n = 1	Cutaneous Basal-cell or squamous-cell carcinoma (n = 4)
		Mucinous colon Adenocarcinoma n = 2	
		Cholangiosarcoma n = 1	
		Breast carcinoma n = 1	
		Liposarcoma n = 1	
		Cutaneous basal-cell or squamous-cell carcinoma n = 3	

Trial	Treatment of antineutrophil cytoplasmic antibody (ANCA)-associated systemic vasculitis with high-dose intravenous immunoglobulin
Substance	Polyspecific 7S-immunoglobulins (IVIG) i. v., 30 g/day for 5 days
	Concomitant medication:
	Trimethoprim/sulfamethoxazole n = 4
	2.5–30 mg prednisone/day at stable dose n = 5
	Cyclophosphamide at stable dose n = 9
	Previous medication:
	Cyclophosphamide n = 10
	Trimethoprim/sulfamethoxazole n = 10
Result	Intravenous immunoglobulins were partially effective, particularly in the skin, ear-nose-throat and arthritis, with some influence on PR3-ANCA levels
Patients	15 patients with ANCA-associated systemic vasculitis
	• Fulfilling the ACR criteria Wegener's granulomatosis and the CHC definitions, with PR-3 ANCA n = 14, with MPO-ANCA positive limited systemic vasculitis n = 1
	• Histologic confirmation of diagnosis n = 13
	• Generalized disease n = 13, initial disease n = 2
	• Pretreatment with different regimens, among others:
	◦ Cyclophosphamide n = 9 (stopped before IVIG because of toxicity n = 2)
	◦ With trimethoprim/sulfamethoxazole n = 10
	◦ IVIG as first treatment n = 1
	• Concomitant therapy with prednisone n = 5
Authors	Richter C, Schnabel A, Csernok E, De Groot K, Reinhold-Keller E, Gross WL
Publication	*Clin Exp Immunol.* 1995;101(1):2–7
Follow-up	4 weeks
Note	*Outcome parameters*:

Note		
Clinically significant benefit (skin, ear-nose-throat findings)	n = 6	
Improvement of conjunctivitis and scleritis, pericarditis or nephritis	n = 0	
Complete remission	n = 0	
Decrease of CRP levels	n = 7 (n = 3 > 50%)	
Decrease of ANCA levels (4×)	n = 5	
DEI baseline (median)	4	
DEI end of study (median)	3	
Repeated courses were no more effective than single courses		

Adverse events	None

Trial	Long-term effectiveness of intravenous immunoglobulin in Churg-Strauss syndrome		
Substance	**Prednisone 1 mg/kg/day** for 1 month Then slowly tapered to 10 mg/day by month 6 (all patients) plus **2 mg/kg cyclophosphamide/day** for 6 months in severe cases plus synchronized cycles with plasmapheresis *Randomization*: And i. v. immunoglobulins (**IVIG, 2 g/kg/month**) for 6 months and every other month for further 3 cycles (group A, n = 9) **No plasmapheresis** (group B, n = 9)		
Result	Treatment with intravenous immunoglobulins in conjunction with plasmapheresis led to complete and long-term remissions with few side effects in all patients		
Patients	18 subjects with new onset Churg-Strauss syndrome • Fulfilling the ACR criteria and the CHC definitions for Churg-Strauss syndrome • Treatment group with plasmapheresis/IVIG n = 9 • Control group with standard therapy without plasmapheresis/IVIG n = 9 • Anti-leukotriene therapy in both groups n = 0 *Major exclusion criteria*: • Serious infections in the past 6 months • Other concomitant severe or uncontrolled disease		
Authors	Danieli MG, Cappelli M, Malcangi G, Logullo F, Salvi A, Danieli G		
Publication	*Ann Rheum Dis.* 2004;63(12):1649–1654		
Follow-up	44 months (median)		
Note	*Outcome parameters*:		
		Group A	Group B
	Remission at 12 months	n = 9	n = 9
	Treatment-free remission	n = 3	n = 2
	Relapses	n = 1	n = 4
	BVAS (median)	2.22	4.2
	Systemic Necrotizing Vasculitis Damage Index	3.78	5.56
	Modified Rodnan skin score	1.11	2.0
	Significant lower CRP levels in the treatment group from month 6 until last evaluation		
Adverse events		Group A	Group B
	Steroid-related osteoporosis	n = 3	n = 8
	Diabetes	n = 2	n = 3
	Arterial hypertension	n = 2	n = 4
	Myopathy	n = 1	n = 2
	Cushingoid habitus	n = 1	n = 1
	Hypogammaglobulinemia	n = 0	n = 2
	Permanent lymphopenia	n = 1	n = 1
	Bacterial pneumonia	n = 1	n = 2

Trial	Prospective study of TNF alpha blockade with infliximab in antineutrophil cytoplasmic antibody-associated systemic vasculitis
Substance	**Infliximab i. v. (5 mg/kg),** at 0, 2, 6, and 10 weeks
	Additive therapy study I:
	Oral 2 mg/kg cyclophosphamide/day for 14 weeks until remission
	Then **switch to 2 mg/kg azathioprine/day** unless inefficient
	Then mycophenolate and prednisolone
	Additive therapy study II:
	Continuation of established therapy, with prednisolone tapered according to clinical status
	Concomitant therapy:
	Sulfamethoxazole/trimethoprim 480 mg three times a week and antifungals continued for 14 weeks in patients on cyclophosphamide
Result	Infliximab was effective at inducing a high rate of remissions and permitted reduction of steroid doses. Severe infections or disease flares were seen in one fifth of patients, respectively
Patients	32 patients with ANCA-associated small vessel vasculitis
	• Wegener's granulomatosis or microscopic polyangiitis fulfilling the CHC definitions; histologic confirmation n = 32
	• ANCA immunofluorescence positive n = 31
	Study I (as adjuvant therapy for induction of remission, n = 16):
	• Patients with acute flares that were not immediately life-threatening BVAS ≥ 10, either initial disease presentation or relapse
	Study II (as additional therapy in persistent disease, n = 16):
	• Patients with active AASV despite ≥ 3 months of combination therapy with
	• Prednisolone plus cyclophosphamide, azathioprine or methotrexate
	BVAS ≥ 4
	Major exclusion criteria:
	• Immediately life-threatening pulmonary vasculitis
	• Untreated infection or previous tuberculosis
	• Cardiac failure
Authors	Booth A, Harper L, Hammad T, Bacon P, Griffith M, Levy J, Savage C, Pusey C, Jayne D
Publication	*J Am Soc Nephrol.* 2004;15(3):717–721
Follow-up	52 weeks

(continued) ➜

Note	Outcome parameters:	
	Remission	88%
		n =14 in both studies
		n = 5 (16%, study I)
		n = 3 (21%, study II) with relapses
	Treatment failures	n = 2 in both studies, respectively
	Change of:	
	BVAS	-10
	CRP	-22.4
	Mean prednisolone dose	-15 mg/day
	Relapse after a mean of 27 weeks	18%
Adverse events	Death	n = 5
		Pulmonary hemorrhage n = 1
		Bronchopneumonia n = 4
	Bronchopneumonia	n = 1
	Urinary tract sepsis, Klebsiella	n = 1
	Leg abscess, surgical drainage required	n = 1
	Endophthalmitis, evisceration of the eye	n = 1
	Skin ulcer/urinary tract infection	n = 1
	Diarrheal illness	n = 1
	B-cell lymphoma, chemotherapy	n = 1
	Pulmonary embolus	n = 1
	Axillary vein thrombosis	n = 1

Trial	Infliximab or rituximab for refractory Wegener's granulomatosis: long-term follow up. A prospective randomized multicentre study on 17 patients
Substance	*Induction of remission*: **3 mg/kg infliximab** i. v. (n = 9) on days 1 and 14 *Response was assessed on day 42*: *Complete remission*: Dose was maintained for the next 6 months Partial remission or absence of a response 5 mg/kg infliximab Response was reevaluated on day 73 Complete/partial response: dose was maintained for the next 12 months Absence of a response: infliximab stopped Or **Rituximab 0.375 g/m^2** i. v. (n = 8) on days 1, 8, 15, and 22. *Response was assessed on day 42*: Complete/partial response: rituximab 375 g/m^2 at months 4, 8, and 12 No response: Rituximab was stopped *Concomitant medication*: Immunosuppressive was maintained Corticosteroids were maintained for 4 weeks, and then tapered or switched to another immunosuppressant *Previous medication*: I. v. pulses followed by oral cyclophosphamide
Result	Infliximab or rituximab were useful to obtain remission of refractory granulomatosis with polyangiitis, with a trend after 12 months favoring rituximab
Patients	17 patients with systemic Wegener's granulomatosis fulfilling the CHC criteria • Refractory to, or intolerant to, steroids and several other immunosuppressives including cyclophosphamide pulses followed by oral treatment
Authors	de Menthon M, Cohen P, Pagnoux C, Buchler M, Sibilia J, Détrée F, Gayraud M, Khellaf M, Penalba C, Legallicier B, Mouthon L, Guillevin L
Publication	*Clin Exp Rheumatol.* 2011 Jan–Feb;29(1 Suppl 64):S63–S71
Follow-up	12 months plus mean 30.6 months follow-up

(continued) →

Note	Outcome parameters:		
		Infliximab	Rituximab
	Complete remission (month 12)	n = 2	n = 4
	Partial remission (month 12)	n = 1	n = 1
	Treatment failure	n = 5	n = 2
	Progressive disease	n = 2	Not shown
	Relapse after 30.6 ± 15.4 months	n = 2	n = 1
	Stop treatment	n = 6	Not shown
	Change of BVAS	-5.6	-9.2
	Five patients unresponsive to infliximab successfully switched to rituximab		
Adverse events		Infliximab	Rituximab
	Death	n = 1	n = 1
	Allergic reactions	n = 2	n = 0
	Severe infections	Not shown	n = 0
	Bronchitis dental abscess	Not shown	n = 3

Trial	Nine patients with antineutrophil cytoplasmic antibody-positive vasculitis successfully treated with Rituximab
Substance	**4 × 500 mg or 375 mg/m² rituximab** i. v., every 4 weeks n = 6
	500 mg, once weeks, for 2 weeks n = 3
	Concomitant medication:
	Mycophenoloate mofetil n = 5
	Azathioprine n = 1
	Cyclophosphamide 5 or 7 weeks, respectively, n = 2
	Prednisolone n = 9
	Concomitant medication:
	Cyclophosphamide n = 9
	Antithymocyte globulin n = 1
	Intravenous immunoglobulins n = 3
	Sirolimus n = 2
	Azathioprine n = 5
	Leflunomide n = 1
	Cyclosporin n = 2
	Methotrexate n = 2
	Mycophenolate mofetil n = 4
	Plasma exchange n = 1
Result	Rituximab was effective and safe in ANCA-positive vasculitis, in addition to other immunomodulatory therapy
Patients	Nine patients with ANCA positive vasculitis
	• PR-3 ANCA n = 7, with a diagnosis of Wegener's granulomatosis
	• MPO-ANCA n = 2, with a diagnosis of microscopic polyangiitis
	• Involvement of organs 4 (median), BVAS 6 (median)
	• All patients resistant to prior immunosuppressants and prednisolone
Authors	Eriksson P
Publication	*J Intern Med.* 2005;257(6):540–548
Follow-up	6 months, duration 6–24 months

(continued) ➜

Note	*Outcome parameters*:	
	Complete remission n = 8 with BVAS 0	At 6 months
	Minor relapses	n = 2 cases, at 12 and 13 months
	Improvement of chest X-rays	n = 4
	Stop progression of gangrene	n = 1
	Remission of neuropathy	n = 1
	Remission of renal vasculitis	n = 2
	Improvement of musculoskeletal pain	n = 1
	Change of:	
	CRP	-18 mg/L
	ESR	-31 mm/h
	PR-3 ANCA levels	No effect
	MPO-ANCA	Not present at study start
Adverse events	Serious adverse events	n = 0
	Respiratory tract infections	n = 2
	Cutaneous herpes infection	n = 1

Trial	Rituximab for refractory Wegener's granulomatosis: report of a prospective, open-label pilot trial
Substance	**Methylprednisolone 3 × 1 g/day** of allowed alternatively as start dose Oral prednisone/day (1 mg/kg, maximum 80 mg/day) Prednisone was tapered and discontinued over 5 months, if no relapse **Rituximab 4 weekly infusions of 375 mg/m²** (RTX) Retreatment in case of relapse (with prednisone) or significant rise of ANCA (without prednisone) and parallel return of B lymphocytes *Concomitant medication*: Discontinuation of immunosuppressive therapies at study start (no washout) 650 mg of acetaminophen p. o. before RTX application 50 mg of diphenhydramine p. o. before RTX application *Previous medication*: Cyclophosphamide n = 10 Corticosteroids n = 10 Azathioprine n = 3 Mycophenolate mofetil n = 1 Etanercept n = 1
Result	Rituximab was effective and safe as the sole remission induction agent for severe refractory Wegener's granulomatosis
Patients	10 patients with active severe ANCA-associated vasculitis • Biopsy-proven or fulfilling the ACR criteria and CHC definitions for Wegener's granulomatosis or microscopic polyangiitis • Wegener's granulomatosis n = 10, PR-3 ANCA n = 10 • BVAS/WG: 6 (median) *Major additional inclusion criteria*: • PR-3 or MPO-ANCA positive at time of enrolment • Active severe (life- or organ-threatening) disease • Resistance to (n = 3) or intolerance of (n = 7), cyclophosphamide • BVAS ≥ 3 or refractory disease *Major exclusion criterion*: • Active infection, HIV, NYHA III/IV
Authors	Keogh KA, Ytterberg SR, Fervenza FC, Carlson KA, Schroeder DR, Specks U
Publication	*J Respir Crit Care Med.* 2006;173(2):180–187

(continued) ➔

Follow-up	12 months	
Note	*Outcome parameters*:	
	Complete clinical remission (activity score, 0) after 3 months	n = 10
	Complete remission at end of trial	n = 9
	Tapered off glucocorticoids by 6 months	n = 10
	Significant drop or disappearance of ANCA	n = 10
	CRP/BSR/serum creatinine in parallel decline to inflammatory disease recurring/rising ANCA titer	n = 5
	Relapse	n = 1 at 9 months
	Effect on quality of life: improvement in all domains of the SF36	
Adverse events	Rigors and chills	n = 1 (first infusion)
	Herpes zoster eruptions followed by postherpetic neuropathy	n = 2
	Influenza	n = 1
	Upper respiratory tract infections	n = 13 in five patients (rhinitis, sinusitis, cough with yellow and green nasal discharge, and phlegm production, with or without fevers)

Trial	Lack of efficacy of rituximab in Wegener's granulomatosis with refractory granulomatous manifestations
Substance	**Rituximab (RTX) 4 × 375 mg/m²** i. v., every 4 weeks
	Concomitant medication: Cyclophosphamide 2 mg/kg/day p. o. Cyclophosphamide 15–20 mg/kg i. v. every 18–21 days Methotrexate 0.3 mg/kg/week
	Previous medication: Cyclophosphamide n = 5 Prednisone n = 8 Infliximab n = 6 Methotrexate n = 1 Leflunomide n = 1 Etanercept n = 2 Mycophenolate mofetil n = 1
Result	No change or progression of granulomatous disease manifestations in the majority of patients with rituximab and additional cyclophosphamide therapy, additional clinical effect in a minority
Patients	8 consecutive patients • Fulfilling the CHC definitions for Wegener's granulomatosis • PR-3-ANCA positive, biopsy proven • Active disease ≤ 3 months despite of therapy with cyclophosphamide/prednisolone and TNF inhibitors
	All patients with granulomatous manifestations: • Retro-orbital granulomata n = 5 • Lung nodules n = 1 • Subglottic stenosis n = 2 • BVAS 1: 7.5 (mean) • DEI 4 (mean)
Authors	Aries PM, Hellmich B, Voswinkel J, Both M, Nölle B, Holl-Ulrich K, Lamprecht P, Gross WL
Publication	*Ann Rheum Dis.* 2006;65:853–858
Follow-up	18 months (median)
Note	*Outcome parameters*:	
	Reduction of disease activity	n = 3
	Complete remission	n.= 2
	No change in disease activity	n = 3
	Progression of disease	n = 2
	No change in ANCA titers	n = 8
	BVAS 1 score after RTX	6.25
	DEI after RTX	3.5
	Change of:	
	CRP	-24 mg/L
	ESR	-28 mm/h
Adverse events	None reported	

Trial	Rituximab for treatment-resistant extensive Wegener's granulomatosis—additive effects of a maintenance treatment with Leflunomide
Substance	**Rituximab 4 × 375 mg/m²** (RTX) i. v. in weekly intervals *Maintenance treatment*: **20 mg leflunomide/day** (n = 5) after the last RTX dose Stop of previous ineffective medication (n = 4) *Concomitant medication*: Increase of prednisolone to 1 mg/kg/day *Previous medication*: Cyclophosphamide n = 6 Corticosteroids n = 6 Infliximab n = 2
Result	Rituximab, along with leflunomide, was an effective and safe remission-inducing agent for patients with Wegener's granulomatosis
Patients	6 patients with Wegener's granulomatosis • Fulfilling the ACR criteria for Wegener's granulomatosis c-/PR-3-ANCA positive n = 6 *Progressive disease despite*: • Cyclophosphamide pulse n = 6 • Cyclophosphamide oral n = 4 • TNF antagonists n = 2 • Corticosteroids n = 6 • Pulmonary involvement n = 6 • Renal involvement n = 3 • Granulomatosis inflammation of the ear, nose, and throat n = 5 • Biopsy-proven, meningeal granulomatous inflammation n = 1 • BVAS/WG (mean): 5
Authors	Henes JC, Fritz J, Koch S, Klein R, Horger M, Risler T, Kanz L, Koetter I
Publication	*Clin Rheumatol.* 2007;26(10):1711–1715
Follow-up	16 months (mean)
Note	*Outcome parameters*: Complete remission at 6 months — n = 5 Persistent sinusitis — n = 1 Mild disease activity at 3 months — n = 2 Major relapse — n = 1 Glucosteroids tapered — -49.9 mg PR3-ANCA (baseline) — 36.8 U/mL PR3-ANCA (end of study) — 4.1 U/mL
Adverse events	RTX infusions were well tolerated

Trial	Efficacy of Rituximab in Limited Wegener's Granulomatosis with refractory granulomatous manifestations
Substance	**4 × 375 mg/m2 rituximab (RTX)** i. v., weekly
	Other therapies:
	Methotrexate n = 7
	Cyclophosphamide n = 6
	Chlorambucil n = 2
	Mycophenolate mofetil n = 1
	Etanercept n = 2
	Infliximab n = 1
	Adalimumab n = 2
	Azathioprine n = 1
Result	Rituximab was safe and effective in limited granulomatous Wegener's granulomatosis
Patients	8 patients with limited, i.e., non-life or vital organ threatening, Wegener's granulomatosis
	• Fulfilling the ACR criteria
	• Failed three immunosuppressive agents (mean):
	◦ Cyclophosphamide n = 6
	◦ Methotrexate n = 8
	• All patients with predominantly necrotizing granulomatous disease manifestations
	• ANCA negative at time of first RTX n = 5
Authors	Seo P, Specks U, Keogh KA
Publication	*J Rheumatol.* 2008;35(10):2017–2023
Follow-up	Minimum 4 months, maximum 3 years
Note	*Outcome parameters*:	
	Remission	n = 7
	Relapse	n = 5
	Successful retreatment with RTX	n = 3
	Time to relapse	14 months
	Time to relapse after B-cell repopulation	5 months
Adverse events	Deaths n = 1 (adenoviral pneumonitis after two courses of RTX and additional therapy with adalimumab for resistant orbital pseudotumor 2 months after last RTX)

Trial	Rituximab is effective in the treatment of refractory ophthalmic Wegener's granulomatosis
Substance	**2 × 1 g rituximab** (RTX) i. v., 2 weeks apart Continuation of standard immunosuppressive and corticosteroids *Second line agents post RTX*: Mycophenolate mofetil n = 3 (6 months), n = 1 (12 months) Azathioprine n = 2 (6 months), n = 2 (12 months) Cyclophosphamide n = 1 (6 months), n = 0 (12 months) Methotrexate n = 2 (6 months), n = 1 (12 months) None n = 2 (6 months), n = 6 (12 months) *Previous medication*: Anti-TNF n = 4 Immunoglobulins n = 1 Azathioprine n = 10 Methotrexate n = 6 Mycophenolate mofetil n = 9 Corticosteroids n = 10
Result	Rituximab was effective in patients with ophthalmic disease refractory to standard immunosuppressive therapy including cyclophosphamide, high-dose corticosteroids and in some cases TNF antagonists
Patients	Retrospective analysis of 10 consecutive patients with refractory ophthalmic Wegener's granulomatosis • Fulfilling the ACR criteria and the CHC definitions • Either biopsy-proven or characteristic disease manifestations of retro-orbital granulomas/necrotizing scleritis • Refractory scleritis n = 3 • Orbital granulomas causing optic nerve compromise n = 4 • Or a combination of both conditions n = 3 • All ≥ 3 previous immunosuppressive agents, including cyclophosphamide and high-dose corticosteroids • Previous treatment with TNF alpha blockade n = 5 • All PR3-ANCA positive n = 10
Authors	Taylor SR, Salama AD, Joshi L, Pusey CD, Lightman SL
Publication	*Arthritis Rheum.* 2009;60(5):1540–1547
Follow-up	36 months
Note	*Outcome parameters*:

Note (cont.)	Beneficial response	n = 10
	Clinical remission	n = 10, within 7 months
	Clinical remission sustained for 6.5 months (median)	n = 10
	Clinical remission for > 12 months	n = 4
	DEI at baseline	~3
	DEI at 24 months	~0
	DEI at 36 months	~0
	Decreased ANCA levels	Positive trend
	Daily prednisolone at 36 months	Almost 0 in all patients
Adverse events	None reported	

Trial	A multicenter survey of Rituximab therapy for refractory antineutrophil cytoplasmic antibody-associated vasculitis
Substance	*Retrospectively analyzed without randomization*:
	Rituximab 2 × 1 g (RTX) i. v. 2 weeks apart (n = 32)
	Rituximab 4 × 375 mg/m² i. v. 1 weeks apart (n = 26)
	Other dosing regimens for RTX (n = 7)
	Second course of RTX (n = 38)
	≥ 3 courses of RTX (up to 6) n = 20
	No immunosuppressive therapy in addition to RTX (n = 22)
	Concomitant medication:
	Mycophenolate mofetil n = 28; 2 g/day (average dose)
	Azathioprine n = 7; av. 75 mg/day
	IV pulse cyclophosphamide (CYC) n = 6
	Oral CYC n = 5; 150 mg/day (average dose)
	Deoxyspergualin n = 4
	Methotrexate n = 3; 20 mg/day (average dose)
	Plasma exchange n = 1
	Enteric coated mycophenolate sodium n = 1; average 2.16 g/day
	Alemtuzumab n = 1; 11 months before RTX
	Combination of 2 or 3 therapies n = 4
	None n = 5
	Oral corticosteroid 12.5 mg/day (average dose)
	I. v. corticosteroids/5 days followed by 1 mg/kg/day p. o. n = 17
	Previous medication:
	Anti-TNF n = 24
	Immunoglobulins n = 17
	Azathioprine n = 49
	Methotrexate 10 n = 18
	Mycophenolate mofetil n = 47
	Other n = 25
	Total no. of previous therapies/patient n = 4
Result	Rituximab was effective and safe in the induction of remission of refractory ANCA-associated vasculitis in this retrospective analysis, without difference in efficacy between the two main treatment regimens. Retreatment was effective and safe after relapses
Patients	Retrospective analysis of 65 sequential patients with refractory ANCA-associated vasculitis
	• Wegener's granulomatosis 71%
	• Microscopic polyangiitis
	• Churg-Strauss syndrome
	• Diagnosis according to the CHC definitions
	• All patients with active disease at time of first RTX
	• Median DEI n = 4 (new disease), n = 2 (persistent disease), at first RTX ANCA (PR3 or MPO) positive n = 33
	• Age ~47 years
	Major exclusion criteria:
	• RTX as first line therapy, follow-up after first RTX infusion ≤ 6 months

(continued) ➔

Authors	Jones RB, Ferraro AJ, Chaudhry AN, Brogan P, Salama AD, Smith KG, Savage CO, Jayne DR	
Publication	*Arthritis Rheum.* 2009;60(7):2156–2168	
Follow-up	21 months (median)	
Note	*Outcome parameters*:	
	Complete remission	75%
	Time to remission (median)	2 months
	DEI (median) at 12 months	0
	DEI (median) at 6 months	0
	Partial remission	23%
	No response	2%
	Prednisolone dose (median, baseline)	12.5 mg/day
	Prednisolone dose (median, 6 months)	9.0 mg/day
	Prednisolone dose (median, 12 months)	7.5 mg/day
	Withdrawal of immunosuppressives	62%
	Relapse after remission	57%
	Relapse before B-cell repopulation remission after second RTX course	48%
	Time to remission (median)	1.5 months
	Decrease in ANCA	84%
	Patients with or without additional immunosuppressives with regard to rate of relapses	No difference
	Between the 2 RTX treatment protocols	No differences
Adverse events	Endo-bronchial disease	7.5%
	Asthma	3.0%
	Peripheral neuropathy	1.5%
	Ear-nose-throat disease	3.0%
	Pulmonary fibrosis, respiratory failure, and death	1.5%
	Retro-orbital granuloma	1.5%
	Pneumonia (organism not specified)	11.0%
	Aspergillus lung infection	1.5%
	Pseudomonas lung infection	1.5%
	Line sepsis	1.5%
	Sepsis	3.0%
	Cellulitis	1.5%
	Pulmonary embolism	1.5%
	Sudden unexplained death	1.5%
	Addisonian crisis	3.0%
	Hip surgery	1.5%
	Aseptic meningitis post-IVIG therapy	1.5%
	Aortic valve replacement	1.5%
	Neutropenia	3.0%
	Failure of B cells to deplete	1.5%
	Ankle surgery	1.5%
	Eye surgery	1.5%

RAVE-Trial	Rituximab versus cyclophosphamide for ANCA-associated vasculitis RAVE: Rituximab in ANCA-associated Vasculitis
Substance	*Induction of remission*: Rituximab group (RTX, n = 99): **Rituximab 375 mg/m²/week i. v. for 4 weeks** *Cyclophosphamide group* (*Cyc, n = 98*): **2 mg cyclophosphamide/kg/day** *Maintenance of remission*: 2 mg azathioprine/kg/day after 3–6 months if remission was achieved *Concomitant medication*: 1–3 × 1'000 mg methylprednisolone Followed by 1mg/kg/day prednisone, tapered
Result	A higher percentage of rituximab-treated patients than those treated with daily cyclophosphamide reached remission and remission without prednisone in this remission-induction trial of severe ANCA-associated vasculitis. Sustained remission rates were high in both groups, and the rituximab-based regimen was not associated with reductions in early severe adverse events
Patients	197 ANCA-positive patients with • Wegener's granulomatosis or microscopic polyangiitis • PR 3-ANCA- or MPO-ANCA-positive • BVAS/WG ≥ 3 (RTX: 8.5, Cyc: 8.2)
Authors	Stone JH, Merkel PA, Spiera R, Seo P, Langford CA, Hoffman GS, Kallenberg CG, St Clair EW, Turkiewicz A, Tchao NK, Webber L, Ding L, Sejismundo LP, Mieras K, Weitzenkamp D, Ikle D, Seyfert-Margolis V, Mueller M, Brunetta P, Allen NB, Fervenza FC, Geetha D, Keogh KA, Kissin EY, Monach PA, Peikert T, Stegeman C, Ytterberg SR, Specks U; RAVE-ITN (Immune Tolerance Network) Research Group
Publication	*N Engl J Med.* 2010 Jul 15;363(3):221–232
Follow-up	6 months

(continued) ➔

Note	Change of:		
		RTX	CYC
	Remission without corticosteroids	64%	53%
	Remission	67%	42%
	BVAS/WG = 0 with ≤ 10 mg prednisone/day	71%	62%
	Estimated creatinine clearances in patients with renal affections (mL/min)	+11.2	+10.5
	Improvement of alveolar hemorrhage	57%	41%
	Flare rate/month	0.011	0.018
	Became ANCA neg.	47%	24%
Adverse events		RTX	CYC
	Adverse events leading to discontinuation	14%	17%
	Total adverse events	n = 31	n = 33
	Adverse events	n = 10	n = 2
	Hospitalized for adverse events	n = 8	n = 2
	Malignant tumors	n = 1	n = 1
	Malignant tumors after the 6 months of follow-up	n = 4	n = 1

RITUXVAS-Trial	Rituximab versus cyclophosphamide in ANCA-associated renal vasculitis RITUXVAS: Rituximab Vasculitis
Substance	*Induction of remission*: **Rituximab, 375 mg/m²/week** i. v. for 4 weeks (RTX, n = 33) **Placebo** (CYC, n = 11) *Concomitant medication*: 2 × i. v. 15 mg/m² CYC pulses (RTX-group) 3–6 x 15 mg/m² CYC (placebo-group) 1 g methyprednisolone i. v., followed by prednisone 1 mg/kg/day, tapered to 5 mg/day after 6 months *Maintenance of remission*: Azathioprine (n = 11 patients, initially treated with CYC without RTX)
Result	A rituximab-based regimen was equally effective, not superior to, as intravenous cyclophosphamide in this remission induction trial of severe ANCA-associated vasculitis with nephritis. Sustained remission rates were high in both groups, and the rituximab-based regimen was not associated with reductions in early severe adverse events
Patients	44 patients with newly diagnosed vasculitis, renal involvement and ANCA positivity • Necrotizing glomerulonephritis on biopsy or • Red cell casts or hematuria (≥ 30 red cells per high power field) on urinalysis
Authors	Jones RB, Tervaert JW, Hauser T, Luqmani R, Morgan MD, Peh CA, Savage CO, Segelmark M, Tesar V, van Paassen P, Walsh D, Walsh M, Westman K, Jayne DR; European Vasculitis Study Group
Publication	*N Engl J Med.* 2010 Jul 15;363(3):211–220
Follow-up	12 months (clinical trial), post-rituximab follow-up 3–52 months

(continued) ➔

Note	Follow-up		
		RTX	CYC
	Sustained remission	76%	82%
	Median weight adjusted doses of prednisolone (mg/kg) at month 12	0.071	0.082
	Remission (BVAS of 0 for 2 months)	93%	90%
	Median estimated GFR increased (mL/min/1.73 m²)	+19	+15
Adverse events		RTX	CYC
	Grade 1 or 2 adverse events	n = 37	n = 14
	Grade 3, 4, or 5 adverse events	n = 31	n = 12
	All adverse events	n = 68	n = 26
	Events requiring hospitalization or life-threatening events	n = 27	n = 9
	Cancer	n = 2	n = 0
	Death	n = 6	n = 2
	All serious adverse events	n = 35	n = 11
	Serious infections	n = 7	n = 3
	All infections	n = 19	n = 7
	All infusion reactions	n = 2	n = 0
	Anemia	n = 2	n = 2
	Neutropenia	n = 2	n = 1
	Thrombocytopenia	n = 1	n = 0
	Hypogammaglobulinemia	n = 1	n = 0

Trial	Prolonged disease-free remission following rituximab and low-dose cyclophosphamide therapy for renal ANCA-associated vasculitis
Substance	**Rituximab 2 × 1 g** i. v. on day 0 and 14
	Cyclophosphamide 2 × i. v. 10 mg/kg (max. 750 mg) day 0 and then every 14 days for a total of six doses
	Followed by 4 × i. v. 10 mg/kg cyclophosphamide (max. 500 mg) every 14 days for a total of six doses.
	1 mg/kg prednisolone p. o. (max. 60 mg)
	Tapered to 10 mg by week 13
	Azathioprine 2 mg/kg/day was commenced at 3 months, at a dose of 2 mg/kg (maximum 150 mg/day)
	Concomitant medication:
	Co-trimoxazole for 3 months
	Proton pump inhibitors
	Calcium/day
	Previous medication:
	No plasma exchange
	No CYP-based regimen
Result	A rituximab-based low-dose cyclophosphamide regimen was effective at inducing long-term disease-free remission
Patients	23 consecutive patients with active renal ANCA-associated vasculitis
	Active renal disease:
	• Presence of circulating ANCA
	• Active urinary sediment
	• Histological evidence of pauci-immune necrotizing glomerulonephritis on renal biopsy
	No serum creatinine > 500 μmol/L
	No pulmonary hemorrhage
	No cerebral vasculitis
Authors	Mansfield N, Hamour S, Habib AM, Tarzi R, Levy J, Griffith M, Cairns T, Cook HT, Pusey CD, Salama AD
Publication	*Nephrol Dial Transplant*. 2011 Oct;26(10):3280–3286
Follow-up	39 months (median)

(continued)

Note	Clinical remission within 6 weeks	n = 22
	BVAS > 0 (week 6)	n = 21
	BVAS = 0 (6 months)	n = 23
	Renal relapse	n = 3
	Change of:	
	eGFR (baseline, mL/min)	24
	eGFR (1 month, mL/min)	33
	eGFR (6 months, mL/min)	42
Adverse events	Multiorgan failure	n = 1
	Hypersensitivity to azathioprine	n = 1
	Cutaneous squamoproliferative lesion	n = 1
	Urinary tract infection	n = 7
	Respiratory infection	n = 3
	Herpes zoster infection	n = 1
	Gastroenteritis (culture negative)	n = 2
	Leucopenia due to azathioprine	n = 3
	Rash related to azathioprine	n = 1
	Gastrointestinal disturbance secondary to azathioprine	n = 1

Trial	Complications of plasma exchange in the treatment of polyarteritis nodosa and Churg-Strauss angiitis and the contribution of adjuvant immunosuppressive therapy: a randomized trial in 72 patients
Substance	**Corticosteroid (1 mg/kg/day)** for 2 months Tapered by 2.5 mg every 10 days for a month Tapered by 2.5 mg every week until half the initial dose was reached Maintenance of this dose for 3 weeks Further reduction by 1 mg/day every week when under 20 mg/day with a 3-week plateau at 10 and 5 mg *Randomization*: **2 mg/kg cyclophosphamide/day** during 1 year (CYC, n = 35) **Without cyclophosphamide** (No CYC, n = 35) *Both groups with plasma exchange*: **Centrifugation was used in 678 plasma exchange sessions** (83.4%) Filtration was used in 128 (15.7%) Every patient with 13 exchanges in 6 months *Replacement fluid*: 4% albumin (n = 698 sessions) Fresh-frozen plasma (n = 68 sessions) Both (n = 47 sessions) Replacement fluid in 745 sessions was 4% albumin and in 115 was fresh-frozen plasma
Result	Plasma exchange was relatively safe in this study of plasmapheresis and corticosteroids in patients with newly diagnosed polyarteritis nodosa or Churg-Strauss syndrome. Additional cyclophosphamide was probably contributed to increased mortality by severe infections while corticosteroids alone resulted in more death due to activity of vasculitis
Patients	72 patients with polyarteritis nodosa or Churg-Strauss angiitis, newly diagnosed based on histologic or angiographic data and without previous treatment
Authors	Lhote F, Guillevin L, Leon A, Bussel A, Lok C, Sobel A, Simon P
Publication	*Artif Organs*. 1988;12(1):27–33
Follow-up	36 months

(continued)

Note	251 complications in 60 patients during 206 (25.3%), of the 813 completed exchanges; 47 sessions (5.8%) were temporarily stopped as a result of complications		
	Data not available in two patients		
Adverse events		CYC	No CYC
	Death	n = 6	n = 6
	Death attributed to the vasculitis	n = 6	n = 4
	Hypotension	n = 26	n = 26
	Allergic reactions	n = 23	n = 28
	Malaise or vasovagal reactions	n = 8	n = 12
	Reactions to citrate	n = 6	n = 5
	Abdominal pain, nausea, vomiting	n = 7	n = 4
	Hypoglycemia	n = 3	n = 3
	Cardiac arrhythmia	n = 2	n = 2
	Fever	n = 1	n = 1
	Voluminous hematoma	n = 0	n = 1
	Hypertension	n = 1	n = 0
	Viral hepatitis B	n = 0	n = 1
	Phlebothrombosis	n = 0	n = 1

Trial	Lack of superiority of steroids plus plasma exchange to steroids alone in the treatment of polyarteritis nodosa and Churg-Strauss syndrome. A prospective, randomized trial in 78 patients
Substance	**Prednisone and plasma exchange** (group A, n = 36)
	Prednisone alone (group B, n = 42)
	No information on type of disease within groups
	Treatment failure:
	Cyclophosphamide 2 mg/kg (Cyc)/day n = 9 (group A),
	n = 5 (group B)
	Prednisone 1 mg/kg/day for 1 month
	Tapered after evidence of improvement by 2.5 mg/week until half of starting dose
	Maintained for 3 weeks
	Then reduction of 2.5 mg/week, to approximately 20 mg/day
	Further tapered in 1 mg/week steps to final 5 mg/day
	Plasma exchange:
	12 treatments during first 2 weeks two treatments in week 3
	The other four treatments spread over a period of 30 days after last treatment in week 3
	Plasma per session 60 mL/kg
	Concomitant medication:
	Corticosteroids < 10 mg/day for asthma
	No high-dose corticosteroids
Result	Combined treatment of polyarteritis nodosa and Churg-Strauss syndrome with prednisone and plasma exchange was not superior to treatment with prednisone alone
Patients	78 patients with polyarteritis nodosa (PAN) or Churg-Strauss syndrome
	• Multiple system involvement
	Major inclusion criteria:
	• Histological or arteriographic evidence of vasculitis, multiple system involvement, activity sufficient for corticosteroid use
	Major exclusion criterion:
	• HBV-related PAN
Authors	Guillevin L, Fain O, Lhote F, Jarrousse B, Le Thi Huong D, Bussel A, Leon A
Publication	*Arthritis Rheum.* 1992;35(2):208–215
Follow-up	7 years

(continued) ➔

	Outcome parameters:		
Note		Group A	Group B
	Completely recovered	n = 27	n = 29
	Prednisolone dose after 1 year (mg/day)	10	13.7
	Additional treatment needed	n = 10	n = 6
	Relapses	n = 10	n = 8
	Disease activity not controlled	n = 14	n = 12
	Steroid dose increased	n = 4	n = 6
	7-year cumulative survival rates	83%	79%
	Cyc was able to control the disease in the 14 patients treated (no further details provided)		
Adverse events	Causes of death:		
		Group A	Group B
	Deaths	n = 6	n = 9
	Bowel infarction	n = 1	n = 1
	Hematoperitoneum	n = 0	n = 1
	Stroke	n = 2	n = 0
	Respiratory failure	n = 0	n = 1
	Cardiac failure	n = 1	n = 2
	Infections	n = 0	n = 1
	Septicemia	n = 0	n = 1
	Pulmonary embolism	n = 0	n = 1
	Unknown	n = 1	n = 1
	Cancer	n = 1	n = 1
	Adverse events due to corticosteroid treatment		
	Osteoporosis	n = 2	
	Aseptic necrosis of femoral head	n = 2	
	Duodenal ulcers	n = 2	
	Pneumonia	n = 1	

MEPEX-Trial	Randomized trial of plasma exchange or high-dosage Methylprednisolone as adjunctive therapy for severe renal vasculitis
Substance	**Seven plasma exchanges** (group A, n = 70) Methylprednisolone 3'000 mg of intravenous (group B, n = 67) *Both groups*: **Cyclophosphamide p. o. 2.5 mg/kg/day** (reduced to 1.5 mg/kg/day after 3 months) **Prednisolone p. o. 1 mg/kg/day** Taper to 0.25 mg/kg/day by week 10 10 mg total/day from months 5 to 12 *Concomitant medication*: Prophylaxis against fungal infection and *Pneumocystis jirovecii* pneumonia suggested
Result	Plasma exchange, in comparison to intravenous methylprednisolone, increased the rate of renal recovery in Wegener's granulomatosis and microscopic polyangiitis presenting with renal failure on a background of oral cyclophosphamide and prednisolone. Patient survival and severe adverse event rates were similar in both groups
Patients	137 patients with a new diagnosis of vasculitis • Wegener's granulomatosis (n = 42) • Microscopic polyangiitis (n = 95) • With biopsy-proven pauci-immune, necrotizing and/or crescentic glomerulonephritis (GN) Serum creatinine 500 mmol/L (5.8 mg/dL) • ANCA negative n = 3 • BVAS 21 (median), Vasculitis damage index 0 (median) *Major exclusion criteria*: • Antibodies to glomerular basal membrane • Life-threatening other organ manifestation • Dialysis for > 2 weeks before entry • Creatinine > 200 mmol/L ≥ 1 year before entry • Previous necrotizing and/or crescentic GN • Previous major or longer immunosuppressive medication
Authors	Jayne DR, Gaskin G, Rasmussen N, Abramowicz D, Ferrario F, Guillevin L, Mirapeix E, Savage CO, Sinico RA, Stegeman CA, Westman KW, van der Woude FJ, de Lind van Wijngaarden RA, Pusey CD; European Vasculitis Study Group
Publication	*J Am Soc Nephrol.* 2007;18(7):2180–2188
Follow-up	12 months

(continued) ➔

Note	Outcome parameters:		
		Group A (%)	Group B (%)
	Alive and independent of dialysis at month 3	69	49
	Patient survival at month 12	76	48
	Reduction in risk for progression to end-stage renal disease (month 12)	24	24
Adverse events		Group A (%)	Group B (%)
	Leukopenia mild	10	52
	Leukopenia severe	11	10
	Recurrent mild leukopenia	3	19
	Recurrent severe leukopenia	6	16
	Infection mild	24	19
	Infection severe	15	25
	Thrombopenia mild	0	3
	Thrombopenia severe	7	4
	Allergy mild	0	6
	Allergy severe	0	8
	Cardiovascular mild	4	3
	Cardiovascular severe	4	1
	Diabetes mild	3	4
	Diabetes severe	1	3
	Gastrointestinal mild	1	0
	Gastrointestinal severe	3	4
	Bone fracture mild	3	0
	Bone fracture severe	3	1
	Thrombosis mild	0	1
	Thrombosis severe	4	1
	Hemorrhage mild	1	1
	Hemorrhage severe	10	11
	Alopecia mild	0	0
	Alopecia severe	0	3
	Vascular access complications mild	1	0
	Vascular access complications severe	11	1

Trial	Plasma exchange for induction and cyclosporine A for maintenance of remission in Wegener's granulomatosis - a clinical randomized controlled trial
Substance	*Induction of remission*: **Prednisolone 80 mg/day** for 3 weeks Tapered to 5 mg and stopped after 9 months Relapse: steroids increase to 40 mg/day **Cyclophosphamide 1.5 mg/kg/day = 100/150 mg/day for 3 months** *Randomized phase*: **Cyclophosphamide 1.5 mg/kg/day** = 100/150 mg/day for 9 months (*n* = 16) **Ciclosporin A 5 mg/kg** for 9 months (CsA, blood-CsA levels: 150–200 μmol/L, n = 16) **Plasma exchange** (PE, performed in 8 patients of every group): Gambro F-1000 filters (Gambro, Lund, Sweden) every other day 4 L of plasma was exchanged with 3% albumin in Ringer's Lactate C-ANCA titers were > 320 or PR3-ANCA > 25 U/m after 6 sessions: additional 3–6 sessions
Result	Plasma exchange improved renal survival at creatinine levels > 250 μmol/L, whereas previous randomized studies had limited plasma exchange to patients with creatinine > 500 μmol/L. Change from cyclophosphamide to ciclosporin did not influence the rate of relapses or time to relapse. All patients who were on dialysis when recruited were dialysis dependent five years later.
Patients	32 patients with Wegener's granulomatosis (WG) • ≥ 2 organ systems involved • Histology-proven WG • Positive c-ANCA/PR3-ANCA • Fulfilling the ACR 1990 criteria for the classification of WG
Authors	Szpirt WM, Heaf JG, Petersen J
Publication	*Nephrol Dial Transplant.* 2011 Jan;26(1):206–213
Follow up	5 years

(continued)

Note

Outcome at 1 month:

	Plasma exchange	Without plasma exchange
Progression	n = 0	n = 6
Remission	n = 16	n = 10
Hemodialysis	n = 0	n = 5
Creatinine < 130 µmol/L	n = 7 (plus 2 patients)	n = 5
Creatinine 130–300 µmol/L	n = 8 (plus 4 patients)	n = 6 (plus 1 patient)
Creatinine > 300 µmol/L	n = 1 (-6 patients)	n = 5 (-1 patient)

Outcome at 3 months:

	Plasma exchange	Without plasma exchange
Progression	n = 1	n = 7
Remission	n = 15	n = 9
Hemodialysis	n = 0	n = 4
Creatinine < 130 µmol/L	n = 9	n = 8
Creatinine 130–300 µmol/L	n = 6	n = 5
Creatinine > 300 µmol/L	n = 0	n = 4

Outcome at 5 years:

	Plasma exchange	Without plasma exchange
Progression	n = 5	n = 11
Remission	n = 11	n = 5
Hemodialysis	n = 2	n = 7
Creatinine < 130 µmol/L	n = 7	n = 5
Creatinine 130–300 µmol/L	n = 5	n = 5
Creatinine > 300 µmol/L	n = 4	n = 6

Relapse rate:

	PE/CsA	PE	CsA	None
No relapses	n = 2	n = 5	n = 4	n = 3
1 relapses	n = 2	n = 1	n = 3	n = 4
2 relapses	n = 1	n = 1	n = 1	n = 0
3 relapses	n = 3	n = 1	n = 0	n = 1
Patients/relapse	6/13	3/6	4/5	5/7

JMAAV -Trial	Severity-based treatment for Japanese patients with MPO-ANCA-associated vasculitis: the JMAAV study. JMAAV: Japanese patients with MPO-ANCA-associated vasculitis
Substance	*Mild form (n = 23):* **Prednisolone 0.3–0.6 mg/kg/day** plus **Cyclophosphamide 0.5–1.0 mg/kg/day** if necessary, or **Azathioprine 25–75 mg/day** *Severe form (n = 23):* **Prednisolone 0.6–1 mg/kg** or i. v. 0.5–1 g/day plus 0.5–2.0 mg/kg oral or 0.5–0.75 g/m^2 i. v. cyclophosphamide/day or 0.5–0.75 g/m^2 i. v. monthly *Most severe form (n = 2):* **Prednisolone 0.6–1 mg/kg** or i. v. 0.5–1 g/day plus **Cyclophosphamide 0.5–2.0 mg/kg/day** (oral) or 0.5–0.75 g/m^2 i. v. monthly plus plasmapheresis 2.0–3.0 L/day for 3 days *Previous medication:* No cyclophosphamide therapy with a cumulative dose of > 10 g
Result	Satisfying results concerning remission, relapse rates, and severe adverse events. The three groups were too small to draw definite conclusions from this open-label trial
Patients	48 patients with MPO-ANCA-positive microscopic polyangiitis, newly diagnosed MPA according to the diagnostic criteria for MPA of the Research Group of Intractable Vasculitis MHLW of Japan • No end-stage renal disease requiring hemodialysis • No respiratory failure with PaO_2 < 60 Torr
Authors	Ozaki S, Atsumi T, Hayashi T, Ishizu A, Kobayashi S, Kumagai S, Kurihara Y, Kurokawa MS, Makino H, Nagafuchi H, Nakabayashi K, Nishimoto N, Suka M, Tomino Y, Yamada H, Yamagata K, Yoshida M, Yumura W
Publication	*Mod Rheumatol.* 2012 Jun;22(3):394–404
Follow-up	18 months

Note	*Outcome:*	
	Remission (6 months)	n = 42
	Relapse	n = 8
	End-stage renal disease	n = 1
Adverse events	Death	n = 5
	Death without remission	n = 3
	Bacterial infection	n = 11
	Fungal infection	n = 6
	Viral infection	n = 7
	PCP	n = 3
	Diabetes mellitus	n = 9
	Bone fracture	n = 3
	Cerebral vascular events	n = 3
	Cardiac vascular event	n = 1

Henoch–Schönlein Purpura

Corticosteroids

Trial	A randomized, placebo-controlled trial of prednisone in early Henoch–Schönlein Purpura
Substance	**Prednisone p. o., 2 mg/kg/day** (n = 21) Tapered over 1 week to 25% of starting dose, then discontinuation or **Placebo** (n = 19)
Result	Early prednisone therapy did not reduce the risk of renal involvement at one year or the risk of acute gastrointestinal complications. There were no cases of intussusceptions in the prednisone group
Patients	40 children with Henoch–Schönlein Purpura (HSP) • Age 2–15 years • ≥ 6 days of disease onset ± *1 of the following*: • Arthritis • Renal involvement (defined as hematuria on urine microscopy ≥ 5 red blood cells per high-powered field, proteinuria ≥ 0.3 g/L) • Hypertension ≥ 90th percentile for age and gender • Gastrointestinal involvement (abdominal pain, gross or occult blood in stool, or a surgical complication, such as intussusception or perforation) *Major exclusion criteria*: • Any corticosteroid treatment within the previous month • Life-threatening complication of HSP Renal involvement n = 4 (prednisone) n = 2 (placebo) Gastrointestinal involvement n = 18 (prednisone) n = 11 (placebo)
Authors	Huber AM, King J, McLaine P, Klassen T, Pothos M
Publication	*BMC Med*. 2004;2:7
Follow-up	1 year

(continued) →

R. Müller, J. von Kempis, *Clinical Trials in Rheumatology*,
DOI 10.1007/978-1-4471-2870-0_13, © Springer-Verlag London 2013

Note		Prednisone	Placebo
	Renal involvement at 1 year	n = 3	n = 2
	Rash duration (median)	7 days	11 days
	Joint pain duration (median)	3 days	6 days
	Abdominal pain duration (median)	5.5 days	2 day
Adverse events		Prednisone	Placebo
	Gastrointestinal complications	n = 2	n = 3
	Intussusceptions	n = 0	n = 2

Trial	Early prednisone therapy in HSP: A randomized, double-blind, placebo-controlled trial
Substance	**1 mg/kg prednisone/day** for 2 weeks n = 84 Followed by 0.5 mg/kg prednisone/day for 1 week Followed by 0.5 mg/kg prednisone/every other day for 1 week **Placebo** n = 87 *Concomitant medication*: Analgetics (paracetamol was permitted)
Result	Prednisone reduced extrarenal symptoms in Henoch–Schönlein purpura patients by prednisone. The general use was not supported
Patients	171 patients with Henoch–Schönlein purpura (HSP) • Age < 16 years • Typically distributed purpura or petechiae • With or without gastrointestinal bleeding • And/or joint pain *Major exclusion criteria*: • Thrombocytopenia • Systemic vasculitis • Established nephritis
Authors	Ronkainen J, Koskimies O, Ala-Houhala M, Antikainen M, Merenmies J, Rajantie J, Ormälä T, Turtinen J, Nuutinen M
Publication	*J Pediatr*. 2006 Aug;149(2):241–247
Follow-up	6 months

Note — *Difference in the improvement of renal symptoms*:

	Month 1 (%)	Month 3 (%)	Month 6 (%)
Prednisone compared to placebo:	-27	-21	-23

Change of:

	Prednisone	Placebo
Increase in weight (kg)	+1.4	+0.4
Systolic blood pressure (mmHg)	109	106
Diastolic blood pressure (mmHg)	64	61
Need for analgesic (days)	2.2	2.7
Abdominal pain score severity	2.5	4.8
Abdominal pain score duration	1.5	2.7
Joint pain score severity	4.6	7.3
Joint pain score duration	3.1	4.4
Improved appetite	n = 26	Not shown
Increased liveliness	n = 7	Not shown

Adverse events	Prednisone	Placebo
Serious adverse events	n = 0	n = 0

Trial	Can Azathioprine and steroids alter the progression of severe Henoch–Schönlein nephritis in children?
Substance	*Azathioprine group (n = 10)*: **Azathioprine/day, at 2 mg/kg,** for 8 months **+ prednisolone**
	Corticosteroid group (n = 10): **Prednisolone alone**
	Corticosteroid therapy: **Oral prednisolone 2 mg/kg/day** on alternate days for 4 weeks Tapered to 1.5, 1.0, and 0.5 mg/kg every other day, each for 2 months Initial pulse 30 mg/kg methylprednisolone for 6 alternate days n = 2 (azathioprine group), n = 0 (corticosteroid group)
	Concomitant therapy: Angiotensin-converting enzyme inhibitors for blood pressure control n = 5 (azathioprine group), n = 7 (corticosteroid group)
Result	There was a tendency for superiority of the combination treatment with azathioprine and steroids, in comparison to steroids alone, in improving the clinical course of severe nephritis in this retrospective analysis
Patients	20 patients with Henoch–Schönlein purpura • Median age 9.3 years • Nephritis with nephrotic proteinuria
	Major exclusion criterion: • Previous treatment with cytotoxic drugs
Authors	Shin JI, Park JM, Shin YH, Kim JH, Lee JS, Kim PK, Jeong HJ
Publication	*Pediatr Nephrol.* 2005;20(8):1087–1092
Follow-up	4.8 years (median)

Note		Azathioprine	Corticosteroid
	Resolution of hematuria	n = 6	n = 4
	Resolution of proteinuria	n = 8	n = 6
	Favorable clinical response	n = 10	n = 6
	Unfavorable clinical response	n = 0	n = 4

Trial	Cyclosporine A therapy for severe Henoch–Schönlein nephritis with nephrotic syndrome
Substance	Prednisolone p. o., n = 5 **Initial pulse 30 mg/kg methylprednisolone** (6×on alternate days i. v. 30 mg/kg; max. 1.0 g/day) Then oral prednisolone, n = 2 **Plus ciclosporin A 5 mg/kg/day,** mean duration 10.6 months *Concomitant therapy*: Angiotensin-converting enzyme (ACE) inhibitors for blood pressure control n = 4 (2.5 mg cilazapril once daily) *Previous medication*: No immunosuppressive therapy
Result	Retrospective analysis of a case series without controls, showing a possible beneficial effect of ciclosporin A plus prednisolone treatment in severe Henoch–Schönlein nephritis
Patients	7 patients with severe Henoch–Schönlein nephritis • With nephrotic syndrome • Hypoalbuminemia < 2.5 g/dL • Urinary protein excretion > 40 mg/m^2/h • Mean age 6.5 years
Authors	Shin JI, Park JM, Shin YH, Kim JH, Kim PK, Lee JS, Jeong HJ
Publication	*Pediatr Nephrol.* 2005;20(8):1093–1097
Follow-up	5.5 years/4.3 years (median) after: disease onset/cessation of ciclosporin A therapy
Note	*Clinical changes*:	
	Proteinuria (g/m^2/day)	-8.9
	No proteinuria at latest observation	n = 6
	Total protein (g/dL)	+2.9
	Albumin (g/dL)	+2.5
	Creatinine (mg/dL)	+0.1
	Creatinine clearance (mL/min/1.73 m^2)	+45
	Histopathologic changes (n = 7):	
	Activity index	-2.9
	Chronicity index	+0.1
	Tubulointerstitial scores	-0.6

Trial	Henoch–Schönlein purpura nephritis: Course of disease and efficacy of cyclophosphamide		
Substance	**Cyclophosphamide, 90 mg/m²/day** (Group A, n = 28) for 42 days **Control** (Group B, n = 28) Group C: **Patients followed concurrently outside trial** (n = 23) *Concomitant therapy*: Diet modifications Diuretics Exchange resins Vitamins		
Result	Cyclophosphamide treatment of severe Henoch–Schönlein nephritis did not result in more full recoveries of nephritis than supportive therapy alone		
Patients	56 patients with histopathologically severe Henoch–Schönlein nephritis • Age 12 weeks to 16 years • Estimated GFR ≥ 35 mL/min/1.73 m² *Inclusion criteria*: • Age between 12 and 16 years • Biopsy-proven HSP nephritis histopathology ≥ Grade III • With heavy proteinuria for > 1 month • Estimated glomerular filtration rate > 35 mL/min/1.73 m² • Purpura + urticaria, affecting lower limbs and possibly buttocks and elbows ± ≥ *1 of the following*: • Joint pain and swelling • Renal involvement • Abdominal pain • Intestinal bleeding *Major exclusion criteria*: • Prior immunosuppressive drugs • Henoch–Schönlein purpura present for > 3 months		
Authors	Tarshish P, Bernstein J, Edelmann CM Jr		
Publication	*Pediatr Nephrol.* 2004;19(1):51–56		
Follow-up	6.93 years (recoveries), 3.71 years (persistent abnormities)		
Note		Group A	Group B	Group C
	Fully recovered	n = 13	n = 14	n = 16
	Persistent mild abnormalities	n = 8	n = 6	n = 0
	Persistent moderate/severe abnormalities	n = 4	n = 4	n = 0
	End-stage renal disease/death	n = 3	n = 4	n = 1

Trial	Efficacy of methylprednisolone and urokinase pulse therapy combined with or without cyclophosphamide in severe Henoch–Schoenlein nephritis: a clinical and histopathological study
Substance	*Retrospectively analyzed without randomization*: *Group A (n = 20)*: **30 mg/kg methylprednisolone/day** i. v. for 3 days followed by oral 1 mg/kg prednisolone/day for 6 months Then tapering of prednisolone until discontinuation over 3 months plus urokinase at 5'000 units/kg/day i. v. for 7 days *Group B (n = 17)*: **30 mg/kg methylprednisolone/day** i. v. for 3 days Followed by oral 1 mg/kg prednisolone/day for 6 months Then tapering of prednisolone until discontinuation over 3 months plus **urokinase at 5'000 units/kg/day** i. v. on 7 days Plus **cyclophosphamide/day at 2.5 mg/kg** for 12 weeks *Concomitant medication*: 1 mg warfarin/day for 24 months Along with 5 mg/kg dipyridamole/day
Result	Methylprednisolone and urokinase pulse therapy, combined with cyclophosphamide, showed improvement of nephritic symptoms and changes in severe Henoch–Schoenlein nephritis, as compared to methylprednisolone and urokinase pulse therapy alone in this retrospective analysis
Patients	37 patients with Henoch–Schoenlein nephritis Grade IVb *Inclusion criteria*: • Age < 15 years • Diagnosed clinically by purpuric rash and abdominal pain without thrombocytopenia • With additional arthritis and nephritis consistent with the diagnosis *Major exclusion criterion*: • Previous treatment with immunosuppressive drugs
Authors	Kawasaki Y, Suzuki J, Suzuki H
Publication	*Nephrol Dial Transplant*. 2004;19(4):858–864
Follow-up	24 months

(continued) ➔

Note	Clinical outcome:		
		Group A	Group B
	Urinary protein excretion (mg/ m²/h)	-140	-175
	Hematuria	-15%	-17% (no hematuria at the end of follow-up)
	Serum albumin (g/L)	+3	+14
	Serum creatinine (µmol/L)	-10	-23
	Mean blood pressure (mmHg)	-4	-11
	Change of renal biopsy staging:		
		Group A (%)	Group B (%)
	Stage 0	+40	+76
	Stage 1	-40	-64
	Stage 2	0	-12
	Stage 3	0	0
Adverse events		Group A	Group B
	Cushingoid habitus	n = 5	n = 5
	Glaucoma	n = 3	n = 2
	Mild growth retardation	n = 1	n = 1
	Mild hypertension	n = 1	n = 1
	Leukopenia	n = 0	n = 1
	Infections	n = 1	n = 1

CESAR -Trial	Addition of cyclophosphamide to steroids provides no benefit compared with steroids alone in treating adult patients with severe HSP CESAR: Randomized Therapeutic Study of Steroid vs. Steroid Plus Cyclophosphamide for Severe Viscera HSP
Substance	**Steroids alone** (n = 29) **Steroids and 0.6 g/m2 cyclophosphamide at weeks 0, 2, 4,8,12, and 16** (n = 25) *Concomitant corticosteroids*: 7.5 mg/kg/day – day 1–3 1 mg/kg/day – day 3–7 0.75 mg/kg/day – day 7–14 0.5 mg/kg/day – week 2–4 0.4 mg/kg/day – week 5–7 0.3 mg/kg/day – week 8–12 0.25 mg/kg/day – month 3–4 0 mg/kg/day – month 4–6
Result	Treatment of adults with severe disease by adding cyclophosphamide showed no benefit compared with steroids alone
Patients	54 adults with biopsy-proven Henoch–Schönlein purpura • Including proliferative glomerulonephritis and • Severe visceral manifestations
Authors	Pillebout E, Alberti C, Guillevin L, Ouslimani A, Thervet E; CESAR study group
Publication	*Kidney Int.* 2010 Sep;78(5):495–502
Follow-up	12-month (primary end point) follow-up of 60.9 months (median)

(continued) ➔

Note		Steroids	Steroids + cyclophosphamide
	Score at day 0, median	28	20
	BVAS score = 0 at month 6	n = 3	n = 3
	BVAS score at month 6, median	12	9
	Change of BVAS from day 0 to month 6, median	-17	-12
	BVAS improvement ≤ −1	n = 26	n = 22
	Unchanged BVAS	n = 3	n = 2
	BVAS worsening > 1	n = 0	n = 1
	Blood pressure > 125/75 mmHg	n = 15	n = 13
	Creatinine (mmol/L), median	98	93
	eGFR (mL/min), median	70	77
	eGFR < mL/min	n = 8	n = 5
	Proteinuria (g/day), median	0.3	0.6
	Proteinuria ≥ 1 g/day	n = 4	n = 3
	Hematuria ≥ 10 RBC/mm^3	n = 3	n = 5
	RAS blockers	n = 14	n = 12
	Renal function improvement > 50%	n = 4	n = 1
	End-stage renal disease	n = 1	n = 1
Adverse events		Steroids	Steroids + cyclophosphamide
	Infection	n = 10	n = 7
	Urinary tract	n = 4	n = 2
	Necrotizing fasciitis	n = 1	n = 1
	Zona zoster	n = 0	n = 1
	Mycobacterium tuberculosis	n = 1	n = 0
	Bronchitis	n = 4	n = 3
	Diabetes	n = 7	n = 6
	Depression anxiety	n = 2	n = 2
	Insomnia	n = 3	n = 0
	Alopecia	n = 1	n = 1
	Acne vulgaris/atrophia striata	n = 0	n = 1 / n = 1
	Vertebral fracture	n = 0	n = 1
	Deaths	n = 6	n = 1
	Hemorrhagic shock	n = 2	n = 0
	Myocardial infarct	n = 0	n = 1
	End-stage liver disease	n = 2	n = 0
	Unknown	n = 2	n = 0

Behçet's Disease

Corticosteroids

Trial	A double-blind trial of depot corticosteroids in Behçet's syndrome
Substance	**Methylprednisolone acetate 40 mg** (n = 42)
	Placebo (n = 44)
	Every 3 weeks for 27 weeks
	Concomitant medication:
	NSAIDs n = 1 (steroid), n = 4 (placebo)
	Low-dose aspirin n = 3 (steroid), n = 3 (placebo)
	Amitriptyline n = 2 (steroid), n = 4 (placebo)
	Colchicine n = 18 (steroid), n = 24 (placebo)
	Previous medication:
	Corticosteroids < 5 mg/day were permitted
Result	Treatment of genital ulcers with low-dose depot corticosteroids did not have any beneficial effect on genital ulcers. Erythema nodosum lesions improved
Patients	86 patients wtih Behçet's syndrome
	• Active disease with ≥ 1 genital ulcers occurring for ≥ 6 months
	• No severe organ involvement
Authors	Mat C, Yurdakul S, Uysal S, Gogus F, Ozyazgan Y, Uysal O, Fresko I, Yazici H
Publication	*Rheumatology* (*Oxford*). 2006;45(3):348–352
Follow-up	27 weeks

(continued) ➔

R. Müller, J. von Kempis, *Clinical Trials in Rheumatology*,
DOI 10.1007/978-1-4471-2870-0_14, © Springer-Verlag London 2013

Note	Treatment period:		
		Steroid	Placebo
	Genital ulcers	0.3	0.3
	Oral ulceration	1.8	1.8
	Erythema nodosum	0.1	0.3
	Folliculitis	1.1	1.0
	Joints with arthritis	0.1	0.1
	Posttreatment period:		
		Steroid	Placebo
	Genital ulcers	0.1	0.1
	Oral ulceration	1.9	2.0
	Erythema nodosum	0.2	0.6
	Folliculitis	1.0	0.9
	Joints with arthritis	0.1	0.1
	Treatment period (females only):		
		Steroid	Placebo
	Genital ulcers	0.2	0.4
	Oral ulceration	1.8	1.8
	Erythema nodosum	0.2	0.4
	Folliculitis	0.7	0.8
	Joints with arthritis	0.2	0.1
	Posttreatment period (females only):		
		Steroid	Placebo
	Genital ulcers	0.0	0.2
	Oral ulceration	1.9	2.1
	Erythema nodosum	0.2	0.8
	Folliculitis	0.6	0.8
	Joints with arthritis	0.2	0.1
	Treatment period (males only):		
		Steroid	Placebo
	Genital ulcers	0.3	0.3
	Oral ulceration	1.8	1.8
	Erythema nodosum	0.1	0.2
	Folliculitis	1.6	1.3
	Joints with arthritis	0.0	0.1
	Posttreatment period (males only):		
		Steroid	Placebo
	Genital ulcers	0.1	0.0
	Oral ulceration	1.8	1.8
	Erythema nodosum	0.2	0.4
	Folliculitis	1.4	1.0
	Joints with arthritis	0.0	0.1
Adverse events		Steroid (%)	Placebo (%)
	Fatigue	42	67
	Increased appetite	17	46
	Weight gain	47	51
	Facial swelling	11	10
	Abdominal pain	22	18
	Hypertrichosis	6	0

Trial	A controlled trial of Azathioprine in Behçet's syndrome
Substance	**Azathioprine 2.5 mg/kg/day** (group 1: n = 12, group 2: n = 13) **Placebo** (group 1: n = 25, group 2: n = 23) *Severe exacerbation*: Methylprednisolone 1´000 mg on 3 alternate days or oral corticosteroid Alternative immunosuppressive agents were permitted *Concomitant medication*: No information provided *Previous medication*: No immunosuppressive agents
Result	Azathioprine was superior to placebo in preventing ocular manifestations

Patients	Turkish men with Behçet's syndrome fulfilling the O'Duffy criteria for diagnosis
	  • Group 1: No history/evidence of uveitis (n = 25)
	  • Group 2: With uveitis (n = 48)
	  • Disease duration ≤ 24 months
	Major exclusion criteria:
	  • No bilateral eye disease
	  • Patients with non-assessable fundi were excluded

Authors	Yazici H, Pazarli H, Barnes CG, Tüzün Y, Ozyazgan Y, Silman A, Serdaroğlu S, Oğuz V, Yurdakul S, Lovatt GE, et al.
Publication	*N Engl J Med.* 1990;322(5):281–285
Follow-up	2 years

(continued) ➔

Note	Outcome parameters:				
		Group 1, without uveitis		Group 2, with uveitis	
		Azathioprine	Placebo	Azathioprine	Placebo
	Necessitating withdrawal	n = 0	n = 0	n = 0	n = 6
	New eye disease	n = 1	n = 8	n = 0	n = 5
	Hypopyon uveitis	n = 0	n = 0	n = 1	n = 7
	Pulse i. v. corticosteroid	n = 0	n = 1	n = 6	n = 10
	Oral corticosteroid treatment	n = 0	n = 0	n = 1	n = 4
	New during drug trial:				
		New during drug trial		Present at 24 months	
		Azathioprine (%)	Placebo (%)	Azathioprine (%)	Placebo (%)
	Oral ulcerations	52	47	12	35
	Genital ulcerations	10	38	3	13
	Erythema nodosum	19	21	0	0
	Papulopustular lesions	79	85	79	74
	Arthritis	3	23	3	9
	Thrombophlebitis	11	26	29	35
	Neurological involvement no change	6	8	3	4
Adverse events		Azathioprine		Placebo	
	Low white cell counts	n = 11		n = 3	
	Gastrointestinal	23%		18%	
	Abdominal pain	6%		3%	
	Nausea	6%		5%	
	Indigestion	5%		1%	

Trial	Azathioprine in severe uveitis of Behçet's disease
Substance	**Azathioprine 2.5 mg/kg/day**
	Concomitant medication:
	0.5–1 mg/kg corticosteroids/day
	Colchicine was permitted
	Topical steroids were permitted
Result	Azathioprine was an effective and safe therapy in patients with severe uveitis
Patients	157 consecutive patients,fulfilling the International Study Group for Behçet's disease criteria
	• With active posterior uveitis or panuveitis
Authors	Saadoun D, Wechsler B, Terrada C, Hajage D, Le Thi Huong D, Resche-Rigon M, Cassoux N, Le Hoang P, Amoura Z, Bodaghi B, Cacoub P
Publication	*Arthritis Care Res (Hoboken)*. 2010 Dec;62(12):1733–1738
Follow-up	≥ 12 months

Note	*During follow-up*:	
	Partial or complete response	n = 146
	Complete response	n = 81
	Partial response	n = 65
	Visual acuity in the better eye	
	Decrease in the mean oral prednisone dosage	-44.8
	Nonresponders	n = 14
	Switched to cyclophosphamide	n = 6
	Cumulative relapse rates of uveitis at 1 year	11%
	Cumulative relapse rates of uveitis at 5 years	32.6%
Adverse events	Withdrawal because of hepatotoxic effects	n = 2
	Withdrawal because of bacterial septicemia	n = 1
	Total patients with adverse events	n = 67
	Gastrointestinal events	19.1%
	Cytopenia	18.4%
	Infections	17.8%

Trial	Double-masked trial of Cyclosporin versus Colchicine and long-term open study of Cyclosporin in Behçet's disease
Substance	**Ciclosporin 10 mg/kg/day** (CsA, n = 47) **1 mg colchicine/day** (n = 49) When CsA was stopped colchicine was introduced *Concomitant medication*: No information provided *Previous medication*: No information provided
Result	Ciclosporin was effective in treating not only the ocular manifestations of Behçet's disease but also oral aphthous ulcers, dermal lesions, and genital ulcerations. Efficacy remained stable during long-term treatment
Patients	96 patients with complete or incomplete Behçet's disease • Ocular lesions • Visual acuity ≤ 20/40 • ≥ 3 occular attacks during 16-week prior randomization
Authors	Masuda K, Nakajima A, Urayama A, Nakae K, Kogure M, Inaba G
Publication	*Lancet.* 1989;1(8647):1093–1096
Follow-up	80 weeks

Note	*Outcome parameters*:		
		CsA (%)	Colchicine (%)
	Improvement of clinical symptoms	91	33
	Dermal lesion improvement	40	15
Adverse events		CsA	Colchicine
	Hirsutism	n = 23	n = 2
	Renal dysfunction	n = 1	n = 2
	Hepatic dysfunction	n = 0	n = 2
	Gingival hypertrophy	n = 6	n = 0

Trial	Colchicine versus placebo in Behçet's disease: randomized, double-blind, controlled crossover trial
Substance	*Cross over of*: **Colchicine 1 mg at night** **Placebo** At 4 months, patients were crossed over for another 4 months *Previous medication*: No treatment for at least 1 month
Result	Disease activity improved in colchicine, but not placebo-treated patients
Patients	169 patients with confirmed Behçet's disease, fulfilling the International Study Group for Behçet's Disease criteria • Without major organ involvement (brain, eye, major intestinal, lung, cardiovascular) • At least one active symptom
Authors	Davatchi F, Sadeghi Abdollahi B, Tehrani Banihashemi A, Shahram F, Nadji A, Shams H, Chams-Davatchi C
Publication	*Mod Rheumatol*. 2009;19(5):542–549
Follow-up	8 months

(continued)

Note	*Change of disease activity*:		
		Colchicine	Placebo
	Joint manifestations		
	IBBDAM = overall disease activity (patients completing study)	-0.24	0.41
	IBBDAM (intention to treat)	0.04	0.2
	Skin lesions		
	IBBDAM (patients completing study)	0.13	0.03
	IBBDAM (intention to treat)	+0.21	0.04
	Genital aphthosis		
	IBBDAM (patients completing study)	-0.33	0.57
	IBBDAM (intention to treat)	0.53	0.38
	Oral aphthosis		
	IBBDAM (patients completing study)	0.57	0.12
	IBBDAM (intention to treat)	-0.35	0.35
	Overall results		
	IBBDAM (patients completing study)	1.03	0.2
	IBBDAM (intention to treat)	-0.8	-0.32
Adverse events		Colchicine	Placebo
	Total adverse events	n = 9	n = 9
	Stop because of nausea and vomiting	n = 1	n = 0
	Diarrhea	n = 4	n = 3
	Elevation of liver enzymes (SGOT–SGPT)	n = 2	n = 0
	Urinary tract infection	n = 1	n = 0
	Abdominal pain	n = 0	n = 1
	Purpura	n = 0	n = 1
	Dysesthesia	n = 0	n = 1
	Hematuria	n = 0	n = 1
	Zona	n = 0	n = 1

Trial	Cyclosporin in Behçet's disease: results in 16 patients after 24 months of therapy
Substance	**Ciclosporin 5 mg/kg/day** (serum level 300–900 ng/mL)
	Concomitant medication:
	No information provided
	Previous medication:
	Previously treated with corticosteroids and/or cytotoxic agents, both stopped ≥ 10 day
Result	Ciclosporin was an effective treatment of ocular and aphthous symptoms of patients suffering from Behçet's disease
Patients	16 Behçet's syndrome patients fulfilling the Nussenblatt criteria
	With all 4 major symptoms:
	• Aphthous stomatitis
	• Genital ulcers
	• Ocular lesions
	• Skin manifestations
Authors	Pacor ML, Biasi D, Lunardi C, Cortina P, Caramaschi P, Girelli D, Botto M, Urbani G, Lombardo G, Bambara LM
Publication	*Clin Rheumatol.* 1994;13(2):224–227
Follow-up	24 months
Note	*Outcome parameters*:
	Clinical remission	n = 14 (6–12 months)
	Change of:
	Visual acuity	+3
Adverse events	Renal dysfunction	n = 1
	Anemia	n = 1
	Increases alanin aminotransferase and alkaline phosphatase	n = 0
	Hirsutism	n = 2
	Gastrointestinal discomfort	n = 1

Trial	Low-dose Cyclosporin A therapy in Behçet's disease	
Substance	**Ciclosporin-A (5 mg/kg/day** as initial dose) *No improvement (after week 2)*: Plus **0.2–0.6 mg/kg/day prednisolone** *Previous medication*: Chlorambucil n = 6 Colchicine n = 2 Cyclophosphamide n = 2 Prednisolone (all)	
Result	Ciclosporin-A treatment lead to an improvement of ocular disease	
Patients	22 patients with Morbus Behçet • Severe ocular involvement • HLA B5 positive: 50%	
Authors	Sajjadi H, Soheilian M, Ahmadieh H, Hassanein K, Parvin M, Azarmina M, Ehyaee V, Amiransari B	
Publication	*J Ocul Pharmacol.* Fall 1994;10(3):553–560	
Follow-up	4–32 months	
Note	*Outcome parameters*:	
	Improvement or stabilization of vision	95%
	Control of intraocular inflammation	100%
	Improvement of visual acuity	+59%
Adverse events	Rise in creatinine	45%
	Rise in bilirubin	27%
	Hypertrichosis	18%
	Increase in uric acid	14%
	Hypertension	4.5%
	Gynecomastia	4.5%
	Gingivitis	4.5%

Trial	Low-dose Ciclosporin A versus pulsed Cyclophosphamide in Behçet's syndrome: a single masked trial
Substance	**Ciclosporin A 5 mg/kg/day** (n = 11) **Cyclophosphamide 1 g intravenous monthly boluses** (Cyc, n = 12) *Concomitant medication*: Corticosteroid together with Cyc (1 month)
Result	Visual acuitiy improved after six months of treatment with ciclosporin in Behçet's uveitis. This was not sustained after 24 months cyclosporin was effective in the treatment of uveitis
Patients	23 patients with Behçet's syndrome • With active, bilateral uveitis • ≥ 3 ocular disease exacerbations within the preceding 6 months • No end-stage disease • No irreversible damage • No blindness
Authors	Ozyazgan Y, Yurdakul S, Yazici H, Tüzün B, Işçimen A, Tüzün Y, Aktunç T, Pazarli H, Hamuryudan V, Müftüoğlu A
Publication	*Br J Ophthalmol.* 1992;76(4):241–243
Follow-up	24 months
Note	*Outcome parameters*:

	Ciclosporin A	Cyclophosphamide
Number of ocular attacks (6 months)	0.48	0.62
Number of ocular attacks (6 months—unmasking)	0.49	0.60
Change of (*6 months*):		
	Ciclosporin A	Cyclophosphamide
Visual acuity	+2.36	-0.63

Trial	Chlorambucil and cyclosporine A in Brazilian patients with Behçet's disease uveitis: a retrospective study
Substance	**Chlorambucil 2 mg/day, increased to 6 mg/day** (n = 13) **and/or ciclosporin A 2–6 mg/kg/day** (n = 9) for ≥ 6 months *Concomitant medication*: 40–60 mg oral corticosteroid/day, therapeutic range (100–300 ng/mL)
Result	Chlorambucil did not induce on long-term remission of uveitis, whereas ciclosporin was effective but side effects limited its use
Patients	22 patients with Behçet's disease uveitis • Meeting the Behçet's Disease Research Committee of Japan Diagnostic Criteria • With ≥ 6 months therapy and ≥ 1 year follow-up
Authors	Zaghetto JM, Yamamoto MM, Souza MB, Silva FT, Hirata CE, Olivalves E, Yamamoto JH
Publication	*Arq Bras Oftalmol.* 2010 Feb;73(1):40–46
Follow-up	13.4 years

Note	*During follow-up*:	Chlorambucil	Cyclosporine A
	Switched to other group	n = 5	n = 1
	Effective regarding flare-up	78.5%	57.2%
	No response	21.5%	28.5%
	Effective regarding prednisone reduction	78.5%	50%

Adverse events		Chlorambucil (%)	Cyclosporine A (%)
	Total	64.2	50.0
	Gonadal dysfunction	25.7	0
	Leukopenia	28.5	0
	Infection	14.2	0
	Nephrotoxicity	0	35.7
	Gastrointestinal complications	0	21.4
	Hypertension	0	21.4
	Gingival hypertrophy	0	7.1
	Paraesthesia	0	7.1

Trial	A double-blind trial of Colchicine in Behçet's syndrome
Substance	**Colchicine (1–2 mg/day, adjusted to body weight,** n = 58) **Placebo** (n = 58) *Concomitant medication*: NSAIDs n = 3 (colchicine), n = 3 (placebo) Intraarticular corticosteroids n = 1 (colchicine), n = 1 (placebo) 1 g methylprednisolone for 3 days n = 0 (colchicine), n = 1 (placebo) 100 mg thalidomide for 1 week and 50 mg for 2 weeks n = 0 (colchicine), n = 1 (placebo) *Previous medication*: No immunosuppressive agents ≤ 6 months
Result	Colchicine was useful in treating some of the manifestations of Behçet's syndrome, especially of women
Patients	116 consecutive patients with Behçet's syndrome, fulfilling the criteria of the International Study Group for Behçet's Disease (60 male/ 56 female) • Active mucocutaneous disease • No eye involvement • No major organ involvement • Disease duration of ≤ 2 years • Minimum presence of oral or genital ulceration or erythema nodosum occurring ≥ 3 times within the preceding 6 months • 18–35 years of age
Authors	Yurdakul S, Mat C, Tüzün Y, Ozyazgan Y, Hamuryudan V, Uysal O, Senocak M, Yazici H
Publication	*Arthritis Rheum.* 2001;44(11):2686–2692
Follow-up	24 months

Note	*Outcome parameters*:		
		Colchicine	Placebo
	Absence of arthritis	91%	64%
	Arthritic joints (total numbers of joints)	Women: 0.3 Men: 2.8	Women: 2.4 Men: 4.4
	Erythema nodosum (total numbers of lesions)	Women: 1.4 Men: 0.7	Women: 6.0 Men: 2.0
	Follicular lesions (mean number)	Women: 4.1 Men: 15.7	Women: 5.9 Men: 13.7
	Free of new attacks of genital ulceration	Women: 89% Men: no difference	Women: 46% Men: no difference

Adverse events		Colchicine	Placebo
	Loss of appetite	38%	34%
	Nausea	26%	39%
	Abdominal pain	41%	30%
	Diarrhea	44%	36%
	Superficial thrombophlebitis	n =1	n = 5

Trial	Long-term effects of Cyclophosphamide and Colchicine treatment in Behçet's disease
Substance	Cyclophosphamide 100–150 mg/day (n = 46) Colchicine 1–1.5 mg/day (n = 18) *Concomitant medication*: 5 mg prednisolone/day *Previous medication*: No information provided
Result	No positive changes of ocular symptoms, e. g. in visual acuity and number of attacks, could be shown when compared with the period after treatment for both medications
Patients	64 patients with Behçet's disease • With ocular disease
Authors	Kazokoglu H, Saatçi O, Cuhadaroglu H, Eldem B
Publication	*Ann Ophthalmol.* 1991;23(4):148–151
Follow-up	9–156 months
Note	*Outcome parameters*:

	Cyclophosphamide	Colchicine
Mean number of attacks during treatment	n = 3.4	n = 1.94
Mean number of attacks after treatment	n = 2.54	n = 1.27
Mean total attacks	n = 7.32	n = 3.22
Mean period post treatment (months)	43.05	51.06
Mean follow-up (months)	84.2	43.05
Macular pigment epithelial alteration	47.6%	46.4%
Optic atrophy	44.6%	50.0%
Perivascular sheathing	26.2%	7.1%
Chorioretinal atrophy	7.6%	3.5%
Branch vein occlusion	1.5%	0%
Cystoid macular edema	1.5%	3.5%
Univisualized fundi	n = 8	n = 2
Posterior synechias	28.7%	46.6%
Complicated cataract	26.0%	21.4%
Seclusio pupillae	6.8%	0%
Rubeosis	4.1%	3.3%
Secondary glaucoma	2.7%	0%
Phthisis	4.1%	0%

Adverse events	Cyclophosphamide (%)	Colchicine (%)
Azoospermia	73.3	0
Hemorrhagic cystitis	10.8	0

Trial	Dapsone in Behçet's disease: a double-blind, placebo-controlled, crossover study
Substance	**Dapsone 100 mg/day** (n = 10) **Placebo** (n = 10) Treatment was crossed over after 3 months *Concomitant medication*: No information provided
Result	Dapsone was effective in the treatment of mucocutaneous manifestations of Behçet's disease
Patients	20 patients with Behçet's disease according to the criteria of the International Study Group • Mucocutaneous manifestations • Joint involvement *Oral aphtae ± 2 symptoms out of*: • Recurrent genital aphtae • Eye lesions • Skin lesions • Pos. Pathergy test *Exclusion criteria*: • Eye/neurological involvement • Anemia • Glucose-6-phosphatase dehydrogenase deficiency
Authors	Sharquie KE, Najim RA, Abu-Raghif AR
Publication	*J Dermatol.* 2002;29(5):267–279
Follow-up	6 months

(continued)

Note	Change of (3 months):				
		Starting with dapsone	Dapsone after placebo	Placebo after dapsone	Starting with placebo
	Count of oral ulcers	-2.7	-2.5	+1.3	-2.7
	Size of oral ulcers	-0.4	+0.2	+1.4	0
	Duration of ulcers	-2.2	-4.7	+2.3	+3.3
	Frequency of oral ulcers	-1.7	-0.7	+1.6	+0.6
	Count of genital ulcers	-0.8	-0.9	+0.4	+0.4
	Size of genital ulcers	+1.1	-2.3	-1.5	+1.3
	Duration of genital ulcers	+0.2	-6.3	-1.5	+0.5
	Frequency of genital ulcers	-0.3	-0.5	+0.3	+0.7

Adverse events	After 3 months:		
		Dapsone (%)	Placebo (%)
	None	26	55
	Nausea	11	10
	Dyspepsia	16	5
	Anorexia	0	0
	Fatigue	16	25
	Anemia	16	5
	Headache	21	5

Trial	Low-dose weekly Methotrexate for progressive neuropsychiatric manifestations in Behçet's disease
Substance	**Methotrexate 5 mg p. o./week** **Increased by 2.5 mg every week up to 10–12.5 mg/week** *Concomitant medication*: Prednisolone ≤ 10 mg/day was permitted Colchicine 1 mg/day was permitted *Previous medication*: Prednisolone n = 4 Colchicine n = 2 Cyclophosphamide i. v. n = 1 Mizoribine n = 1 Azathioprine n = 1 Ciclosporin A n = 1
Result	Methotrexate therapy was beneficial in delaying disease progression of Neuro-Behçet's symptoms
Patients	6 patients with Behçet's disease according to the criteria of the International Study Group • Neuropsychiatric manifestations were judged to be progressive variety of neurological, including meningitis, dysarthria, ataxia
Authors	Hirohata S, Suda H, Hashimoto T
Publication	*J Neurol Sci.* 1998;159(2):181–185
Follow-up	12 months
Note	*Outcome parameters*:	
	Neuropsychological manifestations	Not significant worsening
	MRI scans	Not significant worsening
	Intelligence quotients	Not significant change
	Discontinuation of MTX after 12 months	Mild exacerbation of symptoms
	IL-6 levels decreased	n = 6
Adverse events	Mild liver dysfunction	n = 3

Trial	Low-dose MTX for progressive Neuro-Behçet's disease. A follow-up study for 4 years
Substance	**Methotrexate 5–7.5 mg/week** **Increased to 5–15 mg in steps of 2.5 mg every 2 weeks** *Concomitant medication*: Prednisolone ≤ 15 mg/day was permitted Colchicine 1 mg/day was permitted 5–10 g folate/week was permitted *Previous medication*: Prednisolone n = 4 Colchicine n = 2 Cyclophosphamide i. v. n = 1 Mizoribine n = 1 Azathioprine n = 1 Ciclosporin A n = 1
Result	Low-dose methotrexate had beneficial effects in patients with Neuro-Behçet and was well tolerated
Patients	10 patients, fulfilling the International criteria of Behçet's disease, with neuropsychiatric manifestations
Authors	Kikuchi H, Aramaki K, Hirohata S
Publication	*Adv Exp Med Biol.* 2003;528:575–578
Follow-up	4 years
Note	*Outcome parameters*:

	Neuropsychological manifestations	Findings on MRI scans
	MRI scans	Not significant worsening
	Intelligence quotients	Not significant change
	Discontinuation of MTX after 12 months	Mild exacerbation of symptoms
	Cerebrospinal fluid IL-6 levels	Decreased in all patients
	Wechsler adult intelligence scale	Stable in all but one patient
Adverse events	Mild liver dysfunction	n = 3

Trial	Mycophenolate mofetil is ineffective in the treatment of mucocutaneous Adamantiades-Behçet's disease
Substance	**Mycophenolate mofetil 2 g/day** for 6 months
	If ineffective increased to 3 g/day
	Plus 30 mg prednisolone/day for 1 month
	Concomitant medication:
	No information provided
	Previous medication:
	No information provided
Result	Mycophenolate mofetil was not able to control the signs of mucocutaneous disease
Patients	30 patients, diagnosed by the CART criteria, with active cutaneous disease
Authors	Adler YD, Mansmann U, Zouboulis CC
Publication	*Dermatology*. 2001;203(4):322–324
Follow-up	12 months
Note	*Outcome parameters*:
	The study was discontinued after the sixth patient because of ineffectiveness
	Mycophenolate mofetil/prednisolone treatment ⇨ Reduction of the disease activity index 5.2 ⇨ 1.3
	Withdrawal of prednisolone led to quick relapses
Adverse events	No adverse effects were assessed under mycophenolate mofetil

Trial	A multicenter clinical open trial of FK 506 in refractory uveitis, including Behçet's disease. Japanese FK 506 Study Group on Refractory Uveitis
Substance	**Tacrolimus 0.05 mg/kg/day** (n = 9) **Tacrolimus 0.10 mg/kg/day** (n = 13) **Tacrolimus 0.20 mg/kg/day** (n = 7) For 12 weeks *Concomitant medication*: No information provided *Previous medication*: Colchicine n = 20 Ciclosporin n = 16 Steroids n = 14 Cyclophosphamide n = 1
Result	Tacrolimus was beneficial in patients with refractory uveitis in this open clinical trial
Patients	29 Patients with Behçet's disease • With refractory uveitis • Actively inflamed posterior segment • Age 16–76 years
Authors	Mochizuki M, Masuda K, Sakane T, Inaba G, Ito K, Kogure M, Sugino N, Usui M, Mizushima Y, Ohno S, et al.
Publication	*Transplant Proc.* 1991;23(6):3343–3346
Follow-up	12 weeks

Note	*Outcome parameters*:			
		0.5 mg/kg tacrolimus	0.1 mg/kg tacrolimus	0.20 mg/kg tacrolimus
	Improvement of uveitis	n = 2	n = 6	n = 2
	Dose was increased because of insufficient efficacy	n = 7	n = 4	–
	Improvement after increase of dosage	n = 4	n = 2	–
	All patients			
	Overall efficacy improvement	62%		
	Overall efficacy unchanged	38%		
	Improvement of visual acuity	32%		
	Visual acuity unchanged	50%		
	Visual acuity decreased	18%		

Adverse events	Renal impairment	n = 4
	Tremor	n = 3
	Nausea	n = 2
	Hyperkalemia	n = 1
	Chest discomfort	n = 1

Trial	Thalidomide in the treatment of the mucocutaneous lesions of the Behçet syndrome. A randomized, double-blind, placebo-controlled trial
Substance	**Thalidomide, 100 mg/day** (n = 32) **Thalidomide, 300 mg/day** (n = 32) **Placebo** (n = 31) For 24 weeks *Concomitant/previous medication*: No information was depicted
Result	Thalidomide was effective for treating the oral and genital ulcers and follicular lesions of the Behçet syndrome, independently of dosage
Patients	96 male patients with the Behçet syndrome who met the International Study Group for Behçet's Disease criteria • Mucocutaneous lesions • Without major organ involvement, age 18–35 years • ≥ 2 episodes of oral or genital ulcerations within 3 months. • No severe eye disease
Authors	Hamuryudan V, Mat C, Saip S, Ozyazgan Y, Siva A, Yurdakul S, Zwingenberger K, Yazici H
Publication	*Ann Intern Med.* 1998;128(6):443–450
Follow-up	28 weeks
Note	*Outcome parameters*:

	Placebo	100 mg thalidomide	300 mg thalidomide
Complete response	0%	6%	16%
Sustained absence of ulcerations	n = 0	n = 10	n = 9
Activation in the eye	n = 9	n = 2	n = 3
Visual acuity scoring other than perfect	n = 5	n = 1	n = 0
Arthritis attacks	n = 11	n = 7	n = 4
Epididymitis	n = 2	n = 1	n = 3

Both thalidomide dosages led to significant increases in the number of erythema nodosum lesions

Polyneuropathia developed in four patients

Adverse events	Placebo (%)	100 mg thalidomide (%)	300 mg thalidomide (%)
Sedation	50	84	87
Fatigue	44	66	68
Sleeplessness	16	25	19
Numbness	28	28	23
Tingling	25	34	26
Constipation	25	59	65
Transient rash	0	6	10
Headache	34	38	29

Trial	Short-term trial of Etanercept in Behçet's disease: a double-blind, placebo-controlled study
Substance	**Etanercept 25 mg twice a week** (ETN, n = 20) **Placebo** (n = 20) *Concomitant medication*: Prednisolone n = 2 (ETN), n = 2 (placebo) Indomethacin n = 1 (ETN), n = 0 (placebo) Naproxen n = 0 (ETN), n = 1 (placebo) Topical corticosteroids n = 0 (ETN), n = 4 (placebo) Paracetamol n = 1 (ETN), n = 0 (placebo) Ornidazole n = 1 (ETN), n = 0 (placebo) Azathioprine n = 1 (ETN), n = 1 (placebo) *Previous medication*: Colchicine withdrawal n = 11 (ETN), n = 7 (placebo) Azathioprine withdrawal n = 0 (ETN), n = 5 (placebo)
Result	Etanercept was effective in suppressing mucocutaneous manifestations
Patients	40 male patients suffering from Behçet's disease, fulfilling the criteria of the International Study Group, with age 18–45 years *Active disease, min 1 positive out of*: • ≥ 1 episode with oral or genital ulcerations • Swollen joints • Erythema nodosum within 3 months • Positive Pathergy test
Authors	Melikoglu M, Fresko I, Mat C, Ozyazgan Y, Gogus F, Yurdakul S, Hamuryudan V, Yazici H
Publication	*J Rheumatol.* 2005;32(1):98–105
Follow-up	4 weeks plus 3 months

Note	*Change of (4 months)*:	ETN	Placebo
	Positive pathergy test	-12	-12
	Monosodium titrate (mm^3)	-1,144	-944
	Oral ulcers	0	-0.22
	Genital ulcers	-0.6	-0.43
	Nodular lesions	+0.3	-1.68
	Papulopustular lesions	0	-0.49
	Swollen joints	+0.34	-0.25

Adverse events		ETN	Placebo
	Diarrhea	n = 1	n = 0
	Gastrointestinal symptoms	n = 1	n = 0
	Increased liver enzymes	n = 0	n = 1

Trial	Efficacy, safety, and pharmacokinetics of multiple administration of Infliximab in Behçet's disease with refractory uveo-retinitis
Substance	**Infliximab (IFX) 5 mg/kg** (n = 7) **Infliximab 10 mg/kg** (n = 6) At weeks 0, 2, 6, and 10 *After onset of ocular attacks*: Colchicine was permitted Subconjunctival decadron injection or 20–40 mg of prednisolone administered orally for 1–4 weeks *Previous medication*: 2.36–5.88 mg/kg Ciclosporin/day was discontinued at study entry
Result	Administration of infliximab in patients with refractory uveo-retinitis suppressed the frequency of ocular attacks
Patients	13 patients with Behçet's disease • With refractory uveo-retinitis • Despite ciclosporin treatment
Authors	Ohno S, Nakamura S, Hori S, Shimakawa M, Kawashima H, Mochizuki M, Sugita S, Ueno S, Yoshizaki K, Inaba G
Publication	*J Rheumatol.* 2004;31(7):1362–1368
Follow-up	26 weeks

Note	*Outcome parameters*:	5 mg/kg IFX	10 mg/kg IFX
	Numbers of ocular attacks (mean/14 day, pre/post treatment)	3.5 ⇨ 1.0	3.8 ⇨ 0.2
	Visual acuity improved	n = 5 out of 7 cases	n = 4 out of 6 cases
	Oral aphthous ulceration disappeared	n = 2 out of 2	n = 2 out of 3

Adverse events		5 mg/kg IFX	10 mg/kg IFX
	Patients with adverse events	n = 7	n = 6
	Number of adverse events	n = 43	n = 30
	Diarrhea	57.1%	16.7%
	Common cold	57.1%	0%
	Malaise	42.9%	16.7%
	Nausea	42.9%	16.7%
	Pyrexia	28.6%	33.3%
	Headache	14.3%	33.3%
	Increased systolic blood pressure	14.3%	33.3%
	Epigastric distress	28.6%	0%
	Vomiting	28.6%	0%
	Decreased diastolic blood pressure	28.6%	0%
	Arthralgia	0%	33.3%
	Constipation	0%	33.3%

Trial	Efficacy of Infliximab in the treatment of uveitis that is resistant to treatment with the combination of Azathioprine, Ciclosporin, and corticosteroids in Behçet's disease: an open-label trial
Substance	**Infliximab 5 mg/kg** At weeks 0, 2, 6, and 14 *Concomitant medication*: 5 mg/kg ciclosporin/day was discontinued 2 mg/kg azathioprine/day was prolonged 300 mg isoniazid was added if necessary *Previous medication*: Combination therapy: Azathioprine 2 mg/kg/day Ciclosporin 5 mg/kg/day Prednisolone > 7.5 mg/day
Result	Infliximab suppressed the occurrence of uveitis attacks, had a corticosteroid-sparing effect, and had favorable implications for the visual prognosis of patients with resistant Behçet's uveitis
Patients	13 patients with Behçet's disease who met the criteria of the International Study Group • ≥ 2 uveitis attacks involving the posterior segment in the last 6 months • Despite receiving treatment with the combination of azathioprine, ciclosporin, and prednisolone (> 7.5 mg/day) • No visual loss • No severe manifestations
Authors	Tugal-Tutkun I, Mudun A, Urgancioglu M, Kamali S, Kasapoglu E, Inanc M, Gül A
Publication	*Arthritis Rheum.* 2005;52(8):2478–2484
Follow-up	54 weeks

Note — *Outcome parameters*:

	Previous 6 months	Treatment period	Observation period
Uveitis attacks	n = 2.4	n = 1.0	n = 1.9
Daily prednisone (mg/day)	27.6	14.1	28.1

Mean occurrence of:

	Week 0–22	Week 23–54
Fatigue	0.33	0.55
Oral ulcers	0.13	0.46
Genital ulcers	0	0.05
Papulopustular lesions	1.07	1.31
Erythema nodosum	0	0

Adverse events

	Week 0–22	Week 23–54
Respiratory infections	n = 7	n = 3
Headache	n = 5	n = 0
Hypertension	n = 1	n = 0
Infusion reaction	n = 1	n = 0
Rash	n = 1	n = 0
Dyshidrosiform eczema	n = 1	n = 0
Contact dermatitis, pruritus	n = 1	n = 0
Lower back pain	n = 1	n = 0
Renal colic	n = 0	n = 1
Inguinal hernia	n = 0	n = 1

Trial	One-year study of efficacy and safety of infliximab in the treatment of patients with ocular and neurological Behçet's disease refractory to standard immunosuppressive drugs	
Substance	**Infliximab 5 mg/kg** At weeks 0, 2, 6, and then every 8 weeks for a total of 1 year *Concomitant medication*: Stable doses of prednisone (< 10 mg/day) No immunosuppressants ≤ 4 weeks *Previous medication*: Corticosteroids ≥ 1 immunosuppressant (cyclosporin, methotrexate, azathioprine, cyclophosphamide) No TNF antagonist	
Result	TNF inhibition displayed a dramatic effect on reduction of signs and symptoms of Behçet's disease with ocular and/or CNS involvement	
Patients	21 patients with active persistent Behçet's disease • Diagnosed by the International Study Group for Behçet's Disease criteriaCRP > 1 mg/dL • Failure to respond to corticosteroids and ≥ 1 immunosuppressant *Ocular and/or CNS involvement*: • Cerebral vasculitis (n = 5) • Retinal vasculitis (n = 13) • Posterior uveitis (n = 13)	
Authors	Giardina A, Ferrante A, Ciccia F, Vadalà M, Giardina E, Triolo G	
Publication	*Rheumatol Int.* 2011 Jan;31(1):33–37	
Follow-up	12 months	
Note	Completed the study	n = 18
	Total remission	n = 18
	Partial remission and relapsed after 3 months	n = 2
	Discontinued IFX after 1 year and relapsed after 3–6 months	n = 6
		n = 4
Adverse events	Headache	n = 1
	Dizziness	n = 1
	Non-Hodgkin lymphoma	n = 1
	Tachycardia	n = 1

Trial	Efficacy of combination therapy of anti-TNF-α antibody infliximab and methotrexate in refractory entero-Behçet's disease	
Substance	Infliximab 3–5 mg/kg At weeks 0, 2, 6 and every 8 weeks thereafter *Concomitant medication*: Methotrexate (n = 10) Mesalazine (n = 2) Colchicine (n = 3) Sulfasalazine (n = 1) *Previous medication*: Refractory to conventional therapies	
Result	Infliximab was rapid and excellent efficient in patients with refractory entero-Behçet's disease	
Patients	10 patients with Behçet's disease, diagnosed by the International Study Group for Behçet's Disease criteria • With refractory gastrointestinal tract complications	
Authors	Iwata S, Saito K, Yamaoka K, Tsujimura S, Nawata M, Hanami K, Tanaka Y	
Publication	*Mod Rheumatol*. 2011 Apr;21(2):184–191	
Follow-up	24 months follow-up	
Note	Improvement of gastrointestinal symptoms	n = 10
	Time to improvement	4 weeks
	Disappearance of ileocecal ulcerations 6 months	n = 5
	Disappearance of ileocecal ulcerations 12 months	n = 9
	Change of corticosteroid dose at 24 months	-20.2 mg/day
Adverse events	No severe adverse effects	

Trial	Rituximab in intractable ocular lesions of Behçet's disease; randomized single-blind control study (pilot study)		
Substance	*Rituximab therapy*: **Rituximab 2 × 1´000 mg in 15-day interval** (n = 10) **Methotrexate 15 mg/weekly** *Cytotoxic combination therapy*: **Cyclophosphamide 1´000 mg i. v./month** (n = 10) **2–3 mg/kg azathioprine/day** *Concomitant therapy*: 0.5 mg prednisolone/kg/day (both groups) Tapered upon good results *Previous medication*: No improvement, aggravation, or partial improvement of the eye disease to combined cytotoxic drugs and steroids		
Result	Rituximab but not cyclophosphamide was efficient in severe ocular manifestations		
Patients	20 patients with longstanding retinal vasculitis and edema, meeting the International Study Group for Behçet's Disease criteria • Resistant to combined cytotoxic drugs		
Authors	Davatchi F, Shams H, Rezaipoor M, Sadeghi-Abdollahi B, Shahram F, Nadji A, Chams-Davatchi C, Akhlaghi M, Faezi T, Naderi N		
Publication	*Int J Rheum Dis*. 2010 Aug;13(3):246–252		
Follow-up	6 months		
Note	*Change of*:		
		Rituximab	Cytotoxic combination therapy
	Total adjusted disease activity index improved	+0.3	+0.6
	Posterior uveitis	-0.75	-0.65
	Visual acuity improved	n = 2	n = 3
	Visual acuity worsened	n = 7	n = 6
	Visual acuity (mean)	-0.31	-0.06
	Retinal vasculitis	-0.8	-0.25
	Edema	-0.9	0.08
	Total inflammatory activity index	-8.3	-3.8
Adverse events		Rituximab	Cytotoxic combination therapy
	Conjunctivitis	n = 2	n = 10
	Pneumonia	n = 1	n = 0
	Herpes zoster	n = 1	n = 0
	Urticaria	n = 3	n = 0
	Flushing	n = 5	n = 0
	Severe allergic reaction	n = 1	n = 0

Trial	Interferon alfa-2b, Colchicine, and Benzathine penicillin versus Colchicine and Benzathine penicillin in Behçet's disease: a randomized trial
Substance	**Interferon alfa-2b (IFN) three million units** s. c. every other day for first 6 months (67) **Control patients** (68) *Concomitant medication*: Colchicine 1.5 mg Benzathine penicillin 1.2 million units i. m. every 3 weeks *Attacks*: Prednisolone 1 mg/kg/day Azathioprine 2–2.5 mg/kg/day
Result	Interferon alfa-2b, colchicine, and benzathine penicillin were all effective in treating eye disease and extraocular manifestations
Patients	135 patients with Behçet's disease who met the criteria of the International Study Group • Established disease ≥ 2 months • No previous therapy for Behçet's disease
Authors	Demiroglu H, Ozcebe OI, Barista I, Dündar S, Eldem B
Publication	*Lancet.* 2000;355(9204):605–609
Follow-up	12 months

(continued)

Note	Outcome parameters:		
		IFN (%)	Controls (%)
	Risk of eye involvement	8	27
	Attack rates (mean/year):		
		IFN	Controls
	Eye involvement	0.2	1.02
	Arthritis	0.29	0.87
	Vascular events	0.06	0.24
	Oral ulcers	5.52	6.68
	Genital ulcers	0.72	1.18
	Skin lesions	1.17	1.84
	Visual acuity loss	n = 2	n = 13
	Arthritis episodes, vascular events, and mucocutaneous lesions were also less frequent in patients treated with interferon		
	Pseudotumor cerebri	n = 1	n = 1
	Hemiparesis	n = 0	n = 1
	Bilateral pyramidal tract disease	n = 0	n = 1
Adverse events		IFN	Controls
	Deep-vein thrombosis of the lower extremity	n = 12	-
	Budd-Chiari syndrome	n = 1	-
	Pulmonary arterial aneurysm	n = 1	-
	Mild and asymptomatic neutropenia and thrombocytopenia	Present	-
	A mild and tolerable flu-like syndrome	Present	-
	Transient alopecia	Present	-
	Abdominal cramping	Present	-
	Vomiting	Both groups	
	Diarrhea	Both groups	
	Mild depression	Both groups	

Trial	Interferon alfa-2a in the treatment of Behçet disease: a randomized placebo-controlled and double-blind study
Substance	**Interferon alfa-2a, 6 × 10⁶ IU**, s.c. three times a week (n = 23, +2 who failed to complete the study) **Placebo** (n = 21, +4 who failed to complete the study) *Previous therapy*: No systemic therapy ≤ 12 weeks prior randomization No topical therapy ≤ 4 weeks prior randomization
Result	Interferon alfa-2a was an effective treatment for mucocutaneous, ocular and joint manifestations
Patients	50 patients with Behçet's disease who met the criteria of the International Study Group • No hepatic, renal, cardiovascular, infectious, or other autoimmune disease • No irreversible bilateral eye disease • No active cerebral or retinal vasculitis, age 16–55
Authors	Alpsoy E, Durusoy C, Yilmaz E, Ozgurel Y, Ermis O, Yazar S, Basaran E
Publication	*Arch Dermatol.* 2002;138(4):467–471
Follow-up	3 months

Note — *Outcome parameters*:

	IFN	Placebo
Withdrawal because of severe eye disease	n = 1	n = 2
Withdrawal because of progressive mucocutaneous and articular symptoms	n = 1	n = 1

Patients with ocular symptoms (n = 6):

	IFN	Placebo
Decrease in the severity and the frequency of attacks	n = 5	n = 3
Complete response	n = 2	n = 0
Partial response	n = 13	n = 3
Overall response	n = 15	n = 3

Duration and pain of oral ulcers, frequency of genital ulcers and papulopustular lesions decreased

Frequency and duration of erythema lesions, nodosum-like thrombophlebitis, and articular symptoms were decreased

Adverse events	
Alopecia	4.3%
Mild, flu-like symptoms	78%
Leukopenia	4.3%
Diarrhea	4.3%

Index

R. Müller, J. von Kempis, *Clinical Trials in Rheumatology*,
DOI 10.1007/978-1-4471-2870-0, © Springer-Verlag London 2013

Printed by Printforce, the Netherlands